Praise for *Living Well with Depressio*

"I doubt there is a person in the world who knows these conditions better, inside and out, than John McManamy.... This book is full of studies and personal insights, in about equal measure, leavened with the practical conclusions of its even handed and often humorous author. It breaks new ground." —S. Nassir Ghaemi, MD, MPH, director, Bipolar Disorder Research Program, associate professor of psychiatry and public health, Emory University

"If you read only one book about bipolar disorder, make it this one. Beautifully written, with profound insight and quirky humor, McManamy integrates cutting-edge science with subjective experience— an instant classic." —John Gartner, author of *The Hypomaniac Edge: The Link Between (A Little) Craziness and (A Lot of) Success in America*

"The reader takes a journey with a wise and compassionate guide who offers extremely clear information and—equally important— hope." —Demitri F. Papolos, MD, and Janice Papolos, authors of *The Bipolar Child*

"As he does in his brilliantly written and researched newsletter, John McManamy brings together his outstanding reportorial skills, his great gift for language, and his remarkable insights about his own disorder to create an invaluable resource for anyone living with bipolar disorder." —Ellen Frank, PhD, professor of psychiatry and psychology, Western Psychiatric Institute and Clinic

"Every single page yields a nugget of information or a piece of insider news or a riveting anecdote. I hope this book gets the attention and acclaim it deserves. In a crowded field, it stands out for its clarity, accuracy, liveliness, and overall readability." —Anne Sheffield, author of *Depression Fallout*

"Never in my life have I read a book quite like John McManamy's *Living Well with Depression and Bipolar Disorder*. His approach is fantastic and unique.... Anyone who has ever been diagnosed with a mood disorder, depression, or bipolar disorder really needs to read this book. And those of you who haven't been diagnosed but who confess to 'wondering' at times—this is the book for you, too." —Colleen Sullivan, owner, Bipolar World; www.bipolarworld.net

"This book belongs in the hands of every person who has suffered from depression or bipolar disorder and every mental health professional who treats them. John McManamy has written the most comprehensive and readable guide I've ever read for the many forms of depression and bipolar disorder and their treatment." —Amy Weintraub, author of *Yoga for Depression*

LIVING WELL WITH

Depression and Bipolar Disorder

What Your Doctor

Doesn't Tell You . . .

That You Need to Know

JOHN McMANAMY

HARPER

NEW YORK • LONDON • TORONTO • SYDNEY

HARPER

*To my family, who stood by me in the worst of times,
who were there for me in the best of times . . .
especially my mother, who "gets it."*

*Also, to the many researchers and clinicians and
others cited in this book, plus countless unsung others
who have dedicated their lives to improving ours.*

*Finally, to my virtual family of newsletter and Web site
readers, many of whom have become my dearest friends,
including Colleen Sullivan, who started me on this journey,
and Susan, the special person in my life who joined me on it.*

HarperCollins books may be purchased for educational, business, or sales promotional use. For information please write: Special Markets Department, HarperCollins Publishers Inc., 10 East 53rd Street, New York, NY 10022.

FIRST EDITION

Designed by Joy O'Meara

Library of Congress Cataloging-in-Publication Data has been applied for.

ISBN-10: 0-06-089742-2
ISBN-13: 978-0-06-089742-0

11 12 13 14 15 WBC/RRD 10 9

ACKNOWLEDGMENTS

This book would still be an unread manuscript sitting in the bottom of a someone's pile were it not for my good friend, Janice Papolos, coauthor of *The Bipolar Child*. When she found out what I was up to she took me under her wing. As well as critiquing my first draft, she mentored me in putting together a state-of-the-art publishing proposal, then enthusiastically recommended the manuscript to Debbie Stier at HarperCollins, who in turn saw that the copy found its way into the hands of the one editor in publishing who would do justice to the material, Sarah Durand.

Through the pioneering Living Well series, which gives voice to authors who are patients, Sarah has boldly gone where no editor has gone before. Prior to Sarah, patients had to settle for writing memoirs and polemics. The front of the publications bus, where doctors and other practitioners sat, was strictly off limits.

With this book, Sarah has once again broken new ground. This time she placed her faith—wholeheartedly—in a patient with a mood disorder. Believe me, in moving me to the front of this bus, Sarah became the ultimate stigma-buster.

The people who work with Sarah at HarperCollins deserve special mention: Jeremy Cesarec, Sarah's assistant editor who expertly minded me; and copy editor Jim Gullikson, who so carefully minded my manuscript.

Many thanks also to Danielle Forte, JD, who closed the deal for me and treated me like John Grisham—actually, even better.

Finally, a second curtain call to the people to whom this book is dedicated, including my family, the researchers and clinicians cited in the book, and my virtual family of newsletter and Web-site readers. This second curtain call merits special bouquets to the three women in my life, who have shown me what love is all about: my mother; my daughter, Emily; and my wife, Susan.

CONTENTS

There is no name adequate to describe
the perfect mental storm that rages inside our heads—
be it depression or mania—that leaves in its wake
such a fearsome trail of wreckage and destruction
and ruined lives. May as well call the thing Fred,
as far as I'm concerned. Fred. For most of my life,
Fred has been my constant traveling companion,
even as I denied his existence and tried so hard to
pretend I was a master of my own fate. I'm normal!
I kept insisting over and over,
much to Fred's quiet amusement.

—The author, from a closing address to
the 2002 Depression and Bipolar Support Alliance
annual conference

PART ONE

DIAGNOSIS

1

Getting Acquainted: Me, You, and the Spectrum We Share

I have an MD. It stands for manic depression. In January 1999, at age forty-nine, following a series of severe depressions and a lifetime of denial, I was diagnosed with manic depression's successor label, bipolar disorder, so technically my MD is now BP, which pisses me off no end. After what this illness has done to me, I feel I have every right to call myself an MD.

Screw the medical profession. What do they have on me? Well, they were smart enough to save my life, so I take it back.

My real qualifications are these: I am a former financial journalist with a law degree. My subsequent research into my illness led to me writing about depression for the Web site Suite 101.com, which in turn motivated me to start the only Internet newsletter devoted to depression and bipolar disorder, *McMan's Depression and Bipolar Weekly*. A year and a half after launching my newsletter, I began a Web site, McMan's Depression and Bipolar Web (www.mcmanweb .com), which now has more than three hundred articles.

This book draws from more than six years of research that have gone into my newsletter and Web site. It is perhaps the first book on mood disorders that attempts to integrate expert opinion from a wide range of disciplines—from psychiatry and neurology and genetics to nutrition and spirituality. Equally important, this book acknowledges the wisdom and insight of those who have experienced depression and bipolar disorder firsthand. Many of these people have written to me directly. Others have posted comments on my Web site. Perhaps you are one of them.

"Please," writes Brian, "may I have my life back and start over again?."

Forget for the time being whether it's depression or bipolar disorder my readers are talking about. Simply listen.

"It's humiliating to me," says Bob, "to have to admit that there is something wrong with me mentally. I hate living this way. I have hope that I can be fixed or healed, but how can I face the people I love and apologize for my behavior and ask for forgiveness?"

Says Kali:

I realize that there are worse things out there, but to dream of having one good day let alone a good week, without having to feel anxiety, or wanting to give up, or confusion, short memory, loss of concentration, and no patience with family. I dream and pray to feel peace and happiness every day. And fight against my illness daily.

And from Claire:

I'm a talented person with a master's degree, but I have no partner, no family, no children, no full-time job, no career, no house, etc, etc. I have given in to my diagnosis, which is tragic.

I know if I had better self-esteem, I would like and appreciate myself just the way I am. I would revel in my talents as a writer and artist, and I might even revel in the extreme moods I've had. But the depressions. Oh, the depressions. I don't know why I haven't killed myself yet. I just haven't been suc-

cessful at it. Whether I commit suicide or not isn't even the is-
sue, because I have been dead inside for many years now.
Stagnant and isolated, unable to create, and alone.

Loneliness. The isolation can be worse than the illness. Eleanor
writes: "I ended up losing my job, my boyfriend, making my kids
feel confused and afraid. I am still trying to recover of all of it and
unsure about the future." And in a similar vein, a year after his diagnosis, Kyle writes: "I only just about manage to hold a job down.
I'm frustrated that my boss and my coworkers are unable to understand how I feel and, as yet, have been unable to tell my family for
the same reason—a lack of comprehension. I would just be told to
'pull myself together.' For the most part I feel lonely, isolated and
paranoid of other people."

Then there is the uncertainty. The knowledge that one is leaving
Planet Normal for a destination unknown weighs heavily on the
minds of those considering seeking help. As Leah explains: "I have
my first psych appointment on Monday. I am scared, nervous, and
freaked out about everything. I feel like everyone around me
doesn't care what I am feeling, especially my husband. I mean, I
know he cares, but when I try to discuss things with him it seems
like he tunes me out, looks right through me."

Meanwhile, the fearsome visage of the beast forces many of us to
look away before we are willing to face it head on. In Talia's words:

When I started going through my episodes of depression and
mania, I explained it off. Even five years ago, when I at-
tempted suicide and was committed for a week I wouldn't face
it. As soon as I was free, I tried to pretend it wasn't real. That
all came to a halt last Thursday. On the advice of a friend, I
visited a psychiatrist he knows. He confirmed what I most
feared: I am bipolar. Why did I seek help now? I'm tired. I'm
tired of trying to fighting alone. I'm tired of lying to myself.

Let us not forget the innocent bystanders, the families of those with mental illness. From Anonymous:

My dad quit taking medication about five years ago. He quit cold turkey. Today he says he is Jesus Christ and calls my mom the black eye devil and wants to put her six feet under-ground. He wants to kill her. He prays and shouts and listens to Gospel music and turns it up as loud as it will go. My mom is out of the house now and is safe. We called 911 and they went to his house but did not take him. He needs help. No-body will help.

Then there is the slow-motion suicide of Michelle: "I am more tearful now than ever before, I see no hope in sight. I really believe that I would be better off dead, yet I am too cowardly to kill myself, so I turn to alcohol and drugs I guess to slowly get rid of myself. I am worried for myself, as well as my children."

But Eric, in response to Michelle, offers this valuable insight:

It is a daily war against giving in to the darkness. The impulses, and constant voices in your head saying how un-worthy to be here, how unworthy of life to push into you. But, each day we win, we survive, and those who have not these forces pushing them have no concept of how strong you are, we all are, for winning a war daily against things that would immobilize any of them. I have had family tell me how weak I am, and I know, in my heart anyway, that they would never get out of bed, if for a moment they were shown what really goes on inside. Each day we survive is another victory we can draw on. Don't give up on yourself. You're 37, that means many years of victories. We can't lose sight of what it means to live each day out, when your own body conspires

*against you. We are not weak. We are strong. By surviving
daily, we show how strong we are.*

To that I can add the following (from a closing address I made to
the 2002 Depression and Bipolar Support Alliance [DBSA] annual
conference):

*In the New English Bible translation of the book of Ecclesi-
astes, it says: "In dealing with men it is God's purpose to test
them and see what they truly are." It's the only explanation, in
my opinion, for why bad things happen to good people. For
all the suffering all of us in this room have endured—all the
pain, tragedy, humiliation, hardship, and loss—I know we are
far better beings as a consequence. We may hate our illness,
but we can hardly hate what our illness has made of us.*

Depression and bipolar disorder can be considered a gift, but
only when we are well enough to appreciate the insights we have
gained from viewing the world through different and often tortured
eyes. So numerous are the artists, writers, musicians, and other
bright sparks with depression or bipolar disorder that a shorter list
may well be creative people with no mental illness. Think Michelangelo, Beethoven, van Gogh, Tchaikovsky, Lord Byron, Hemingway,
and Woolf. Think also how most of them wound up. Would
Beethoven have traded in his Ninth to shut down the raging mental
storms that tormented him so? What would van Gogh have given up
to enjoy but one day of peace and tranquillity? Yes, there are the
door prizes—a mystical third eye, creative wings, sparkling wit,
moral muscle—and we will be discussing these at length later on.
But it is the destructive and incapacitating nature of our illness that
demands our immediate attention.

Depression and bipolar disorder are treatable, but getting help is not as straightforward as simply throwing Prozac or lithium down the hatch. If only life were that simple. When I walked into my first support-group meeting not long after I was diagnosed, Moe, who ran the group, told me that meds are only one part of the equation. Getting well and staying well, he said, also involves eating right and sleeping right, diet and exercise, as well as a wide range of intangibles, which may include getting out of the house, volunteer work, spiritual practice, developing a support network, and a whole bag of survival tricks one starts to pick up.

To this day, this is the best advice I have ever received. What we are now learning about the brain is truly mind-boggling, but psychiatry still remains more of an art than a science. Treatments tend to be hit or miss, and patients can endure weeks and months and even years of frustration and heartbreak before striking oil. Compounding matters is that a medical treatment or lifestyle practice that appears to work for others may have no effect on you. Conversely, a much-maligned remedy may be your salvation.

"Whatever works" is my two-word credo, even if that applies to something that gets only 10 percent of us 10 percent better. For one, you could be one of the lucky 10 percent. For another, a 10 percent improvement may be all that it takes to help you turn the corner to full recovery.

There are two major qualifications to this 10 percent rule. First, it is foolhardy to risk prolonging your suffering and jeopardizing your safety at the outset by rolling the dice on a long-shot treatment. Second, the potential benefits of any treatment need to be carefully weighed against the possible dangers of that same treatment.

But simple math dictates that you will have several "ten-percenters" and even "one-percenters" in your arsenal. You may, for instance, find yourself on four different meds, taking a multivitamin, drinking a daily power smoothie, doing yoga and exercise, seeing a talking therapist, attending a support group, pursuing a hobby, and attending religious services.

Add to this the 101 informal things that you find yourself doing every day—from a relaxing soak in the tub to listening to Maria Callas to watching SpongeBob SquarePants to hugging your child, and you can see why there is nothing surgically precise about treating a mood disorder.

Chances are that most of the weapons in your arsenal won't even directly relate to mood. One of your meds, for instance, may help you sleep while another serves double duty for depression and anxiety. Your multivitamin may be more relevant to maintaining mental and physical function, the talking therapy may be for coming to terms with earlier trauma, the yoga may be for dealing with stress, while attending religious services may give you a sense of connection to something greater than your individual self.

Then there is the question of timing. One particular antimania med may quickly calm you down, but a different one may better serve you over the long haul. An antidepressant is another long-distance med, while sleep aids tend to be prescribed on an as-needed basis. Good lifestyle choices need to be regarded as constants while SpongeBob is strictly a short-term fix.

Blind faith is your worst enemy. Whether it's the pharmaceutical industry, the psychiatric and talking-therapy professions, or natural-health advocates, all are guilty of overselling their products and services and downplaying their own failings. The negative campaigning that goes on would put a politician to shame.

Yes, we need to listen to the professionals who treat us, but they also need to listen to us. They are the ones with the specialist knowledge, but we are the ones living in our own skins with access to the complete picture.

It is my fervent belief that learning about our illness equates to better outcomes. "Knowledge is necessity" has been my mission since Day One of my newsletter and Web site, and it applies with equal force to this book. The more we know, the better we will understand our illness and the smarter the choices we will make in its management, in partnership with our treating professionals. Patients who are motivated to build partnerships with their doctors have a better chance of achieving a successful outcome. An editorial in the March 27, 2004, issue of the *British Medical Journal* (BMJ) reports that two Stanford University studies found that so-called expert patients with chronic diseases felt better and had 42 to 44 percent fewer doctor visits than the other patients in the studies.

"Patients who have the resources to find out about their illness and want to take an active part in managing their own care are to be welcomed as allies and partners," concludes the *BMJ*. "Long live [quite literally, one presumes] expert patients . . ."

This book is not intended as medical or any other type of professional advice, but it should offer you some insights into working with your psychiatrist or therapist or physician or other professional. Ultimately, though, the responsibility for managing your illness lies with you.

Depression and bipolar disorder are classified as separate illnesses, but psychiatry is increasingly viewing them as part of an overlapping spectrum that also includes anxiety and psychosis. Accordingly, perhaps for the first time, depression and bipolar disorder are allotted equal space in one book. To me, it's a no-brainer: Many patients with bipolar disorder spend much of their lives depressed. Conversely, some people with clinical depression may be bipolar cases waiting to happen. Then there are the tweeners.

The Spectrum Project is an international consortium of academic researchers led by Giovanni Cassano, MD, of the University of Pisa. In the summer of 2004, I sat down with one of Dr. Cassano's collaborators on the project, Ellen Frank, PhD, professor of psychiatry and psychology at the University of Pittsburgh and director of the Depression and Manic Depression Prevention Program at the Western Psychiatric Institute and Clinic. Says Dr Frank: "What we've been arguing is that even isolated symptoms that don't cluster together to create episodes may be important."

This contrasts to the current approach of assigning clinical significance generally only if a certain number of symptoms are lumped together in a fixed period of time. What tends to distinguish clinical or unipolar depression from bipolar disorder, for example, is an episode of hypomania (think of mania lite, for the time being). Thus, if a person has enough hypomanic symptoms to come to the attention of a clinician, that person is diagnosed as having bipolar disorder. If not, that person is considered to have unipolar depression.

But an article published by the Spectrum collaborators in the July 2004 *American Journal of Psychiatry* illustrates where psychiatry may be headed. First, the researchers drew up a long list of hypomanic symptoms—far more than clinicians generally use—and surveyed a population of 117 adult patients with recurrent unipolar depression with no history of hypomanic episodes, and 106 patients with a severe type of bipolar disorder known as bipolar I. Predictably, the bipolar I patients had a lot more manic or hypomanic symptoms over their lifetimes than the unipolar group. Nevertheless, there were 12 items associated with hypomania (from high mood to irritability) that were each present in at least 40 percent of the depressed patients.

Intriguingly, the study's investigators found a relationship between the hypomanic/manic symptoms and the depressed symptoms. Patients with a higher number of lifetime manic/hypomanic symptoms had a higher number of lifetime depressed symptoms (and vice versa), a finding that held for both the bipolar and unipolar patients.

Perhaps the most important finding to emerge from the study was that even one symptom can have significant repercussions. In the group with unipolar depression, each manic/hypomanic item increased the likelihood of suicidal thinking by 4.2 percent. For ten items, this would equate to a 42 percent increased risk.

Approaching the spectrum from the bipolar end is Hagop

Akiskal, MD, of the University of California, San Diego, who has proposed that the illness be broadened to include "softer" criteria. This may include, for instance, a depressed person who cycles up into a state of simply feeling good rather than to a manic or hypomanic episode before cycling back down into depression.

In a 2003 study with his university colleague Lewis Judd, MD, Dr. Akiskal reexamined data from the landmark Epidemiological Catchment Area study from two decades ago. The original study found that 0.08 percent of the population surveyed had experienced a lifetime manic episode (the diagnostic threshold for bipolar I) and 0.05 a hypomanic episode (the diagnostic threshold for bipolar II).

Successor surveys have found a much higher bipolar population in the United States (more on this in Chapter 3), but the data from this survey gave Dr. Akiskal and his team plenty to work with. By tabulating survey responses to include criteria below the diagnostic radar, such as one or two symptoms over a short time period, the authors of the study recalculated the data to arrive at an additional 5.1 percent of the population, adding up to a total of 6.4 percent of the entire population who could conceivably be thought of as having bipolar disorder.

In other words, arguably one-half of patients who have or have had major depression, using Dr. Aksikal's reasoning, may be bipolar patients waiting to be reclassified.

Raymond DePaulo, MD, chair of the Department of Psychiatry and Behavioral Sciences at Johns Hopkins, tackles the mood spectrum from a genetic viewpoint. What his Johns Hopkins team and others are doing is slicing and dicing their study populations into various family subgroups in order to try to tease out elusive genes. Thus, the broader the spectrum, the more diverse the patients, who tend to pass on their particular spectrum traits to their offspring. This means looking for unusual connections that defy current diagnostic logic while paradoxically finding many degrees of separation. Dr. DePaulo and his Johns Hopkins team, for instance, have uncovered a possible genetic association between bipolar disorder and panic disorder (the manic-panic connection, which an editorial in the *American Journal of Psychiatry* called "striking") while also turning up convincing evidence that bipolar I and bipolar II each cluster in separate families.

The spectrum approach cannot be overstated. Although Dr. Frank cautioned in our interview, "I don't think we know yet whether [our findings have] treatment implications," and that "this is a new area of research, relatively speaking, and we don't know exactly where it will lead us," she also advised: "I think patients need to be aware of what might be softer expressions of both hypomania or mania, and try to the fullest extent possible to get their doctors to listen to their concerns that there may be something more going on here than unipolar depression."

Long before I began to appreciate the subtleties of the mood spectrum, it was clear to me that depression and bipolar disorder could not be artificially separated. So it was in June 1999 that I launched a newsletter to reach what I saw as two distinct but largely overlapping audiences. I had been diagnosed recently as having bipolar disorder, but what originally brought me to the emergency room was suicidal depression, and what I had been struggling with for most of my life was low-grade chronic depression.

It did not take me long to find out that many of the medications for both illnesses are interchangeable. Antidepressants are used (with a considerable degree of controversy) for both clinical depression and the depressed phase of bipolar disorder. Zyprexa, an antipsychotic medication for treating schizophrenia, has a Food and Drug Administration (FDA) indication for treating bipolar mania. When combined with the antidepressant Prozac under the trade name Symbyax, the drug can treat bipolar depression. Lithium, a common salt used for controlling the mood swings of bipolar disorder, is also used to kick-start an antidepressant to battle difficult-to-treat depression.

On and on it goes . . .

But a full appreciation of the spectrum also demands looking at what makes each of us different. In his National Book Award—winning *The Noonday Demon: An Atlas of Depression,* Andrew Solomon observed that depression is like a snowflake in that no two are alike. Ironically, however, by failing to consider his own depression in the broader context of a spectrum that also embraces bipolar disorder, and by focusing his book exclusively on depression, Mr. Solomon failed to recognize anomalous symptoms within his own depression. A few years after publication of his highly acclaimed depression magnum opus, Mr. Solomon was diagnosed with bipolar disorder.

Thus, even if you see yourself in the context of just one illness, it is strongly recommended that you cast your gaze outward to the other.

This book will look at both depression and bipolar disorder in terms of classical diagnostics, as there can be no discounting the convenience of psychiatry's separate but equal approach. Nevertheless, at all times these two separate illnesses and their many manifestations will be considered against the backdrop of a unifying spectrum. In addition to the overlap between depression and bipolar disorder, this includes looking at anxiety, psychosis, and alcohol and substance use—all of which are related to mood—as well as behaviors such as anger and temperaments such as introversion and exuberance, plus environmental-biological triggers such as stress and trauma. This book will also take an extended look at physical symptoms that are usually merely mentioned in passing in relation to mood, such as pain and eating and sleeping irregularities, as well as cognitive anomalies that can cause our minds to run on rocket fuel one minute and molasses the next.

We will also work our way out from the brain to examine how mood can affect the heart and other organs and body functions. Only after we have developed a basic appreciation for the intricacies of the spectrum and how it affects our complete being can we begin to deal with how we can cope, from numerous lifestyle options and natural remedies to various medical treatments and talking therapies.

We will also consider such serious topics as suicide prevention, how our illness affects special populations such as children, and relationship issues.

I was going to save the best stuff for last—brain science and genetics. Then again, why wait? Many of you may be intimidated by the subject matter, but I urge you to approach this section with the enthusiasm of a good beach read.

Along the way, I include interludes from my own lifelong struggles with depression and mania, as well as some idle musings. I also quote liberally from reader accounts on my Web site.

Let us proceed . . .

2

Depression

Introduction

Depression is a very common term. People say that they are depressed without meaning they are clinically depressed, leaving clinically depressed people to wonder if they're depressed in the first place. So let's start with some people who know they are depressed. Writes Charlene, on my Web site:

> I have been dealing with depression for so long I can't remember when it started. I spent most of my life thinking if I had more money, a better house, a better marriage, etc then everything would be okay. I have those things and nothing is better. I am so tired of fighting. I often believe my family would be so much better off without me, and on the days when I don't believe they would be, I still feel like I am only

*here for them and just surviving life waiting to die so I can fi-
nally have peace.*

Says Dove:

*Crying up to God to please take me home. I see friends pass
and envy them, or at least wish I could give them my time. I
go to the doctor and he will say "well how are we feeling today." If I was feeling good or happy enjoying life I would not
be in his office. I want death so bad, but what stops me from
doing it myself is how will God see what I've done. I feel
trapped, damned if I do damned if I don't. So life goes on
trapped in a world and body I wish to have no part of.*

Jason, age thirty-seven, despairs:

*I have no friends and haven't had any for at least 10 years.
The last time I danced was when I was 16. I am too self conscious and worried about what a fool I will make of myself to
dance. I don't and never did enjoy socializing, sports, muse-
ums, art, the movies. The things I like doing—science, math,
computers, electronics—are activities I like doing by myself. I
don't like to talk about them. I don't like to share them.*

*I'm pathetic. I haven't had sex with someone I haven't paid
in over two years.*

*I don't want to live. I know it's a joke. There is no real pur-
pose to life other than to procreate. I don't have any children.
I can't remember what it feels like to be idolized/loved the
way a man does a woman or vice-versa. Things don't really
happen for a reason. Events and outcomes are just some part
of some statistical distribution, normal, well take your pick.*

*I've come to the conclusion that I'm not depressed. I've re-
alized that I am supposed to feel this way. I am a loser. Like*

*the lion who can no longer win the pride back. Or like the al-
pha male who's been dethroned, I'm supposed to fade away
and die and not live a meager existence.*

Oh what joke and what a tragedy this life has been.

Strangely enough, you don't have to feel depressed to have clinical
depression. The *Diagnostic and Statistical Manual of Mental Disorders,* fourth edition, text revision *(DSM-IV-TR),* the diagnostic bible
put out by the American Psychiatric Association, in its criteria for
major depression lists *either* feeling depressed most of the time for
two weeks *or* abnormal loss of interest or pleasure most of the time
for two weeks. This dichotomy effectively divides depression into an
either-or choice of exaggerated sadness on one hand or lack of emotion on the other.

Are you *both* feeling depressed *and* having no pleasure? Don't
worry. The *DSM-IV* has thoughtfully provided a nine-item menu
choice that gives you a second crack at the first two, namely (in
slightly edited form):

■ Abnormal depressed mood (or irritable mood if a child or
adolescent)
■ Abnormal loss of all interest and pleasure
■ Appetite or weight disturbance, either weight loss or weight
gain
■ Sleep disturbance, either abnormal insomnia or abnormal
hypersomnia
■ Activity disturbance, either abnormal agitation or abnormal
slowing (observable by others)
■ Abnormal fatigue or loss of energy
■ Abnormal self-reproach or inappropriate guilt
■ Abnormal poor concentration or indecisiveness
■ Abnormal morbid thoughts of death (not just fear of dying) or
suicide

The *DSM-IV* mandates having at least five symptoms, though in actual clinical practice having only three or four is hardly going to rule out treatment.

At an Ask the Doctors session at the 2004 Depression and Bipolar Support Alliance (DBSA) annual conference, David Kupfer, MD, chair of the Department of Psychiatry at the University of Pittsburgh, said he "doesn't like the Chinese menu approach" of the *DSM-IV*. The number of symptoms, he said, is not as important as impairment in functioning, even if that involves relatively few symptoms.

And the impairment in function can be substantial. According to the World Health Organization, major depressive disorder is the leading cause of disability in the United States and established market economies worldwide. A 2000 DBSA survey reported that prior to being treated, 76 percent said that depression limited them in sleeping, 70 percent in social activities, and 69 percent in lifestyle. Sixty-two and 58 percent, respectively, reported that physical activities and work motivation were affected, and 52 percent said that depression had a negative effect on their loving relationship.

Dr. Kupfer was responding to an anecdote related by Lydia Lewis, then president of the DBSA, who reported on how Dennis Charney, MD, former head of the Mood and Anxiety Disorders Research Program at the National Institute of Mental Health Program (NIMH), tracked down the doctor who oversaw the *DSM* and asked how they arrived at five symptoms for depression. "It sounded like a good number," he was told.

Numerology apparently rules in psychiatry.

What is striking about the list of symptoms is that four of them can be considered physical in nature. Had the person responsible for the *DSM* had a yen for, say, the number 17, we might have had a lot more.

Speaking of seventeen, that's the number of symptoms listed in one version of the Hamilton Depression Rating Scale (HAM-D), used by clinicians and researchers to assess the severity of one's depression and to measure one's improvement (if any) over the course of treatment or a clinical trial. The HAM-D includes the *DSM-IV* symptoms (some listed more than once), plus anxiety (including physical anxiety symptoms, such as heart palpitations or sweating), sexual dysfunction, and general aches and pains, such as backache. These symptoms should arguably be included in the *DSM*, and perhaps in the next edition one or more of them will. Consider Jillian's narrative of her depression on my Web site.

> *There were nights I was not able to sleep, and then there were days when that's all I did. The most frustrating thing was that all the tools I had been using for years to deal effectively with my life just didn't work. I tried to tell myself that "this too shall pass," or, "look, you've handled worse than this." But to no avail . . . I ended up in hospital with chest pains. They thought it may have been a heart problem . . . just kept getting worse and worse. I had absolutely no energy, and I sometimes would have a hot flash that lasted all day. The doctors began thinking menopause. . . . It was like I was in this huge black hole and there was no life and no hope. . . .*
>
> *Finally, it got so bad that I decided to try a new doctor. I walked into her office and told her what was happening, and she said: "Jillian, I don't think this is menopause. I think this is depression." I really believe she saved my life.*

If only depression just made you feel sad or robbed you of pleasure. On my Web site, I describe it this way:

> *It's like a cardiac arrest, only it happens in the brain—something responsible for holding the gray mass together abruptly shifts, there is a sickening feeling of something terri-*

ble about to happen, and next thing your head is experiencing the awful sensation of being emptied out. From somewhere inside the power goes down and the body seems to collapse into itself like a marionette being folded into a box. You look for a way out, and what's left of your broken brain does its best to oblige with images of high bridges and frozen ponds and nooses dangling from balconies.

A person who had failed nearly every treatment and who identified herself as Patient 012 from Site 050 in 2004 testified before an FDA panel in support of an experimental surgical implant she had received in a clinical trial. "I ask you to imagine the unimaginable," she pleaded to the panel. "To think the unthinkable. To experience second-degree emotional burns with third-degree prognosis. All you experience is pain, but with no cure. In fact, there is no viable treatment. You can attempt to salve it. Only death solves it."

She went on to say:

But the medical community does not accept death as a cure. It asks us to continue to hang on and to continue to live, yet offers us no viable treatments. Trust me, it's not that we don't want to live. It's that we don't want to live "like this." Our illness is embedded in our physical bodies, our cells; we are prisoners there and our sentence is life.

Menacing insomnia; isolation; fear; anxiety; sadness; hopelessness; general malaise; malingering fatigue; physical exhaustion; apathy; lack of motivation, concentration, and focus; absence of pleasure; amplification of pain; agitation; sensitivity to criticism; thoughts that life isn't worth living. You are familiar with this short-sheeted laundry list of symptoms. Now imagine having them all at once. Imagine passing from one room to another in the House of Pain where some

symptoms are more prevalent than others, sometimes exacer-
bated by the very medications that were meant to alleviate
them.

Now we begin to see a commonality in all the stories, replete
with jarring descriptions and tortured thoughts: tired of fighting,
crying up to God, the power going down, house of pain . . .

Depression isn't the word for it. Brain crash is more like it. It is a
total assault of the body as well as the brain, every bit as much a
physical illness as mental. Our ancestors had every right to confuse
mental illness with demonic possession. This is an illness that lays
waste to the body as well as the mind. You can't think, you can't
move, you can't function.

Small wonder people can't take it. "Well, my own work," Vincent van Gogh wrote in his last letter to his brother Theo, "I am
risking my life for it, and my reason has half foundered." Six days
later, he would be dead, a bullet to his chest, an act of suicide.

Virginia Woolf couldn't bear the thought of going under once
more. One cold day in 1941—her body wasting from neglect, her
thoughts racing, and hearing voices—she wrote: "I feel certain now
that I am going mad again. I feel we can't go through another
of those terrible times. And I shan't recover this time. . . ." Then she
walked down to the riverbank, filled her pockets with stones, and
left her walking stick on the ground. Children would discover her
body three weeks later.

Sylvia Plath put her kids to sleep upstairs, then went down into
the kitchen and turned on the gas.

Those who never had depression cannot possibly comprehend.
When they tell us to snap out of it, we must forgive them for their
ignorance. This is an illness one must have lived through to truly understand. Far too many of us, unfortunately, wind up taking that
understanding to the grave.

However bad you are feeling, it is critically important to note that depression is an illness rather than an attitude or personal weakness, and thus is not your fault. Although having an upbeat manner would do wonders for your depression, the very nature of the illness militates against this happening.

If you are experiencing depression right now, the important thing to know is that you are not alone. It's not just you. As terrible as you are feeling, as hopeless as your situation may appear, things will get better, despite your brain trying to trick you into thinking otherwise.

As to what causes depression, the short answer is that we don't know. It is convenient to say that it is the result of a chemical imbalance in the brain, but this is not entirely accurate, especially since we cannot pinpoint the exact chemicals. Scientific consensus so far indicates that depression, as well as bipolar disorder, is the result of genes, biology, and the environment interacting with one another. We have yet to identify the mood genes, though experts expect we will find several, each making a small contribution.

The biology largely concerns how neurons in the brain communicate with one another, plus the chemical actions that take place inside the neuron.

The environment interacts with biology in the form of the body (which includes the brain) responding to stress or trauma or other triggers, resulting in the release of excess cortisol and adrenaline, which leads to the type of cellular breakdown that can result in depression and a host of other ills. Studies have shown, for example, that victims of childhood sexual abuse, war refugees, low-income women, and the poor are all particularly vulnerable. While it is true that all these populations have more to be depressed about, these studies indicate a lot more is going on.

A 2005 National Comorbidity Survey (NCS) Replication survey of 9,282 U.S. residents found that the prevalence for lifetime major depression was 16.6 percent, equating to 35 million U.S. adults, and for the previous twelve months was 6.7 percent, representing

14 million U.S. adults. Thirty percent of the episodes were serious. Half of the individuals with depression in the previous year had received care for their depression, but treatment was only adequate less than half the time.

According a 2001 National Mental Health Association survey, only 18 percent of the U.S. adult depressed population has ever received a diagnosis. Forty-two percent of those with a formal diagnosis said they were embarrassed by or ashamed of their symptoms, and 16 percent were afraid to talk to their friends. Only 55 percent of diagnosed individuals expected treatment would provide even initial relief.

Part of the problem is that people literally don't know what has hit them. The *DSM-IV* gamely attempts to break down different types of depression according to symptoms or circumstances, but until we can do it according to biology and genes, even the experts are flying in the dark. Even in the same individual, no two depressions are alike. A 2003 Columbia University study examined seventy-eight inpatients with major depression during two separate episodes and found there was little association between the symptoms across episodes. The authors of the study used the word *pleomorphic* to describe the illness's uncanny ability to assume different forms in the same person.

What psychiatry has been able to do is distinguish situational from clinical depression, so let's begin with the obvious.

Situational versus Clinical Depression

The best way to explain depression to a friend is to ask that person to recall what it was like when a loved one died. But grief is a normal response to the death of someone close to you and is not regarded as pathological. Only when bereavement lasts for two months or more, says the *DSM*, should we reconsider the diagnosis.

The same thinking goes into the *DSM*'s requirement that a depressive episode go on for two weeks or more. As an example, psychiatrists noticed a lot of their patients reporting depression soon following the 2004 election (it is fair to say they would have received similar reports from a different set of patients had the results gone the other way).

Perhaps, if you were on the losing side, you handled your disappointment well. But there were some, no doubt, who began to think like classic depression cases, despairing, with dark thoughts, and perhaps with no will to go on. Such an individual—let's call him Ishmael—may have taken to his bed, not showered or shaved, lost his appetite, canceled appointments, not returned calls, and snarled at his kids.

But it's difficult to imagine this going on for two weeks. The cause of Ishmael's despair is situational, and his reaction, though worrisome, is understandable (to Democrats, anyway). He may still entertain a beef about politics, but within a few days he will be back to looking forward to better times, such as perhaps walking his daughter down the aisle.

Now compare Ishmael to the real-life example of Terry Bradshaw, Hall of Fame football quarterback and sports announcer known for his boyish exuberance. In 2003, Terry astounded everyone by publicly acknowledging he had depression all his professional life. "I didn't understand that after every Super Bowl victory, I could never find pleasure in what I'd done," came the stunning revelation.

Instead of seeking help, Terry admitted to spending lots of money to feel better, buying horses for his ranch, then more horses when he still wasn't happy. It wasn't until the breakup of his marriage that he finally sought help, starting therapy and taking an antidepressant.

What Terry Bradshaw went through clearly wasn't normal. True, fame and fortune can't buy you happiness, but even an existentialist knows that you're supposed to feel elated after leading your team to a Super Bowl victory.

For lack of a better term, Terry was suffering from clinical depression, a medical condition thought to be caused by a physical malfunction in the brain. If you think of Terry's brain as a computer, his software was basically filtering out all that should have brought him any sense of accomplishment and joy. On my Web site, Lucinda describes it this way:

> *I am so lethargic and cannot find anyway out. . . . I cannot seem to make myself do anything. All I want or seem to be able to do to get out of bed is get the newspaper and try and read it, smoke, or open a can of something or eat a box of ice cream, watch TV or surf the Internet, and now a new addiction—buying things on eBay! Getting expensive!!! . . .*
>
> *I make jewelry and used to love it, but now can't complete anything and am in such a mess with my beads I don't think I'll ever get them straightened out. I've gained forty pounds, don't care about my appearance, can't clean the house, etc etc. I feel I have all the symptoms of depression, plus I can't feel any excitement about seeing loved ones, can't think of anything, or anywhere I want to be but in my bedroom.*

The Prize Patrol could probably show up on Lucinda's door with a check for $25 million and she would still feel miserable. Or even if she levitated to the ceiling in exultation, it wouldn't be long before she went back to her current life in a darkened room, even if that room happened to be part of a new mansion in the Hamptons.

But situational and clinical depression can be related. Let's go back to Ishmael's case. Let's suppose that Ishmael's brain has been biologically predisposed to depression since birth, and that the condition had remained dormant all his life, waiting for the right trigger to set it off. This time, instead of recovering in a few days, Ishmael continues to feel like a dead man walking. He manages to drag himself to work, but he's just going through the motions. Several months pass. He walks his daughter down the aisle, but he is as indifferent as Terry Bradshaw after winning a Super Bowl.

Call me Ishmael. In 1997–1998, my life was unraveling in slow motion. I had suffered from depression from childhood, but now, with nothing going right in my life, I was well on my way to buying a one-way ticket out of it. Then, in the fall of 1998, came a crushing series of rejections. I simply had no oxygen. My run of bad luck had propelled me into the Mount Everest Death Zone from which there was only one way out.

In previous years, around Christmastime, I had made gifts for my niece and nephews. One year it was watercolors of dinosaurs playing basketball (try to imagine a brontosaurus dribbling downcourt on a fast break). Another year I did an illustrated book. Yet another year I made papier-mâché masks, and the next it was a seven-foot-tall cardboard-and-papier-mâché totem pole that you could take apart and reassemble. My pièce de résistance was a miniature golf course with interchangeable putting surfaces for reconfiguring the holes.

I can't begin to describe the hours of pleasure those projects brought me, and how I much I looked forward to my once-a-year excursions from life as usual, where I would plot and scheme and plan and draw and buy new materials and go to the pantry where I had my art supplies stowed away in an old roasting pan. Then, out on the kitchen table, I could get down to the serious business of pretending I was Leonardo da Vinci.

But this year, I couldn't be bothered. The pencils stayed in their drawers, the art supplies remained in the pantry. I recall going over to the next-door neighbors for Christmas Eve drinks. The previous year, they had coaxed me into croaking out my rendition of "Ol' Man River." This time, I could barely pretend I was enjoying the finger food. I can't recall how Christmas went.

By now, suicide was a constant in my thoughts. I couldn't help but think of "Ol' Man River":

> *Ah gits weary*
> *An' sick of tryin'*
> *Ah'm tired of livin'*
> *An' skeered of dyin' . . .*

I clearly didn't want to live, but death was so permanent, so irrevocable. If I could have opted for being dead for a little while, I would not have hesitated. Perhaps that was why I found myself sleeping so much. It was the closest living experience to being dead. And I enjoyed it. I liked being dead. I looked forward to being dead. Being dead gave me the walking dead man's equivalent of unequivocal pleasure.

It was only a question of working up the courage. But the way things were going, courage would no longer enter into it. Just a little deeper into the Mount Everest Death Zone, I knew, and it wouldn't be a matter of me committing the act. The act, instead, would commit me. The rope would tie its own noose, the pond's frigid waters would warmly embrace me, the bridge would obligingly throw me off . . .

But at the last minute I chickened out. I chickened out. That's how I felt at the time. I stood in my mother's kitchen, back to her, hands clutching the sink, and called out for help. The total illogic of the decision stunned me. It made no sense to a person in my condition. I had chosen life over death.

Would things have been different had those rejections from several months earlier been acceptances? To be sure, my life would have played out a lot differently, but in the overall scheme of things, the good news would have been a stay of execution, nothing more. My biology made me an emergency-room case waiting to happen, only waiting for the right situation. My time came two days into

1999. There was snow outside, there were bowl games on TV. My brother showed up and calmly urged me to get in the car. He was taking me to the hospital.

I don't kid myself. I will always be an emergency-room case waiting to happen. Once you have emerged from the Death Zone and lived to tell the tale you are never the same. On one hand, I am amazed at my strength in surviving the ordeal; on the other, I am humbled by the fact that I am no more than a leaf in a tornado to my condition.

Back to the *DSM*

The *DSM* classifies the different types of depression—either as subtypes of the illness, part of another illness, as specifiers, or as separate disorders—including melancholic depression, atypical depression, bipolar depression, dysthymia, psychotic major depression, seasonal affective disorder, and postpartum depression. Bipolar depression and postpartum depression will be discussed at length later on in the book.

Melancholic and Atypical Depression

In an article in the March 15, 2004, *BMC Psychiatry,* Konstantinos Fountoulakis, PhD, and colleagues at Aristotle University of Thessaloniki report that melancholic and atypical depression occupy opposite poles. In melancholia, say the authors, "the autonomous nervous system and the stress response seem hyperactive. Patients are anxious, dread the future, lose responsiveness to the environment, have insomnia, lose appetite . . . with depression at its worst in the morning."

Patients with atypical depression, by contrast, tend to be "lethargic, fatigued, hyperphagic [leaden], hypersomniac, reactive to the environment, and [are] . . . best in the morning." The stress response may be dampened.

Back when depression was called melancholia, its poster boy could have been the great Romantic composer and pianist Frédéric Chopin. In his own words: "Why do we live on through this wretched life which only devours us and serves to turn us into corpses? The clocks in the Stuttgart belfries strike the midnight hour. Oh how many people have become corpses at this moment!"

Take out the reference to the belfries and one could easily mistake that passage for something straight out of Ecclesiastes and the book of Job. Chopin's depressive temperament was a constant leitmotif throughout his life. The crushing of the Polish revolution devastated him. An early engagement ended in sorrow. The breakup of his relationship with the novelist George Sand and the failure of the revolutions of 1848 left him a broken man. Undoubtedly, depression contributed to his ailing health, and he died not long after in 1849, having seemingly given up on living.

Then there is our presidential poster boy, Abraham Lincoln.

"I am now the most miserable man living," the thirty-one-year-old man confessed in early 1841. "Whether I shall ever be better I can not tell; I awfully forebode I shall not. To remain as I am is impossible; I must die or be better." Concerned friends removed all sharp objects from his room and maintained a close vigil.

In an article in the *New York Times,* historian Doris Kearns Goodwin relates how historians regard a broken-off engagement to Mary Todd as the trigger to his famous depression, but it was his perceived failure as politician, she maintains, that fed Lincoln's black dog. As a state legislator in Illinois, young Lincoln had championed various public-works projects, but a sustained economic recession resulted in his beloved projects being scrapped in midcompletion and the state fell into bankruptcy, with Lincoln cast as a scapegoat. So bleak was his depression that his best friend, Joshua Speed, warned Lincoln he would die if he did not rally.

Assuming the presidency in 1861—as perhaps the most inexperienced person to ever hold that office—during the nation's gravest crisis would pose an extreme challenge to Lincoln's well-being. But in 1862, he surprised his cabinet with a proposal for freeing the slaves in Union-held Southern territory, the first step to universal freedom and enfranchisement.

Soon after the signing of the Emancipation Proclamation, Joshua Speed visited his old friend and they recalled their earlier conversations about his depression twenty-two years earlier. Referring to his historic document, Lincoln told his friend, "I believe that in this measure my fondest hopes will be realized."

But our melancholic poster boy was also renowned as a masterful storyteller who loved to laugh, even while he was depressed. The only reason photographs show Lincoln appearing somber is because the technology of the day required him to hold his pose for thirty seconds. So did the sixteenth president actually have atypical depression? Perhaps his depressions "pleomorphically" shifted from one to the other.

Don't be fooled. "Atypical" depression is actually the most common subtype of depression in outpatients, according to Andrew Nierenberg, MD, and his colleagues at the Depression Clinical and Research Program at Massachusetts General Hospital, affecting anywhere from 25 to 42 percent of the depressed population.

According to the *DSM-IV*, as opposed to major depression, the patient with atypical features experiences mood reactivity, with improved mood when something good happens. In addition, the *DSM-IV* mandates at least two of the following: increase in appetite or weight gain (as opposed to the reduced appetite or weight loss of "typical" depression); excessive sleeping (as opposed to insomnia); leaden paralysis; and sensitivity to rejection.

A 2003 multicenter study identified a group with atypical depression, representing 36.4 percent of the depressed sample in the U.S. National Comorbidity Survey. The study found that those with atypical depression were mostly women, had higher rates of depressive symptoms, more co-occurring psychiatric illnesses, more suicidal thoughts and attempts, greater disability and restricted activity days, more use of some health-care services, greater paternal depression, and more childhood neglect and sexual abuse than the other depressed individuals in the survey.

The fact that depression has an atypical face takes many of my Web-site readers by surprise. In response to an article on my site, Lorraine writes: "I was struck by the description of atypical depression as it appears in my life. I have had 75-plus pound weight gain, bouts of crying, suicidal thoughts and bleak moods, yet I can still laugh at a really good joke. I thought I was just plain crazy because I wasn't depressed all of the time." Says Annette: "I feel I have finally found a name for what I've been suffering from ever since I was a teenager."

The same treatments that work for "typical" depression also work for atypical depression, but the difference between merely getting somewhat better and much better may depend on your ability to communicate to your psychiatrist and therapist. Matters that don't seem important to you at the time, such as how you sleep, may make all the difference in devising medications and talking-therapy strategies that really work.

Dysthymia

If we think of major depression as a spectacular brain crash, milder chronic depression (dysthymia) can be compared to a form of mind-wearing water torture. Day in and day out, it grinds us down, robbing us of our will to succeed in life, to interact with others, and to enjoy the things that others take for granted. The gloom that is generated in our tortured brains spills outward into the space that surrounds us and warns away all those who might otherwise be our friends and associates and loved ones. All too frequently, we find ourselves alone, shunned by the world around us and lacking the strength to make our presence felt.

The symptoms are similar to major depression, with feelings of despair and hopelessness, and low self-esteem, often accompanied by chronic fatigue. This can go on for years, day in, day out.

The *DSM-IV* mandates the same symptoms as for major depression, except for suicidality, but requires only three symptoms in all, so long as they have persisted over two years.

Still, we are able to function, a sort of death-in-life existence that gets us out into the world and to work and the duties of staying alive, then back to our homes and the blessed relief of flopping into our unmade beds.

All too often, we are told to snap out of it, that the invisible water torture we carry in our heads is our own fault. Thus shamed into thinking something is wrong with our attitudes, we fail to seek help. Or, if we do, it's our family physician who sends us out the door with a prescription and no follow-up care.

On my Web site, Mac describes his unremitting sense of living a kind of no-life.

If this is a "minor" depression, anything worse is hard to contemplate. There is nothing interesting. Friends, work, music, play, sex, God—these are things that others experience. (And even enjoy, or so you're told.) Or if you experience them, it is as though you are doing it through a thick fog, dulling the sensation to the point of meaninglessness.

Yet you keep on. You have to. Others depend on you. There are bills to pay, children to raise, laundry to do, a lawn to mow. You put off what you can, doing only what is absolutely necessary. Because just existing takes such effort, and you are so bone-weary all the time.

Sooner or later, it happens: the brain crash. Major depression. That's how most of us wind up, according to the experts— sometimes with a double depression, a depression on top of a depression that never had to be.

I won't even begin to estimate how many years I've lost to a disorder predicated by the modifier *mild to moderate*. The least they could have done was assign the name of a Shakespeare character— Hamlet's disease, Lear's disease, anything, really. Just so long as it doesn't imply I was cut down in my prime by some invisible stupid nerf bat pounding against the inside of my brain. For the rest of you: You can end it right now. You don't have to endure the mental water torture any longer.

Psychotic Major Depression

With psychotic major depression, one's thoughts of guilt and worthlessness and hopelessness cross the line into the realm of delusion. The *DSM* cites examples of "mood congruent" features, including holding oneself responsible for the death of a loved one or deserving to be punished for some moral transgression or personal inadequacy. One can also experience delusions of illness or poverty.

Less common are "incongruent" features that include delusions of persecution and the belief that one's thoughts aren't one's own. Those in a state of psychotic depression can also experience hallucinations such as hearing voices.

Not surprisingly, individuals with psychotic depression are more likely to wind up in the hospital than their nonpsychotic counterparts, accounting for 25 percent of hospitalized depressed patients. Recurrences are common, and treatment is problematic, though we are learning more, especially since the advent of a new generation of antidepressants and antipsychotics, which can be effective when taken as a combination.

Seasonal Affective Disorder

In the fall of 1975, I had moved to Vancouver to be with my fiancée. There, in Kitsalano, where the hippies hung out, one could wake up to a breathtaking view of the ships in the harbor and the snow-capped mountains behind North Vancouver. But nine days out of ten, the clouds dropped to treetop level, discharging a light mist that carried the intoxicating scents of the nearby forests into the city, but also creating a filmy shroud that settled over every landmark in the vicinity.

"They took away the mountains," I would half-joke to my fiancée, not used to a force that could turn mighty peaks invisible. Then December approached, and with it a Stygian darkness that descended at four in the afternoon and snuffed out the murky gray that passed for light in this part of the world.

So it came as a welcome relief to spend Christmas with my folks in Connecticut, where the temperatures were much colder, but where there was light in abundance. How resplendent it was reflected off the snow, in brilliant blues with gold highlights. Light, light, glorious light. I drank it in the way a dehydrated person might immerse himself in water.

Then it was back to the gloom of Vancouver, one that lasted through the summer. I felt my own lights going out. It got so bad that I actually flunked a driver's test twice. As the darkness settled in, I could feel the whole city turning against me. It was as if everyone in the phone directory had entered into a secret pact to make my life miserable. Every time a Canadian said, "Eh," I knew it was a personal insult directed at me and me only.

"I hate this city!" I screamed in the rain to my fiancée.

Thankfully, though, I could now see light at the end of the tunnel—literally. We were moving to New Zealand and into a Southern Hemisphere spring. I could actually feel the clouds lift as I boarded that plane. And down at the other end of the world, I landed on my feet. I had been delivered. I was going to make it.

Little did I know that nearly the whole time I spent in Vancouver, I was experiencing a winter depression known as seasonal affective disorder (SAD). Even science was stupid about the phenomenon back then.

To make matters worse, I had undiagnosed bipolar disorder, which made me a sitting duck. People with mood disorders are far more likely to be affected by the change in seasons, with estimates of likelihood ranging as high as 38 percent. Looking back, it was amazing my relationship survived that year in Vancouver. It almost certainly wouldn't have lasted a second year there.

A year or two after my experience, a South African psychiatrist, Norman Rosenthal, MD, moved to New York, where he experienced the same kind of mood change I went through. With the assistance of a colleague, he began to expose himself to artificial light, and almost immediately noticed a marked improvement in his mood.

The *DSM-IV* does not list SAD as a separate disorder but rather as a "seasonal pattern" for depression and bipolar disorder. According to the *DSM,* there must be a "regular temporal relationship" between the onset of major depression and the time of year (fall or winter), accompanied by a full remission (or change to mania or hypomania) in the spring. People with SAD often experience symptoms associated with atypical depression.

Approximately 4 to 6 percent of the population experiences SAD. Women are four times more likely to be affected than men. People with a long history of depression or bipolar disorder need to be especially mindful of the change in seasons; many patients await the turning of the leaves with a trepidation that borders on terror.

SAD is most likely to affect people in higher latitudes and coincides with the darkest months of the year, making the seasonal reduction in light the obvious culprit. But how this registers on the brain is still a matter of speculation. One theory is that serotonin levels drop off in winter. Another is that melatonin secretion may be the cause. Yet another theory posits that circadian rhythms are thrown out of whack. Since serotonin, melatonin, and circadian rhythms all interact, the true answer is likely a combination of all three.

One thing that science agrees on is that light therapy is the treatment of choice, and that the eyes and not the skin respond to the light. Going for winter walks outdoors will save you the $200 or $300 cost of a light box, while buying a light box for indoor use will spare you the necessity of freezing outdoors in the cold. (More on light therapy in the "Complementary Treatments" chapter of this book.)

A few of my Web site readers point out some very interesting variations to the seasons and weather theme. Aura (gotta love the irony of the name) describes herself and her husband as "severe weather gauges," whose moods begin to change for the worse with a storm on the horizon, so much so that "I have developed a phobia about driving in the rain." LuAnne reports on her case of "reverse SAD," which compels her to wear dark glasses and have heavy drapes in the bedroom. "I HATE Spring," she writes; "it fills me with foreboding. Summer renders me stupid, indecisive, and ravenous for carbohydrates." Finally, Woody reports that two years of living in constant summer in southern Florida triggered severe depression, which abated with the change of the seasons when he moved back north. "For some of us," he reports, "the tropics can be very destructive. The sameness of the weather and foliage was very numbing and enervating."

Things to Consider for the Next *DSM*

The *DSM* was never meant to be regarded as cast in stone, though I came away with that impression when I found myself unexpectedly seated at a dinner symposium next to one of its principal architects at the 2003 American Psychiatric Association's annual meeting. In fairness, no one ever told Harley Earl, the legendary auto designer, what to do with the shape of his fins.

The next edition of the *DSM* is scheduled for 2010 at the earliest, and there are bound to be changes based on what we have learned about depression since the *DSM-IV*, which came out in 1994; the revised edition of the *DSM-III (DSM-III-R)*, which is very similar, came out in 1987; and the groundbreaking *DSM-II* of 1980 (the equivalent of the '55 Chevy), which influenced everything that came after.

But, by nature, the *DSM* is a conservative document, so there will always be a certain disconnect between clinical reality and diagnostic formality. It appears that some kind of anxiety component will be built into the next edition, but borrowing pain and other items from the HAM-D appears problematic.

In an article in the May 2001 *Neuropsychopharmacology and Biological Psychiatry,* Herman van Praag, MD, of Maastricht University, has proposed there be a new subtype of depression called anxiety/aggression–driven depression, with treatment zeroing in on different chemical targets.

Along a similar line, at the 2001 Fourth International Conference on Bipolar Disorder, Athanasios Koukopoulos, MD, of the University of Rome, made a case for agitation as a separate subtype. Agitation is a symptom, but subtypes get more respect. As Dr. Koukopoulos explained: "Major depressive episodes with or without agitation are treated in the same way, and the result is disastrous in many cases of agitated depression."

Then there is the matter of gender. According to conventional wisdom, twice as many women suffer from depression as men, at least using the current *DSM* as a measure. Adding new criteria to account for male behavior, however, could even the score. (The Harley Earl of the *DSM* positively hated hearing about this.)

A critical issue that psychiatry is not addressing is apathy, or lack of motivation. Your "get up and go just got up and went." Life, the universe, everything—nothing matters. The *DSM* is halfway there in its "loss of pleasure" criterion, but stops short of the emotional numbing that also incorporates a deadening to grief. If one thinks of depression as too much emotion, apathy is too little. We may have to wait until the *DSM-XXVII* before the experts get around to reconciling these opposites.

One cautionary note to this discussion is that depression is already difficult enough to define without piling on yet more symptoms and adding subtypes. A good case can be made that the clinical conception of depression is so wide as to be absolutely meaningless. Imagine if we assigned the same name to cancer, diabetes, and broken bones and treated them all the same way. Imagine if we could not understand why the patients with broken bones and diabetes failed to respond to radiation. Imagine if we were unaware entirely of the broken bones.

Adding new symptoms to depression, then, is justifiable only in the context of breaking down an impossibly amorphous phenomenon into more clearly defined illnesses or illness subtypes. The next *DSM* may pass on this challenge, but your clinician cannot afford to—and neither can you.

That Spectrum Thing Again

The pioneering diagnostician Emil Kraepelin did not distinguish between depression and bipolar disorder. Hagop Akiskal, MD, the leading proponent of widening the bipolar end of the mood spectrum to include more patients currently classified as having unipolar depression, has urged a return to Kraepelin (though obviously to incorporate what we have learned since then).

The *DSM-IV* fails psychiatrists and their patients in two key areas: (1) its criteria for bipolar depression are exactly the same as its criteria for unipolar (clinical) depression; (2) its criteria for bipolar hypomania read as a simplistic form of mania lite.

Not surprisingly, depressed patients who have never sung at karaoke bars (or only thought about it) are likely to wait many years before psychiatrists figure out what's wrong (ten years for more than one-third of patients, according to a 2000 DBSA survey).

Some of you with difficult-to-treat depression may be bipolar cases waiting to happen, especially if a future *DSM* comes up with softer criteria for the illness. But a good many of you may find yourselves along a gray area in the spectrum, inhabiting a sort of no-man's-land between depression and bipolar disorder—clearly depressed, but with inexplicable surges of anger, agitation, and even occasional giddiness.

As mentioned earlier, a Spectrum Project study found that 40 percent of patients with recurrent unipolar depression had hypomanic symptoms typical of bipolar patients—not enough to qualify as an episode and rate a change in diagnosis but clearly sufficient to make a clinical impact.

Unfortunately, no-man's-land is virtual terra incognita to psychiatry. Even just over the border in the land of bipolar II there are almost no studies. Thus we have no conclusive findings on whether treatments that work for bipolar I can be successfully applied to bipolar II, much less to what can best be described as novel depressions.

A competent clinician in this situation may simply throw out the *DSM* and any treatment guidelines and work with you as an individual, labeling you only for the sake of filling out insurance forms, but treating your symptoms rather than your so-called illness. A psychiatrist may try using bipolar meds, and a talking therapist may work on ways of managing your anger or impulsivity.

But even an expert needs your help, a point that will be stressed in this book again and again. So as well as confiding to your psychiatrist or therapist about how miserable you are, come prepared to talk about those times you felt agitated and irritable and even a little hyper and happy. In other words, give your clinician something to work with. We're still learning as we go, but what you say can make all the difference in the world.

3

Bipolar Disorder

Introduction

Consider the following scenario:

A person visits his doctor or psychiatrist in a state of near suicide. After probing for other possible causes of the patient's condition, the psychiatrist concludes the culprit is clinical depression and prescribes a standard antidepressant. The pill works uncommonly fast. Within two or three days the patient's energy has returned, his dark mood lifts, and for one brief shining moment he knows what it's like to feel normal, and even better than normal.

His mind is racing now. He starts making grand plans. Meanwhile, his mind keeps racing. He thinks this is just a side effect that will go away, so he takes another pill. After all, the very last thing he wants to happen is to crash back into that horrible depression of his, knowing full well that next time there may be no return.

But his racing mind refuses to stop. Instead, it cranks into an even higher gear. He cannot sleep, his heart is pounding, he is talking a mile a minute, and soon he is vividly hallucinating. "Roller coaster" is totally inadequate to describe the experience. One is not driving the brain. Rather, the brain is driving the person. In extreme cases, the victim will rage completely out of control. In one extraordinary situation, a person on an antidepressant actually robbed a bank and was acquitted.

That, my friends, is the closest modern medicine has come to a laboratory test for a psychiatric condition. The illness is bipolar disorder, also known as manic depression. Toss an antidepressant at a person with bipolar disorder—with no mood-stabilizing medication to hold the antidepressant action at bay—and watch him flip out.

Ping! Flip City. Totally manic.

The reason I happen to know so much about this is that it happened to me. Thankfully, I did not rob a bank, but I know from my experience how it could happen. For the crisis-intervention psychiatrist who later saw me, it was a no-brainer.

"Bipolar mixed," she wrote on the script with no comment. With those two words, my life changed. I was branded. By the same token, I was also relieved. After a lifetime of denial, I finally knew what I was up against. Having identified my adversary, I could begin to fight it, and I stood an excellent chance of winning.

So how come my first psychiatrist did not pick it up? I consider myself lucky. According to a 2000 DBSA survey, 69 percent of bipolar patients were misdiagnosed on their first professional visit, and of these, one-third waited ten years to achieve a correct diagnosis. Unfortunately, unless we happen to land in the hospital in the midst of a wildly manic episode, there is not much for the doctor to go on.

I was depressed. At the time, I had no knowledge of bipolar disorder in the family (since my diagnosis, I have discovered it exists on both sides). All I talked about was my depression. All of them—

my depression within a depression, my depression following a depression, my depression following the depression on top of the depression, and so on. My "ups" were what I mistook for normal behavior, so I did not feel compelled to bring them to my psychiatrist's attention. Besides, considering the state I was in, he wasn't about to mistake me for the type who danced on tables.

I consider myself one of the fortunate ones. After one false start I found a treatment that worked, soon started my own business, and five years later remarried. Years of going untreated virtually wrecked my life, but I've been able to pick up the pieces. Others do not share my good fortune. Check out the frustration of Marcy, writing on my Web site shortly after being denied disability:

> *Come, join me as I take six medications. Watch me as I enter a manic mood and decide that I will try to go to college and live a happy, normal life. Watch me as, hours later, I lay sobbing and crumbled on the floor because I am depressed now and have just been brought back into the realization that college isn't going to happen for me right now. Watch me as I call my sister and talk about her college studies and friends. Watch me as I watch "Friends."*
>
> *Well, you see, Claims Officer, it's terribly hard for me to make and keep friends because they don't like they way I go from being energized to being suicidal. Well, neither do I! Watch me as I choke down yet more large, expensive pills that never seem to work.*

Says Shelly:

> *I have been on every medicine known to man and I have never had any relief. I can't hold a job or care for myself correctly. Yet, I have an IQ of 151. Do you know what it's like to be smarter than 98.9 percent of the population, but yet somehow*

not be able to be a productive member of society? It just seems like such a waste. Up and down, down and up. That is my life. I have to deal with all on my own because very few people, including my parents and my ex-husband, care what happens to the mentally ill in our country. The stigma is just too much to people. My parents do not have a picture of me in their home. So many people do not understand that we are real people too that need love and need help.

Adds Francine: "At age 56, I keep thinking the madness will ebb soon; that the days will start to look brighter. I try to see the blessings in my life. There are a few. Then why is it so hard to get out of bed every day? Why can't I keep a job? Why do I cry all the time? Why do I feel that God is away at an important meeting so he's not there for me?"

Cheryl observes: "Living the life of a bipolar person is the greatest challenge I will ever face. Each is a new day. I face death each day that I live. And each day, I try to find a reason to live."

And Meow gets right to the point:

A small poem on Bipolar. . . .
SCREEEEEEEAAAAAAMMMMMM
Did you hear that?
That was me;
Inside my head.
I wish I was dead

The quick definition of bipolar disorder—the one I would give standing on one foot while juggling plates—is that it is an illness of the brain characterized by extreme shifts in mood from depressive lows to manic highs. One of my Web site readers, Trisha, calls the illness the really reallys, in reference to her being "either really really happy or really really sad."

Lest we convey a false impression, people with bipolar disorder do not necessarily shuttle exclusively from pole to pole. Long periods in the temperate and equatorial zones are common. Having said that, symptoms and their aftereffects have a way of persisting even during so-called normal states. Accordingly, the term bipolar is a misleading one. Nevertheless, it is a useful reference for initiating discussion.

The ups—let's talk about the ups for a while. We all have our moments of elation, giddiness, or bliss. This is perfectly normal, as are those days when we get up on the "right" side of bed and the world seems to spin in our direction. If someone has hit the genetic jackpot, he or she can feel something like this nearly every day, with fame and fortune and friends gravitating to him or her like iron filings to a magnet.

"When you look across the entire bipolar spectrum, you find that maybe 10 percent to 15 percent of these people never get depressed. They're just up," Ronald Kessler, PhD, of Harvard and the head of the National Comorbidity Survey, said in an article in the *New York Times*. These are your classic American success stories, according to John Gartner, PhD, of Johns Hopkins, author of *The Hypomanic Edge: The Link Between (a Little) Craziness and (a Lot of) Success in America*.

When these people get depressed, it's only because they have been sidelined (usually as a consequence of their exuberance). But then it's back to a new project.

The rest of us should be so lucky. Depression is often our next stop. Other times, that intoxicating sense of elation starts escalating out of control. One may start talking fast, spending money, and engaging in inappropriate activities. Or the magic may start to wear off, as winning behavior deteriorates into crass and embarrassing caricature. Sometimes the elation turns sour, into a dysphoric rage that makes work and social and family life hell for all concerned.

Generally, someone in a state of sustained elevation is said to be "hypomanic."

Full-blown mania turns up the heat. If one hasn't wrecked his life while in a state of hypomania, he or she is a prime candidate going into mania. These tend to be your 911 cases, bordering on and breaking through into psychosis. Nevertheless, an antipsychotic medication or tranquilizer can bring down a person with mania in a matter of hours or less, though long-term stabilization can be a lot more problematic.

Yet even with our brains firmly held in place by the best medical science has to offer, there is no peace of mind. At any minute, any second, at the slightest provocation, we are all too aware that the insides of our skulls can break loose from their pharmacological moorings and indiscriminately tear down what took us a lifetime to build.

Simply losing a night's sleep may trigger a manic episode, not to mention the stress from work or a relationship breakup. And past trauma, bad lifestyle choices, and failure to manage stress conspire to set us up like sitting ducks.

Hence the need for vigilance. Many people with bipolar disorder are encouraged to keep mood journals, which they and their psychiatrists track like meteorologists keeping watch on hurricanes in the Caribbean.

Now let's talk about those depressions, the flip side of bipolar disorder. In one way, there is nothing to distinguish bipolar depression from "unipolar" depression, from mild to severe, with similar suicide rates of about 15 percent. But now we are beginning to discover that bipolar depression may be an entirely different animal, involving different biological processes and treatments (more on this later in this chapter and Chapter 11).

Sadly, the depressive side of bipolar disorder has been overlooked by the experts. As Michael Thase, MD, of the University of Pittsburgh, observed at the 2002 American Psychiatric Association annual meeting: "Although manic episodes are often more the emergent and notorious phase of bipolar affective disorder, depressive episodes last longer, are typically harder to treat, and result in the high ultimate risk of suicide." The course of the illness accelerates in some people, so that they are known as "rapid-cyclers." These are the people who can go up and down and back again, sometimes in a matter of hours. Since rapid-cyclers represent a moving target, treatment is especially difficult. Antidepressants can induce mania, and antimania medications can induce depression.

Then there are those with "mixed states," who can be up and down at the same time, with what can be best described as either agitated depression or dysphoric mania. Some people with unipolar depression can also experience some of these symptoms, and here is where depression gets especially dangerous—for if one is feeling suicidal while in an agitated or manic state, then one has the energy to carry out the deed.

According to the 2005 National Comorbidity Survey Replication, bipolar disorder affects 3.9 percent of the U.S. population; these cases are about equally divided into bipolar I and bipolar II. Adopting slightly softer criteria pushes the figure to 4.3 percent. Over the course of twelve months, the rate is 2.6 percent, of which 83 percent of these cases are serious.

Men and women are affected in equal numbers.

A 2003 University of Texas Medical Branch at Galveston survey found that only 19.8 percent of those with positive screens reported receiving a diagnosis of bipolar disorder from a physician, while 31.2 percent reported a diagnosis of unipolar depression.

Bipolar disorder is no picnic. Two recent Stanley Foundation Bipolar Network surveys revealed that just 11.2 percent of the patients in their participating clinics remained virtually well for 12 months. A 2003 Case Western Reserve mail survey of 85,458 adults found that more than half of those with symptoms of bipolar disorder were at high risk of being fired or laid off, with nearly half reporting poor job performance. In addition, symptomatic individuals were only half as likely to marry and twice as likely to separate or divorce.

So terrible is the havoc that bipolar disorder can bring on that a 2001 University of Texas Medical Branch at Houston study has estimated the present value of lifetime cost of the illness for an individual ranges from $11,720 for those with a single manic episode to $624,785 for those nonresponsive or with chronic episodes. This includes medical care, as well as unemployment and reduced earnings.

Make no mistake: this illness is a major career and home wrecker.

The Bipolar Time Warp

To me, bipolar disorder is the equivalent of being stuck in bumper-to-bumper traffic in a race car. The world is simply too slow and people too dull-witted to accommodate you. The initial advantage over one's fellow man inevitably gives way to frustration and occasional rage. Sure, at first you experience the exuberation of weaving in and out of traffic as you leave the world behind in your rearview mirror, but now there are more cars, all closer together, backed up for miles on end. Your engine is revving hard, but you find yourself banging your head against the dash in utter despair because you are desperate to pop the clutch and floor it, yet all you can do is hopelessly idle and suck other people's fumes.

Or it can be the very opposite. This time you are the one standing still. The mind, once engaged in a certain activity, finds it impossible to switch off into another one. One finds oneself staying in the shower until the water in the tank runs cold or staring off into space as if in a trance. As for getting out of bed, forget it—one is effectively bound to the mattress.

We may associate bipolar disorder with mood swings back and forth from mania to depression, but in truth the major characteristic of this illness is its capacity to bend time in ways that even Einstein failed to comprehend. When everything is going right, the optimum ratio of their time to your time is something like 1 to 2. You can think faster, react faster, and produce faster. If I were a batter facing a pitcher, I would be able to see the seams of the ball coming at me and calculate the trajectory of the object as I leisurely brought my bat around in anticipation of a satisfying smack.

Ah, the manic high, that satisfying smack.

But things never stay the same. Inevitably, the clock speeds up or winds down. In speedy mode, this time as a batter, I swing at the ball way too early, but I have time to swing at it again and yet again. "What's the matter with you, ball!" I rage in a white heat. "What's taking so goddamn long?" By now I have completely forgotten about the ball as I take out my anger on the bat, the ground, or, heaven forbid, the person nearest to me.

Nothing goes right in this state of time. Every rock, every tree, everything God has placed on earth has turned against me and me alone. People conspire to make my life miserable, computers find new ways to throw up error codes, numbers and their values change right before my very eyes, and being placed on hold is enough to reduce me to tears.

But then we have those time-standing-still moments—those times in the shower and under the covers. Yet time also stands still in the midst of feverish activity. When I am on a creative writing streak, I note at the end of this book, "the sun takes its leave, booming music falls mute, and the steaming hot cup of tea by my side is stone cold when I pick it up a minute later."

Walking into company in this frame of time can be an out-of-world experience, for you are there, completely in your own moment, but not theirs.

So what state of time will it be today? Forget about the terms *manic depression* and *bipolar disorder.* Instead, let's give this thing a name that truly represents its characteristics—bichronicity.

Yes, I am proud to say, I am bichronic. I experience the full spectrum of time, from warp speed to standing still. In the past, I never knew which state of time I would turn up in, day to day, minute to minute. This tended to make my life somewhat unpredictable. I recall being a law student kicking the pants off of the slickest lawyer in town, and in other situations being unable to respond to a simple question. I've gone from recluse to life of the party to social embarrassment, from hyperproductive to plain lazy, from being totally on top of the situation to being completely out of it.

These days, my medications tend to hold my time in check and make my life more predictable. Sure, I would love to have my optimum time back, but they haven't invented a pill that can keep it in place forever. I still have my still time, which is a great advantage when I write, but it is my bane when I try to get out of bed. Thankfully, those frightening warp-speed times have largely receded. Still, learning to live on other people's time requires a bit of adjustment.

All in good time, though, all in good time.

Reader Reactions

My observations on bichronicity first appeared in the form of an article on my Web site, and no article there has drawn such an immediate and direct response. Writes Sarah:

> *I have tears in my eyes. I call the times when time doesn't exist my catatonic times. I can sit there, perfectly still, not reacting to my surroundings because to me, they don't exist. I am in a time bubble when that happens. I thought I was the only one that happened to and never mention it to my psychiatrist because sometimes I am embarrassed to ever admit, even to him, that my own perceptions of the multiverse are so profoundly skewed.*

Says Louise: "I have not seen a more exact way of describing how a bipolar feels. I have often tried to explain what it is like but have never been very successful." And from Amanda: "This article made me want to scream 'FINALLY!'"

Cleo writes: "This is dead on. I always thought that the 'time standing still moments' were me procrastinating and being lazy. On the other hand, I'm a person who decides on a Tuesday that I want to change my hair and I need an appointment that day."

And Toby had this totally cool, occult take:

My "illness" came with a gift. A gift or a curse, not sure which. Its name is Arithmancy Divination. Here is a sample. Bipolar or Bichronic? BICHRONIC = 2 9 3 8 18 15 14 9 3 = 81 = 8+1 = 9 Nine is the complete number in numerology. There is much concerning this practice that is not understood, and I understand it more than others, but even I don't have a complete understanding of arithmancy divination. By the way, BIPOLAR IS A 10. 1 2 9 16 15 12 1 9 = 64 = 10 = 1.

Being bipolar is a number one problem, but at the same time the high is definitely a 9!

Finally, Skyler brings us back to earth: "Unfortunately the police did not accept my psychiatrist's supporting letter about why I was speeding. I should have produced a copy of your article in court."

Back to the Boring Stuff

The *DSM-IV* divides bipolar disorder into two types, rather unimaginatively labeled I and II. "Raging" and "Swinging" are far more apt.

Bipolar I and Mania

Raging bipolar (I) is characterized by at least one full-blown manic episode lasting at least one week or any duration if hospitalization is required. This may include inflated self-esteem or grandiosity, decreased need for sleep, being more talkative than usual, flight of ideas, distractibility, increase in goal-oriented activity, and excessive involvement in risky activities.

The symptoms are severe enough to disrupt the patient's ability to work and socialize, and may require hospitalization to prevent harm to himself or others. The patient may lose touch with reality to the point of being psychotic.

The other option for raging bipolar is at least one "mixed" episode on the part of the patient. The *DSM-IV* is uncharacteristically vague as to what constitutes mixed, an accurate reflection of the confusion within the psychiatric profession. More tellingly, a mixed episode is almost impossible to explain to the public. One is literally "up" and "down" at the same time.

Depression is not a necessary component of raging bipolar, though it is strongly implied, for what goes up must come down. The *DSM-IV* subdivides bipolar I into those presenting with a single manic episode with no past major depression, and those who have had a past major depression (corresponding to the *DSM-IV* for unipolar depression).

In an article on my Web site, Billy O writes:

It seemed so logical at the time. I went to Mexico to convince the local government that I could help them set up a community for recovering alcoholics. I was going to solve their social problems single-handedly. I recall driving to the auxiliary border crossing in southeast San Diego. It was closed due to the late hour. There was no one in sight and nothing but a metal bracket sticking out of the road to prevent passage. Well this wasn't going to stop me. I had urgent business to attend to. I hit that thing at full speed and it gave under the force of impact. It bent forward to an angle and converted itself from a barricade to a ramp. I must have sailed twenty feet through the air before bashing back down onto the road. I continued on into Mexico completely unimpeded feeling pretty proud of myself.

Probably the best way to describe mania is by making reference to five comics whose work is driven by a certain manic engine. Only two have openly acknowledged bipolar disorder, the late Spike Milligan and Jonathan Winters. John Cleese, Robin Williams, and Jim Carrey, however, have made excellent livelihoods by passing themselves off as certifiably manic. All of them, even when they play it straight, extrude a certain mad edge through the pores of their beings. It's as if they can't help it. Catch John Cleese doing his silly walks or Robin Williams in full (m)ad-lib flight during a live performance or Jim Carrey's tour de farce in *The Mask,* and you be the judge.

But there is nothing funny about the real thing. Naomi, in an unpublished diary entry, wrote the following in a state of mania, five weeks prior to tying one end of a bathrobe cord to a tree limb and the other around her neck (miraculously, she survived):

My head. My head. The lunatic is in my head. The lunatic is in my head. I am hearing voices that aren't there. I am seeing things that aren't there. I am . . . oh god, am I going crazy.

The moon is outside. The moon. Lunatic. Where the word comes from. They want to put me in the hospital. I don't want to go. I cannot sleep. I cannot eat. I hear voices. The doctor puts me on more and more medication. I vomit. I shake, I sweat, I see things. I don't like this. . . .

I have to calm down. I cannot calm down. I need to sleep.
I cannot sleep. My skin feels like it's peeling off.
. . . Stop my brain. Stop my brain from thinking. Stop my
brain stop my brain stop my brain stop stop stop stop stop
stop stop stop stop stop stop stop stop stop stop . . .

In his classic 1921 work, *Manic-Depressive Insanity and Para-noia,* the pioneering German psychiatrist Emil Kraepelin divided mania into four classes: hypomania, acute mania, delusional or psychotic mania, and depressive or anxious mania (i.e., mixed). Researchers at Duke University, following a 2001 study of 327 bipolar inpatients, have refined this to five categories.

The first one, comprising 20.5 percent of the sample, resembles Kraepelin's hypomania (which in turn corresponds to the threshold hypomania for bipolar II), with euphoric mood, humor, grandiosity, decreased sleep, psychomotor acceleration, and hypersexuality. Absent was aggression and paranoia, with low irritability.

The next category (24.5 of the sample) turns up the heat—it's a very severe form of classic mania, similar to Kraepelin's acute mania (corresponding to the threshold mania for bipolar I), with prominent euphoria, irritability, volatility, sexual drive, grandiosity, and high levels of psychosis, paranoia, and aggression.

Eighteen percent (corresponding to Kraepelin's delusional mania) experienced the extreme end of mania, with high ratings of psychosis, paranoia, delusional grandiosity, and delusional lack of insight, but hardly any of the pleasures.

The last two groups (37 percent) were unequivocally mixed, with high levels of depression, anxiety, irritability, and psychosis. What distinguished one mixed group from the other was that one had more symptoms of euphoria and fewer of dysphoria.

The authors of the study noted that while the last two groups comprised 37 percent of all manic episodes in their sample, only

13 percent of the subjects would qualify under current *DSM* criteria for a mixed bipolar episode, leading the authors to conclude that the *DSM* is too restrictive.

With the Duke study, we once again witness the spectrum phenomenon in action, this time from a different perspective—of depressive symptoms in mania, rather than manic symptoms in depression. As with novel depressions, the treatment implications are enormous.

If one thinks of either pure or mild mania as the music of Duke Ellington and Louis Armstrong on a cool, clear summer night, mixed mania is heavy metal and rap in a thunderstorm, the blast of jackhammers, the frizzle-frazzle of shorted-out power lines, and the elbows on the black keys of every neuron in the brain vibrating to extinction.

In 1988, I woke up from a drunken stupor in a strange city in a strange country, jobless and friendless and nearly penniless, with my psyche playing host to the type of cold-fusion nuclear reaction that demanded instant release. "Rage—Goddess, sing the rage"—a line from Homer. My high had turned on me. I was now a nonperson, a pariah.

I'M NORMAL! I wanted to shout. I've always been normal. And just to prove it, I didn't seek help. It was by no means my first round of Russian roulette with my brain. Why I'm not dead is a mystery to me.

At the 2004 APA annual meeting, Stephan Heckers, MD, of Harvard, shed further light on mixed states by identifying three "domains" of bipolar disorder: mood, thought, and psychomotor activity. These regularly cycle up and down in bipolar patients, but not necessarily in perfect sync. Mood, thought, and psychomotor activity can be out of phase with one another, which may explain why so many of us are walking anomalies much of the time.

Psychosis

A patient arriving at the emergency room vividly hallucinating, hearing voices, and uttering gibberish can easily be misdiagnosed as having schizophrenia, especially if that person is Afro-American, given a cursory examination, and is sedated and sent back onto the street a day or two later, as is all too often the case in this modern era of drive-by psychiatry. In bipolar disorder, psychosis may adapt to the person's mood. Thus, someone going through a manic episode may believe he or she is Superman or God or have powers similar to a god or Superman (psychiatrists refer to this as grandiosity and ascribe it to nonpsychotic behavior, as well).

The *DSM-IV* has given delusional or psychotic mania its own separate diagnosis as schizoaffective disorder—a sort of hybrid between bipolar disorder and schizophrenia—but this may be an artificial distinction, at least until we are able to single out this population for specialized treatment. Fifty-eight percent of patients with bipolar disorder experience at least one psychotic symptom, according to Frederick Goodwin, MD, and Kay Jamison, PhD, in their definitive work on bipolar disorder, *Manic-Depressive Illness*, while preliminary findings from psychiatric geneticists such as John Kelsoe, MD, of the University of California, San Diego, indicate that a common set of psychosis genes may play a role in both bipolar disorder and schizophrenia.

A 2004 Institute of Psychiatry (London) study of postmortem brains of subjects with bipolar disorder and schizophrenia (all of whom had experienced psychotic symptoms) turned up a possible biological basis for the overlap. In that study, researchers found that the brains exhibited similar white-matter deficiencies, but gray-matter irregularities appeared in different brain regions. The authors of the study speculated that psychosis may be caused by a white-matter abnormality that interferes with connectivity between two regions of the cortex.

Yet another indication of the overlap is that both old- and new-generation antipsychotics work for treating both mania and psychosis, for people with bipolar disorder and schizophrenia alike. As Terence Ketter, MD, of Stanford, told the 2001 DBSA annual conference, "it may be inappropriate to have a discrete cut between [bipolar disorder and schizoaffective disorder] when both may represent part of a spectrum."

Ah, that spectrum thing, again. Earlier, we talked about the overlap between depression and bipolar disorder. Now we see the spectrum stretching into schizophrenia territory, a frightening thought for many. The NIMH paints a grim picture of the illness, reporting on its Web site:

> *People with schizophrenia often suffer terrifying symptoms such as hearing internal voices not heard by others, or believing that other people are reading their minds, controlling their thoughts, or plotting to harm them. These symptoms may leave them fearful and withdrawn. Their speech and behavior can be so disorganized that they may be incomprehensible or frightening to others. Available treatments can relieve many symptoms, but most people with schizophrenia continue to suffer some symptoms throughout their lives; it has been estimated that no more than one in five individuals recovers completely.*

Schizophrenia's most famous poster boy, John Nash, of *A Beautiful Mind* fame, thought he was the king of Antarctica, but he also produced a brilliant body of work that resulted in a Nobel Prize. Unfortunately, he acknowledged he lost a full twenty-five years of his life to schizophrenia.

The legendary clinician Emil Kraepelin distinguished bipolar disorder from schizophrenia, referring to the latter as dementia praecox to indicate what he saw as the brain in a process of irreversible deterioration (which successors changed to its current name to indicate this wasn't necessarily so). Dr. Kraepelin also categorized schizophrenia as more chronic in its course compared to bipolar disorder, which he saw as more episodic. The *DSM* still preserves this distinction, mandating that schizophrenia symptoms persist for six months or more, as opposed to one week for a manic episode, though the lingering effects from a bipolar episode may cause experts to reconsider (see below).

It is important to emphasize that the best evidence we have indicates that bipolar disorder and schizophrenia occupy two sides of a biological chasm, but that the separation grows uncomfortably narrow in some places.

Thinking

Kay Jamison, PhD, of Johns Hopkins University writes in *Touched with Fire: Manic-Depressive Illness and the Artistic Temperament*: "[Bipolar disorder] encompasses the extremes of human experience. Thinking can range from florid psychosis, or madness, to patterns of unusually clear, fast, and creative associations, to retardation so profound that no meaningful activity can occur."

This inability to think clearly is a feature of both depression and mania, as well as psychosis, and its effects are often felt long after an episode has abated, leading experts to question the long-held belief that bipolar disorder is episodic in favor of the idea that its course may be truly chronic.

A lengthy review article by Carrie Bearden, PhD, and others at the University of Pennsylvania, published in the June 2001 *Bipolar Disorders,* cited "findings of persistent neuropsychological deficits" in long-term bipolar patients, even when tested in symptom-free states. The relationship between these deficits and length of illness led the authors to suggest that "episodes of depression and mania may exact damage to learning and memory systems."

These deficits, said Deborah Yurgelun-Todd, PhD, of Harvard, at the 2004 APA annual meeting, include attention, concentration, and psychomotor speed; abstract reasoning and executive control; verbal fluency; and verbal memory performance. Some one-third of the bipolar population, she said, are affected by these residual impairments. Accordingly, Dr. Yurgelun-Todd argued, cognitive deficits should be regarded as a core feature of the illness.

My Web site readers know all about the problem. Writes Valerie:

I have earned my associate's degree and am going into my second year at a university. I can only handle 10 credits at a time, despite having a high to genius level IQ. I cannot remember things and at times cannot even take notes in class because I have no attention span. My mind is my only "trump card" I have to play in life and I am desperate to overcome and to be a resource in this life, to help others. I want to work again. I am 34. . . . I feel like an idiot at times and despair. Friends mention things I don't remember, so I say, I forgot. "Did we have a good time?" I am easily confused and disoriented and study 80–90 percent of my waking hours during school taking only 10 credits at a time. . . . I used to be the household dictionary, thesaurus, phone directory and address book, with little effort. Now I have to paste my PIN numbers in code on the backs of my cards and then hope I remember the nature of my codes. Passwords and user names are the bane of my existence.

Says Jason:

I am only a junior in high school, and the symptoms of lack of concentration, inability to pay attention during class, too much sleep, and memory loss has been going on since 9th grade. I am seriously worried. My GPA is a 3.99 and it is be-

coming ever so harder to study. I cannot find the right words
when I write up my reports. I do not know how to do the
math problems I've learned in 8–10th grade. I don't remem-
ber a lot of things. I feel that my brain is dying. I feel that I'm
losing brain cells. I cannot use my brain like I used to. I was
spelling bee champion in 6th grade. Whatever happened?

One of the best-known tests to measure the ability of the brain to process tasks (commonly referred to as executive function) is the Stroop Color-Word Task, where various colored words representing colors, but not necessarily matching colors, are displayed with the clock running. Thus the word *Green* may appear in blue text. Rather than calling out "Green," which the mind reads instantly and almost automatically, the subject being tested needs to respond with "Blue," which requires being on top of one's cognitive game.

In a study published in 2004, Dr. Yurgelun-Todd and her colleagues scanned the brains of eleven stable bipolar patients while undergoing the Stroop task, and found significant delays in their ability to respond with correct answers compared to ten healthy controls. The study also found decreased activation of the brain region responsible for processing the task compared to the controls.

A 2003 Dalhousie University study of bipolar adolescents with their illness in remission found they took significantly longer than remitted depressed youths and healthy kids in completing a math test. Only 9 percent of the bipolar kids scored above average. The bipolar kids also scored significantly lower on spelling and reading.

Other recent studies have found deficits in working memory, visual processing, long-delayed free recall, and verbal organization.

Unfortunately, these deficits have severe real-world implications. A 2004 Sheppard Pratt study that ran 117 individuals with bipolar disorder through a battery of tests found that "current employment status was significantly associated with cognitive performance."

The prospect of losing brain function is as frightening as being buried alive—just ask any senior citizen who has misplaced his car keys. But never underestimate the brain's unending capability to remap its seemingly limitless neuronal pathways. A cognitive deficit from bipolar disorder is not the same thing as Alzheimer's. You are not a helpless bystander. There are things you can do to keep your brain sharp. The Mayo Clinic recommends:

- Exercising your mind. This includes crossword puzzles, reading, and interacting with people.
- Staying physically active, which improves blood flow.
- Maintaining a healthy diet.
- Developing a system of reminders and cues, such as keeping a diary.
- Learning relaxation techniques. Stress and anxiety interfere with concentration.

Racing Thoughts

Our illness is one defined by polar opposites, and this applies with equal force to thinking as it does to mood. Imagine a chronic physical illness that has you bedridden one week and running a sub-four-minute mile the next. In its criteria for mania, the *DSM* refers to "flight of ideas or subjective experience that thoughts are racing." Believe me, there is nothing subjective about these racing thoughts. The only reason that the word *subjective* made it into the *DSM* is that science has no way to objectify the phenomenon.

Researchers only have the capability to get us into a room and put us through tests that make us look stupid. These are the parts of our brains that function like busted laptops. We droop on the Stroop.

What the experts have yet to figure out is how to set up an experiment that can record the birth of a creative thought or take a snapshot of a breakthrough idea. These are the parts of our brains that run like Cray supercomputers. We rule in this school.

Our minds are literally processing data so fast that we make the type of connections and associations that lead to Eureka! moments, often at a rate that astounds people who do not share our illness. If there is anything subjective about our thinking, it is only after our brains have delivered the mental goods, when a solution miraculously reveals itself or a revelation floors us.

Society has benefited enormously from this aspect of our illness, from Newtonian physics to the Sistine Chapel. A good case can be made that we would all still be living in caves were it not for our supercomputers. In Darwinian terms, this would explain why our illness—terrible as it is—is seen as a positive trait worth passing down to the next generation.

Like our cognitive deficits, one need not be in an episode to experience racing thoughts. For this writer, they are a constant in my life. Since these thoughts are often running in the background as I am performing other tasks and at speeds usually quicker than the conscious mind can capture, one might call the process subconscious. Ideas simply pop out of the brain.

Paradoxically, my brain can run like a supercomputer and a clapped-out laptop at the same time. I can go to Google to follow up on a brilliant thought only to forget momentarily why I am on the page. Since I am not a math whiz, my supercomputer is not going to outperform Stephen Hawking. It is only as good as what I put into it, from the books I read to the people I meet to the problems I focus on.

Racing thoughts can be a liability. The mouth can find itself articulating an errant thought before the rest of the brain has had a chance to process it. The intoxication of a latest revelation can distract one from current projects—ironically, ones initiated by previous moments of inspiration. And many bright ideas turn out to be plain stupid ones. Our rational minds can usually protect us here, but in a state of mania we are not thinking rationally. It is one thing to come up with a brilliant idea for dog mascara, for instance, but it is another to quit your day job and sink your entire 401(k) in pursuit of such a venture.

No doubt, a future *Business Week* cover will feature the entrepreneurial genius who succeeded in convincing millions of dog owners that they were abusing their pooches by neglecting their mutts' eyelashes. That person could well be you, but only if you possess the skills to marry reason and persistence to inspiration and enthusiasm. Be advised: Our supercomputer is both a rare gift and potentially devastating liability. Act wisely.

Bipolar II and Hypomania

Swinging bipolar (II) presumes at least one major depressive episode, and for this reason alone it should not be thought of as "bipolar lite." Since those with bipolar II tend to be depressed far more often than those with bipolar I, those who fall into this camp may be at greater risk than the "raging" bipolar crowd.

For bipolar II, the *DSM-IV* mandates at least one hypomanic episode over at least four days. The same characteristics as mania are evident, with the disturbance of mood observable by others, but the episode is not enough to disrupt normal functioning or necessitate hospitalization, and there are no psychotic features.

Those in a state of hypomania are typically the life of the party, the salesperson of the month, and more often than not the best-selling author or Fortune 500 mover and shaker, which is why so many refuse to seek treatment. But the same condition can also turn on its victim, resulting in bad decision making, social embarrassments, wrecked relationships, and projects left unfinished.

In an article on my Web site, Sophy Patterson writes:

One night, I decide to call a very good friend of mine, who lives on the opposite coast. The next morning when I call him,

I am witty, I am humorous. I am flirty. And I proposition him. He and I are good enough friends he knows something is wrong, the last thing you could ever say about me is I would do something like that. And although he is flattered, he tells me no, and talks to me. But I am off laughing, nothing can go wrong. Everything is lovely. I feel good. Every part of me feels great, it's like I am a Christmas tree, all lit up and beautiful and I want to show everyone how bright and pretty I am.

This is how Cindy described her hypomania on my Web site:

Thursday night I was so angry it was difficult to keep from throwing and breaking everything within reach. Friday I was elated, giddy, fun to be around. Saturday seemed fine, happy but calm. Sunday morning I woke up and started cleaning the apartment. . . . I moved furniture, on hands and knees I scrubbed every bit of carpet and floor, I vacuumed, I mopped, I took the vacuum and cleaned out all the vents and heaters, I reorganized my closets . . .

Hypomania certainly has its advantages. Vincent van Gogh executed 189 paintings in one incredible twelve-month run, and 143 in another—unfortunately, without a single buyer to be had. "What am I in the eyes of most people," he wrote his brother not long after embarking on his career in painting in 1882, "a nonentity, an eccentric, or an unpleasant person—somebody who has no position in society and will never have; in short, the lowest of the low."

Crows in the Wheatfields turned out to be his final opus. Even van Gogh acknowledged the work was an expression of "sadness and extreme solitude." There was that little bit of sky pressing down on the fields, as if of a heavier substance than earth, and there were the fields trying to crowd the sky out of the canvas, as if vaster than the heavens. And there were the crows, hedging their bets, represented by stark black flicks. There were no two ways about it. It wasn't just a landscape. It was a picture of van Gogh's horribly bleak world closing in on him. Even as the wheat rose high and the sun shone hot and bright, one can't help but gaze into that canvas and feel night falling.

"I generally try to be fairly cheerful," he wrote his brother Theo, "but my life is also threatened at the very root, and my steps are also wavering."

Then night would fall for good. One day he went out for a walk and shot himself in the chest with a pistol, then managed to stagger home to his bed. Theo was sent for, and he climbed in bed alongside his beloved brother and cradled his head in his arms.

"I wish I could pass away like this," Vincent told his brother, apparently feeling an inner peace he had never known. Minutes later he got his wish. He was thirty-seven.

Then there was Beethoven, whose life could fill up a segment on *Oprah:* an abusive father who tried to exploit him as a child prodigy, an infatuation for women who were totally out of reach, a tragic deafness that defies imagination, the comical frequency in which he shifted residences in Vienna, his disillusionment with Napoléon, his unkempt appearance and lack of personal hygiene. He was a man with a vision of universal brotherhood who was increasingly withdrawing into himself.

In *Manic Depression and Creativity,* Jablow Hershman and Julian Lieb, MDs, report that Beethoven's hypomania seemed to stoke his creativity, as he crashed and banged on his pianoforte, taking the instrument to its limits, scribbling on walls and shutters if paper wasn't available, dousing his head with water that ran through to the rooms below.

A friend describes one Beethoven session: "He . . . tore open the pianoforte . . . and began to improvise marvelously. . . . The hours went by, but Beethoven improvised on. Supper, which he had purported to eat with us, was served, but—he would not permit himself to be disturbed."

His highs also had their flip side, as he destroyed relationships with raging quarrels and psychotic delusions. On one occasion, he flung a gravy-laden platter of food at a waiter's head. His friends called him "half crazy," and when enraged, "he became like a wild animal."

Ultimately, Beethoven medicated himself with the only available drug besides opium—alcohol. He literally drank himself to death.

What psychiatry has failed to address is the type of person least likely to come to its attention, that of someone in a perpetual state of hypomania. John Gartner's *Hypomanic Edge* lists many examples of history-changing "unipolar hypomanics," ranging from Christopher Columbus to Alexander Hamilton to geneticist Craig Venter.

But hypomania is not all fun and games. People called Columbus mad for better reasons than his just wanting to sail west to reach the east. Alexander Hamilton recklessly stopped a bullet, and Craig Venter's antics resulted in the company he had founded firing him.

Hypomania can also occur in those with raging bipolar, and may be the prelude to a full-blown manic episode. In addition, there may be more to hypomania than mere mania lite. While working on the American Psychiatric Association's latest *DSM* version of bipolar disorder (*IV-TR*, which was a mere technical update), Trisha Suppes, MD, PhD, of the University of Texas Southwestern Medical Center in Dallas, carefully read its criteria for hypomania and had an epiphany. "I said, wait," she told a UCLA grand rounds lecture in April 2003, "where are all those patients of mine who are hypomanic and say they don't feel good?"

Dr. Suppes had in mind a different type of patient—say, one who experiences road rage and can't sleep. Why was there no mention of that in hypomania? she wondered. A subsequent literature search yielded virtually no data.

The *DSM* alludes to mixed states where full-blown mania and major depression collide in a raging sound and fury, but nowhere does it account for more subtle manifestations, often the type of states many bipolar patients may spend a good deal of their lives in. This would include patients just over the arbitrary diagnostic divide between depression and bipolar disorder (think spectrum, again), with enormous potential treatment implications. Dr. Suppes referred to a 2003 secondary analysis of a study of patients with acute mania on lithium or Depakote that found that even two or three depressed symptoms in mania were a predictor of outcome.

Clinicians commonly refer to these under-the-*DSM* radar mixed states as dysphoric hypomania or agitated depression, often using the terms interchangeably. Dr. Suppes defines the former as "an energized depression," which she and her colleagues made the object of a prospective study of 919 outpatients from the Stanley Foundation Bipolar Network. Of 17,648 patient visits, 6,993 involved depressive symptoms, 1,294 displayed hypomania, and 9,361 were euthymic (symptom-free). Of the hypomania visits, 60 percent (783) met her criteria for dysphoric hypomania. Females accounted for 58.3 percent of those with the condition.

None of the major treatment guidelines (more on these in Chapter 11) offer specific recommendations for treating dysphoric hypomania, such is our lack of knowledge. Clearly, the day will come when psychiatrists will probe for depressive symptoms or mere suggestions of symptoms in mania or hypomania, knowing this will guide them in the prescriptions they write, thus adding an element of science to the largely hit-or-miss practice that governs much of meds treatment today. But that day hasn't arrived yet.

A 2001 University of Chicago–Johns Hopkins study makes a strong case for a genetic distinction between bipolar I and bipolar II. That study found a greater sharing of alleles (one of two or more alternate forms of a gene) along the chromosome 18q21 in siblings with bipolar II than mere randomness would account for.

Nevertheless, for many people, bipolar II may be bipolar I waiting to happen.

A 2003 NMIH study tracking 135 bipolar I and 71 bipolar II patients for up to twenty years found both had more lifetime co-occurring substance use than the general population. Those with bipolar II had "significantly higher lifetime prevalence" of anxiety disorders, especially social and other phobias. Bipolar Is had more severe episodes at intake, while bipolar IIs had "a substantially more chronic course, with significantly more major and minor depressive episodes and shorter interepisode well intervals."

In her UCLA grand rounds lecture, Dr. Suppes observed that bipolar II is the object of only about twenty review papers. None of the treatment guidelines, in their recommendations, distinguish between treating a patient with bipolar I and bipolar II, as there is precious little research to go on. At the time of her talk, bipolar II was estimated to be present in 0.5 percent of the U.S. population (now it is about 1.5). "That's a lot of people," she concluded, "not to know anything about."

Bipolar Depression

Major depression is part of the *DSM-IV* criteria for swinging bipolar (bipolar II) and is also present in most people who have bipolar I, but the next edition of the *DSM* may have to revisit what constitutes the downward aspect of this illness. At present, the *DSM-IV* criteria for major unipolar depression pinch-hit for a genuine bipolar depression diagnosis. On the surface, there is little to distinguish between bipolar and unipolar depression, but certain "atypical" features may indicate different forces at work inside the brain.

According to Francis Mondimore, MD, of Johns Hopkins and author of *Bipolar Disorder: A Guide for Patients and Families*, addressing the 2002 Depression and Related Affective Disorders

Association (DRADA) annual conference, people with bipolar depression are more likely to have psychotic features and sloweddown depressions (such as sleeping too much), while those with unipolar depression are more prone to crying spells and significant anxiety (with difficulty falling asleep).

A 2003 GlaxoSmithKline-funded study carried out by Robert Hirschfeld, MD, of the University of Texas in Galveston, and others found that those with bipolar disorder fared significantly worse in their depressions than those with unipolar depression. According to the study, individuals with bipolar depression "were more likely to report that they did their work poorly, felt ashamed of their work, had arguments outside the home, felt upset, and never found their work interesting compared to those with unipolar depression. The bipolar depression group also reported significantly more disruption in work, social and family functioning, and significantly more symptom days versus those with unipolar depression."

In an article on my Web site, Sophy Patterson describes her bipolar depression:

I want to drink tonight. I want to take a bottle of vodka and take a long hot bath in my pajamas. Drink the bottle in the bath tub. Toast the New Year's. And when the bottle is empty, crash it against the bathtub, shattering it. And taking the shards and slitting my wrists, my ankles, my throat. Watching the blood ebb out. I want the pain to stop. I want the loneliness to stop. I feel all alone. I feel empty. I feel worthless. I feel like I should have been born dead. I don't know why I was conceived in the first place.

I feel hollow. I do not feel alive anymore. I feel like a basilisk. I feel dead.

I cannot sleep. I just took a handful of sleeping pills. I am tired. I will sleep. If I die before I wake, I have said my prayers. If I wake before I die, then maybe the feeling will pass by then. If it doesn't perhaps I may get a bottle anyway and die. If I do not drink, maybe I can still die. I can throw myself under the train. I can die. I can crawl into the car and die that way.

I am not afraid of dying. That is easy. It is living that is hard and living sucks. I feel the loneliness, the despair and it's choking me. I do not know who to ask for help. I don't think I want help. I want to curl up and never wake up again.

According to a 2003 Stanley Foundation Bipolar Network survey of 258 of its bipolar patients, this population was depressed three times more often than they were manic, despite being treated with an average of 4.1 medications. Bipolar I patients were depressed 32 percent of the weeks over a 12.8-year period, as opposed to being manic or hypomanic for 9 percent of those weeks and mixed or cycling for 6 percent of those weeks. For bipolar II patients, the same study found depression present in 50 percent of the weeks over 13.4 years, as opposed to 1 percent of those weeks for mania or hypomania and 12 percent of those weeks for mixed or cycling.

The same study also found that dysthymia (minor depression) and subsyndromal (not full-blown) depression dominated, with bipolar II patients more likely to have major depression and a more chronic course. Meanwhile, early data from the NIMH-underwritten Systematic Treatment Enhancement Program for Bipolar Disorder's (STEP-BD) first five hundred patients found 80 percent of relapses were into depression. At the 2000 APA annual meeting, Alan Swann, MD, of the University of Texas at Houston, observed that those with bipolar depressions are characterized by greater episode frequency, earlier onset, greater co-occurring substance use, and a more equal gender ratio. Significantly: "The differing biological properties of unipolar and bipolar depression suggest that treatments that were originally intended for unipolar depression may not be optimal for bipolar depression."

Cyclothymia

A likely candidate for the *DSM-V* as bipolar III or bipolar IV is "cyclothymia," listed in the current *DSM* as a separate disorder, characterized by swings from symptoms of hypomania to symptoms of mild depression. The use of the term *symptoms,* rather than *episodes,* is what differentiates (at least for the present) this illness from true bipolar disorder. Nevertheless, one-third of those with cyclothymia are eventually diagnosed with bipolar disorder, lending credence to the "kindling" theory of bipolar disorder: that if left untreated in its early stages, the illness will break out into something far more severe later on. Sadly, cyclothymia is often not taken seriously by people who should know better. Writes Jenna: "I asked my psychiatrist about cyclothymia recently (I read about it and it sounded just like me) and he said that I probably do have this and there isn't really any treatment for it. This is very frustrating. It's like people don't consider it a problem just because it isn't full-blown bipolar disorder. It is an absolute nightmare to live with and hard to maintain friendships and stick with one idea/course."

Fortunately, another reader, Braveheart, found the right psychiatrist: "I've been on lithium for a year now and feel wonderful. I still have mild ups and downs, and sometimes feel paranoid, but nothing at all like before. I do not have my creative 'highs,' but my creative 'middles' have become very reliable and in the end I am producing more steadily than ever."

Rapid-Cycling

On my Web site, Anonymous writes: "One day this, a couple days that, a couple more days back to this . . . back and forth back and forth. My boyfriend now, well, he can't handle me. . . . Sometimes I feel like I will never be able to have a relationship because my feelings keep flip-flopping. Well, that's what is happening now. I think I have worn him out."

Nowhere is the *DSM* more out of touch with reality than in its criteria for rapid-cycling, this despite the fact that up to 20 percent of those with bipolar disorder may rapid-cycle. The *DSM* specifies at least four episodes of mood disturbance over the last twelve months to at least two months in remission and back or by a switch from one pole to the other. Rapid-cycling can occur in patients with both bipolar I and bipolar II, as well as unipolar depression.

For an illness defined by its ups and downs, however, cycling in and out of four mood episodes a year seems perfectly normal and downright leisurely. True, four episodes a year is four episodes too many, particularly when just one represents a life-threatening situation, and especially if the episodes come on suddenly. But poor Anonymous has to contend with the emotional whiplash of lurching from one extreme to the other every couple of days. Ironically, because the *DSM* requires a minimum of two weeks for a depressive episode, one week for a manic episode, and four days for a hypomanic episode, this unfortunate woman's condition is technically unrecognized as such by psychiatry.

In an article in the fall 2003 *Journal of Child and Adolescent Psychopharmacology,* Rebecca Tillman, MS, and Barbara Geller, MD, describe the example of a bipolar child who cycles up and down twice a day for one year. "With the terminology currently in use," they report, "it is unclear whether this should be described as a single episode that had a duration of 365 days or as approximately 730 episodes . . . each less than 24 hours in duration."

Unofficially, psychiatry recognizes ultrarapid cyclers (occurring every few days) and ultradian cycling (occurring during the course of a day). Unfortunately, there is virtually no data providing insight into clinical distinctions, much less treatment. We do know that rapid-cyclers are more difficult to treat and that they are particularly sensitive to mood triggers, from bad encounters at work or with family to medication side effects to being overstimulated to too much caffeine to losing a night's sleep. We also know that rapid-cycling is more prevalent in those with bipolar II, that hypothyroidism is associated with rapid-cycling, and that more women rapid-cycle than men.

Because, unfortunately, our knowledge stops right about there, rapid-cycling represents the true dark side of the moon of our illness.

In Conclusion

The *DSM*'s artificial time minimum for episodes may exclude many true bipolar patients. The British Association for Psychopharmacology's 2003 *Evidence-Based Guidelines for Treating Bipolar Disorder,* for instance, notes that when the four-day minimum for hypomania was reduced to two in a sample population in Zurich, the rate of those with bipolar II jumped from 0.4 percent to 5.3 percent.

Meanwhile, the cause and workings of the illness remain a mystery to science, though there are lots of theories. We do know that the illness tends to run in families. Family studies have shown the approximate lifetime risk of a first-degree biological relative of a person with bipolar disorder to be 5 to 10 percent, far higher than for adopted relatives. Studies of identical twins show that their risk of contracting the illness is as much as seventy-five times greater than that for the general population.

So little is actually known about the illness that the pharmaceutical industry has yet to develop a drug to treat its symptoms. Lithium, the best-known bipolar med, is a common salt, not a proprietary drug. Drugs used as mood stabilizers—Depakote, Tegretol, Lamictal, and Trileptal—came on the market as antiseizure medications for treating epilepsy. Antidepressants were developed with unipolar depression in mind, and antipsychotics such as Zyprexa and Risperdal went into production to treat schizophrenia.

Inevitably, a "bipolar" pill will find its way to the market, and there will be an eager queue of desperate people lining up to be treated. Make no mistake, there is nothing glamorous or romantic about an illness that destroys up to 1 in 5 of those who have it, and wreaks havoc on the survivors, not to mention their families. The streets and prisons are littered with wrecked lives.

Bipolar disorder has so intimately influenced how I think and feel and perceive and relate that it has defined who I am from day one, both for better and for worse. One brutal cold day in early 1999, a psychiatrist confirmed what I had known but what I had been afraid to face up to all my life—that I wasn't like the other 96 or 97 percent of the population. I wasn't normal. Never was. I had been lying to myself all these years.

Ironically, having accepted that I'm different, it's much easier these days for me to pass myself off as normal. But first I had to get through grieving the loss of the person I could never be. Only then could I experience the dual terror and pleasure of meeting myself for the first time.

4

Behavior

Between the "I" that is us and our illness that presumes to establish dominion over the "I" is a battle played out on the field of behavior. Everything is fair game, from our likes and dislikes to how we relate to people to having sex to how we experience our surroundings.

In some instances, we need to accept who we are and adapt accordingly. In others, we need to learn to control that which puts our families, livelihoods, reputations, and lives at risk. Finally, we can give thanks for those parts of us that are true gifts.

Poison-ality

Every bit as bad as our illness is the isolation and despair it leaves in its wake. In May 2003, I asked my newsletter readers to take an online Myers-Briggs personality test and e-mail the results, along with their diagnosis. Although this was strictly a readers' poll and not a scientific study, and bearing in mind the risks inherent in pigeonholing personalities, the findings were striking enough to indicate I might be on to something.

The Myers-Briggs Type Indicator (MBTI) begins with eight personality functions in contrasting pairs—Introversion (I) or Extroversion (E), Intuition (N) or Sensing (S), Thinking (T) or Feeling (F), and Judging (J) or Perceiving (P).

The introversion/extroversion dichotomy relates to people drawing their energy from being alone or with people rather than simply being either shy or outgoing. Thinking and Feeling are self-explanatory. Sensors tend to focus on the here and now, while Intuitives look for meaning and possibilities. Judgers prefer structure in their lives over the messy flexibility of Perceivers.

Combining six of the functions yields four temperaments: Guardians (SJ), who value tradition and seek security; Artisans (SP), who are sensation-seekers and hands-on people; Idealists, (NF), who are abstract and conceptual; and Rationals (NT), born scientists and engineers.

Falling within these four temperaments are sixteen distinct personality types, defined according to the eight paired personality functions, thus INFP, ESTJ, and so on.

Approximately 150 responses were received, and of these the first 100 were analyzed (a nice even number for this math-challenged individual). Most readers also sent in their diagnosis, nearly all depressive or bipolar. Since most people with bipolar disorder are depressed more than manic, it is safe to conclude that this poll was dealing with a mostly depressed population, without further breaking down the figures. Approximately three-quarters of the respondents were women, which about matched the newsletter's readership.

The first eye-popping result was 83 percent of those who replied were introverts, which sharply contrasts with the 25 percent to be found in the general population. According to one reader, who had a strong extrovert score four years ago and a much weaker one when responding to this poll: "Over the last four years I've sunk into a very isolated existence. The mania has worsened despite changes in medication/dosages and I spend most of my time sleeping and avoiding large social functions. I do slightly better in small social gatherings, but up until just a couple of months ago I didn't go anywhere or see anyone other than my immediate family within our house." A confounding variable could be that loners who are drawn to the Internet are not representative of the wider population of those who have depression or bipolar disorder, but a legitimate scientific study supports my findings (more on this in a minute).

Several readers commented that their results varied on circumstances and phase of illness. Georgie wrote that "when manic I'm as sociable as Bette Midler on cocaine and when I'm depressed, seriously come not near me." Steven reported that in 1995 when he took the test at work, in a stimulating environment, he was an extrovert; but at home, where he could relax away from people, he was an introvert. Another reader, who rapid-cycles, reported different results on the same day.

Another eye-opener was that 41 percent of those responding reported being idealists, who comprise but 8 percent of the general population. Among the idealists were 17 INFJs and 14 INFPs, the largest populations in this survey, the "mystics" and "dreamers," respectively, who only account for 1 percent each of the general population.

Among the extroverts, possibly because it was just one letter off INFP, there were seven ENFPs, "visionaries" who would fit right in with the introverted mystics and dreamers, the only category of extrovert overrepresented in this poll. Since other extroverts go by such monikers as "enforcers," "adventurers," "helpers," and "jokers," you can see what we are missing.

All this begs the question of whether psychiatry or psychology is addressing itself to what may be a patient's most pressing need, once the more severe symptoms are resolved.

One of the few psychiatric studies using the MBTI, by David Janowsky, MD, of the University of North Carolina, and others appearing in the October 2002 *World Journal of Biological Psychiatry,* also found a preponderance of introverts and feelers among a depressed population (74 percent introverts and 84 percent feelers). Another study by Dr. Janowsky and others found that 84 percent of the sixty-four suicidal patients examined were introverts, leading him and his coauthors to observe: "The introverted individual almost certainly has trouble reaching out to others, especially in times of stress and need. Thus the social isolation of introversion may set the scene for suicidality."

In a 2001 article appearing in the December 2001 *Current Psychiatry Reports,* Dr. Janowsky cited various studies to support the proposition that "increased introversion predicts the persistence of depressive symptoms and a lack of remission" (and, conversely, that extroversion can improve outcomes).

One of my respondents, Carol, who came up ENTJ back in college and again a couple of years ago when working for a mutual-fund company, offered this advice: "If I may draw a conclusion, those of us who can break through isolation and make contact with others, could be better able to keep the depression at bay."

This is generally more easily said than done, given the nature of our illness, but the stakes are enormous in what could very well be the most important aspect of our treatment.

Unfortunately, even healthy people are too busy to take time out for each other. In his 2000 book, *Bowling Alone: The Collapse and Revival of American Community,* Harvard professor of public policy Robert Putnam cites stacks of *Roper Reports* and DDB Needham Life Style Surveys to point out that we are fast becoming a society of loners. Attendance at local public meetings is down by 60 percent since the seventies and families entertain at home half as much as they did thirty years ago.

We are cutting ourselves off, Dr. Putnam maintains. As a society we are losing our social capital.

Could this be why we are we are so depressed? A 2003 World

Values Survey of more then sixty-five countries ranked Nigeria number one in terms of happiness. How could this be? According to the World Bank, the average Nigerian earns $300 a year and has a life expectancy of 45.3 years. Nearly 6 percent of the young female population there has HIV, and only 7.1 in a thousand have a computer. Electricity and other services are luxuries, and the country is drowning in $31.1 billion of debt.

But the happiness finding was no fluke. In 2004, a major World Health Organization survey of fourteen countries and two Chinese cities found the impoverished but exuberant Nigerians putting the affluent but angst-ridden Americans and Europeans to shame with a twelve-month prevalence of mood disorders of 0.8 percent, far less than any of the surveyed nations. The United States had the dubious distinction of leading the pack at 9.6.

When I reported this Nigerian mood puzzle on my Web site, one of my readers, Anna, had this to say: "What do the Nigerians have that we don't? The answer: COMMUNITY."

Who's going to tell her she is wrong? Is sense of community yet another victim of modern life, and is the resulting isolation driving us to hopelessness and despair? Could the antidote be as simple as getting out the door and making an effort to be with people?

Maybe, maybe not. After I published my survey results on my Web site, one of my readers, Mel, challenged me:

A point that seems to be missed here is that idealists—that is to say mystics and dreamers—are not like the other 99 percent of the population because we DO see a different perspective and that our depression stems from the inability to relate to the general values of the mass population.

As an intelligent and creative artist, visionary, thinker and compassionate human, I find most extroverts obnoxious, self-centered narcissists who have little respect for topics which do not serve them in some way.

Idealists BECOME depressed after years of not caring about the simple-mindedness of sports, trivia, pop culture and fashion, but being surrounded by it every day like a disease. We ARE NOT like others and do not want to be. The advice that we would be better off somehow by getting out more often and mingling with the very people we can't relate to makes no sense at all.

Fair enough—and, no doubt, many of us can relate to Mel—but another reader, Avatar, who has spent long periods of time in monasteries, replied: "There I was in a true community, no longer alone, eating, prayer, and working, no longer isolated, but alone together. I hope this makes sense. Community is vitally important to sanity."

Think Nigeria, again.

I, myself, am an INFP, a dreamer. I am a loner by nature who takes comfort in and draws strength from my own inner world. But many mood episodes have taught me the value of community, which is as powerful as any medicine. Yes, the world may be full of the kind of jerks Mel finds so revolting, but that should not stop us in making the extra effort to seek out our own communities that nourish and sustain us. I have found it among the people I share this illness with, and this may well be the most important part of my wellness program.

Call it a coincidence, but within four months of reporting in my newsletter on the dangers of isolating oneself I got engaged to a very lovely woman, and three months later I was married for the second time. No longer alone, but connected.

Exuberance

We have "given sorrow many words," Kay Jamison, PhD, of Johns Hopkins, said at the 2002 DRADA annual conference, "but passion for life few." Exuberance, she went on to say, "takes us many places," with "delight its own reward, adventure its own pleasure." But exuberance and joy are also fragile—"bubbles burst, cartwheels abort," all part of the yin and yang of emotion, as "joy with no counterweight has no weight at all."

Dr. Jamison was reading from a draft of a book she was working on at the time, *Exuberance: The Passion for Life,* which was published in 2004.

Dr. Jamison's book starts out with Teddy Roosevelt, the youngest U.S. president, whose life, according to a friend, was the "unpacking of endless Christmas stockings." Said Rudyard Kipling, after a meeting with him: "I curled up on the seat opposite and listened and wondered until the universe seemed to be spinning around and Theodore was the spinner."

In her DRADA talk, Dr. Jamison described TR as "hypomanic on a mild day," an observation that did not make it into her book. John Gartner, PhD, also of Johns Hopkins, did not evince the same reticence in his 2005 book *The Hypomanic Edge: The Link Between (a Little) Craziness and (a Lot of) Success in America.*

The theme of Dr. Gartner's book is that America was founded by go-getters and visionaries crazy enough to leave their settled existences for new and dangerous lives on a strange shore. These were outrageously behaving boat-rockers such as Alexander Hamilton and Andrew Carnegie, whose genes live on in our present generation of entrepreneurs, creative artists, and religious zealots.

In this context, without the depression, hypomania is a temperament rather than an illness. Hypomanics, as Dr. Gartner is free to acknowledge, do tend toward reckless and irrational behavior, even the successful ones, so judicious treatment may be appropriate.

Alexander Hamilton, for one, could have benefited from a one or two-second period of sober reflection before posting that fateful letter to Aaron Burr.

Still, be it exuberance or hypomania, we should regard this aspect of our illness as a gift. Think of all those who have never seen a sunset through our eyes. They're the ones to be pitied.

Creativity

Back in the seventies, a *New York Times* piece quoted Kurt Vonnegut to the effect: "I would suffer like Van Gogh to paint like Van Gogh. I would not suffer like Van Gogh, however, to paint like Gauguin."

Depression and mania may have a way of coaxing out the most noble and creative and visionary in us, but I also think of the promising lives cut tragically short: Virginia Woolf's body fished out of the water, weighted down by stones; van Gogh cradled in the arms of his brother at age thirty-seven, a thousand *Starry Night*s never to be painted; Sylvia Plath with the gas on and her kids in the upstairs room; Marilyn Monroe found in a state of partial rigor mortis, forever young.

Then I think of all our close calls. Suppose Abraham Lincoln had had one of his colossal depressions as Lee was marching on Gettysburg? What if Winston Churchill had decided to stay in bed as the Battle of Britain was being fought?

Then I think that if we are to give this beast credit for, say, the Sistine Chapel and *The Starry Night* and the Choral Symphony, perhaps we are compelled to admit that we are little more than mere puppets on a string, yanked back and forth by the whims of some unseen hand, incapable of emotions of our own volition.

Which means many of us are setting ourselves up to be disfranchised of our own joy and anger and grief and everything in between. It means knowing looks from our close friends and significant others, as if to say, that's really your illness talking, not you.

Finally, I think of all the unknowns out there, the ones who never made any list, some thirty thousand of us a year in the United States, all told, who take their lives by their own hand. That's one Vietnam Wall every two years. The rest of you, you can play your celebrity games, if you like. Me, I'm going to have a brief moment of silence for all those unsung others.

More Thoughts on Celebrity

All right already! Dig down into the brains of a creative individual and you're bound to find some mood genes. Is there any artist or writer or composer NOT on the list? Well, Shakespeare and Vermeer and the highly prolific Anonymous, but only because next to nothing is known about them, especially Anonymous.

Kay Jamison was by no means the first to notice a strong association, but her 1993 book, *Touched with Fire: Manic-Depressive Illness and the Artistic Temperament,* put the issue front stage center. Says Dr. Jamison, in her introduction: "The fiery aspects of thought and feeling that initially compel the artistic voyage—fierce energy, high mood, and quick intelligence, a sense of the visionary and the grand, a restless and feverish temperament—commonly carry with them the capacity for vastly darker moods, grimmer energies, and, occasionally, bouts of 'madness.'" Individuals with bipolar disorder, she maintains, possess the rare ability to think along unrelated tangents, then put the pieces together ("making connections between opposites") into a grand visionary whole. Unbridled self-assurance and manic energy fuel the creative fire.

Mild melancholia, on the other hand, she maintains, allows a deeper tapping into emotional pools.

Dr. Jamison's artistic bipolar poster child is the great Romantic poet Lord Byron. Suicide was a frequent conversational topic, while his episodic promiscuity, violent rages, and sheer reckless behavior made him a walking, talking *DSM*. At Trinity College, Cambridge, when rules forbade him to keep a dog, he acquired a tame bear, which he kept in a tower and walked through the streets of town. In Greece, during his grand tour, he wrote, "I have outlived all my appetites and most of my vanities."

His fellow poet Shelley wrote that Byron was "an exceedingly interesting person, but as mad as the wind."

Hershman and Lieb's *Manic Depression and Creativity* provides further insight into our warped and twisted muse. The book zeros in on Isaac Newton, Ludwig van Beethoven, Charles Dickens, and Vincent van Gogh from a viewpoint many of us know too disturbingly well: Newton, whose existence alternated between that of the hypomanic life of the party to dysphoric manic feuding with his colleagues to long spells of depressive seclusion; Beethoven, who so desperately lived for those ultimate highs that he sought to freeze into music; Dickens, whose inexhaustible manic engine ultimately wore the rest of him out; and van Gogh, who was fated to be van Gogh.

Rounding out the book are the authors' passing insights on creative minds as disparate as Michelangelo, Mozart, Marilyn Monroe, Nikola Tesla, Pablo Picasso, Chopin, and Elvis.

In the end, that long list of wildly diverse and singular characters provides us with the ultimate affirmation of ourselves. We are not just our illness any more than we are clones. We are individuals, each of us with highly unique temperaments. How we channel our moods is a matter of personal choice. We can write a Choral Symphony or open an animal shelter or make our loved one an omelet. Our contradictory capacity for passion and despair is as confusing to us as outsiders. Far from being mere puppets on a string, we all have personality in abundance, tons of it. Some or most of us would trade it away in a heartbeat, with just cause. But at what price?

That is the never-ending—and next—question.

Gift and Curse

What is there to like about having bipolar disorder? Beth represents a lot of us when she writes: "The world is a different place to me than it is to 'them.' As a bipolar, I am artistic, creative, articulate, brilliant, comedic, cynical, energetic."

In a similar vein, Annabelle observes: "I have learned to appreciate the deeper things in life, and I have become a good person because of the changes that I have been forced to make. . . . Bipolar is a part of me, and I cannot imagine life without it."

In early 2004, I posted on my Web site this question: "We know that bipolar disorder is a horrific illness. But do you also regard it as a gift that you would not trade to be normal?"

Predictably, there were no unconditional takers. Beth confesses that for all her creativity, she is unable to hold down a job, and Annabelle admits: "About every two years, I have some sort of breakdown . . . I am so fragile that anything that most folks deal with, like harassment, or being treated badly at work or other hardships of life seem to 'bowl me over.' " Susan, who says her illness has taken her to Mount Olympus and Hades, can muster at best a disquieting affirmative: "I've had this illness since I was four. I don't know what it would be like not to have it. And that scares me. I don't want to know."

Those who regard their illness or that of their loved one as a curse, by contrast, are decidedly less equivocal. Writes Amy: "A 'gift?' Are you having a laugh? My mother has just ended her life after struggling with an illness that robbed me of the most beautiful person to ever walk the earth." MJ, who has never experienced the highs others "so glowingly describe," says that "if it is a gift, then I must thank Satan, because only he could be so gracious and generous." And Flo, who has been to Hell and back more times than she can count and fears her children will inherit her illness, concludes:

"I will gladly return this gift if someone will point me in the direction of the Customer Service Counter of life."

Barbara, forty-three, describes herself as a talented person with a master's degree, but as having no partner, no family, no children, no full-time job, no career, and no house. "My greatest wish," she says, "would be if the world changed, instead of me. If I could find a place where people would like me for exactly who I am, and not be afraid or treat me differently for being eccentric or unusual. I have been treated like a scary criminal a few too many times in my life."

Certainly no one wants to suffer, but a number of readers took pains to point out how their struggles have imbued their lives with a deeper insight and sense of purpose. Says John: "The Buddha regarded life as suffering. He was certainly onto something!"

But John also adds: "Suffering, if survived, can be a life-transforming experience leading to deep compassion for other beings. . . . A year and a half ago if I had been asked this question I would have said, "can you be serious, I would trade everything to be free of this curse." However, everything can change. Burning self-transformations do happen.

Says Jane: "Bipolar is not the problem. The problem is the problem. If you suffer with bipolar, you will suffer. If you merely cope, you will merely cope. If you live with bipolar, you will live."

Abigail writes:

My bipolar is such an integrated part of my being that it is impossible for me imagining trading it anymore that I could imagine trading my voice. It has shaped my spirituality and helped me to live, love, and have gratitude. Because I know it will sometimes feel unbearable, I fill my world with reminders that I am responsible for my health and personal growth. I accept responsibility to do the best I can and always strive to learn more and do better.

And this final word from Christina: "The best reason for not wanting to trade my disorder for normalcy is that two people who were likely bipolar cared enough to bring me into this world and let me experience it. It's a wild ride, but it's mine."

Spirituality

Many spiritual beliefs teach us that we pick the lives we're born into, and many times I have played the scene in my head, of me a half century ago ready to disembark the godly planes as I negotiate with my cosmic broker the terms for my upcoming earthly existence. I have been singled out, he informs me. I can have all the worldly success of Diamond Jim Brady, he lets me know. The catch is I will *be* a Diamond Jim Brady (the proto Donald Trump, heaven forbid). The other path, he tells me, leads to a deeper humanity and spirituality through a trail of a thousand sorrows.

I am clearly being honored. Precious few souls, I realize, are presented with such spectacular options. Nevertheless, I find myself trying to strike a better deal.

Can't I have the spirituality and humanity, I ask, with the Diamond Jim success, without the sorrows? And the cosmic broker only laughs. He sees my hesitation, then presents me with another choice—of a successful but modest professional life, a family, security, perhaps a light karmic obligation or two. He catches the wistful look in my eyes, of a simple dream denied by someone who has already made up his mind. He reaches over and hands me the thousand-sorrows documents, which I sign without reading.

Denise writes:

I entered the class about 10 minutes late and the professor had already started a discussion on mood disorders. As I was looking for a seat, he said jokingly to the class, "You'll know a person with bipolar disorder because he'll tell you he believes he is God." This brought laughter from the class and, immediately following class, I dragged my deflated self to his office to tell him, "I think I am God. Can you tell me what I do now?"

Denise may have been delusional at the time, but she also notes, following her diagnosis and recovery: "I am at peace with all aspects of my spirituality and have complete faith in my own ability to touch the part of God which lives inside of me and find what brings me wellness."

In 2003, I posted this question on my Web site: "Do you feel that you are a more spiritual person as a result of your depression or bipolar disorder?" The replies from Denise and others—as well as posts on other pages of my site—offer excellent insights into the blessing and curse that is our illness. As Katie puts it: "To have lived (and survived) the highest elation and lowest depression has been an awakening of my spirit I would not otherwise have known. Persons not affected cannot imagine nor will they ever be able to understand how this affects our spiritual lives as much as it controls and twists our physical lives." On the flip side of the coin, Carla notes: "I used to have a profound belief in God and was raised Roman Catholic. But as my depression took hold in childhood and got worse through my teens, and some truly horrible life events happened, well I just didn't believe anymore."

But depression also has a spiritual upside. As Paul puts it: "Suffering has its own way of getting you closer to God and being more spiritual; it is just a natural response." In a similar vein, Bobbie writes: "Years of suffering brought me to the realization that comfort was closer at hand than I could have imagined. Spirituality is calming; it lets me know that I am not in this mess alone."

Stella reports that when manic: "My life priorities shift from materialism, negativity, pettiness, self-centeredness and self-indulgence to an enlightened plane of existence where I want to help those in need, feel a direct line to God, have absolute clarity and absolute certainty of my purpose in life."

But Mandy argues: "When manic, I think you move in the wrong direction. It's a spiritual high but you spend and waste your spirit on delusion."

Following his diagnosis, Frank felt compelled "to question the authenticity of my every experience." Likewise, William, a fourth-year seminarian, confesses: "I used to empathize with the spiritual turmoil of the likes of St. Augustine in his *Confessions,* but now doubt whether we are on an equal footing. Are we dealing with the same 'demons,' or am I just a chemical imbalance on legs?" Perhaps both.

In a severe depression, it seems that God has turned his back on us. Paradoxically, in our need to heal, we reach out to embrace and ultimately feel that embrace returned. Appropriately, God is beyond all human understanding. *I am who I am* is all God told about himself to Moses—or simply, *I am.*

Spirituality focuses on personal meaning, a reason for living, for getting up in the morning, says Patricia Mulready, MD, who runs a practice in Connecticut that combines conventional and complementary medicine. There is an interconnectedness with others and an emphasis on goodness.

One of the most powerful forces on earth is fear. We know how paralyzing it is. Hope, on the other hand, activates us, gets us going. If that flicker of hope goes out, so do you, but it is faith that is the ultimate conqueror of fear, trusting in things we can't see.

But do we put our faith in God? People uncomfortable with the idea of God need go no further, says Dr. Mulready, than the unconscious mind. Here, you will find the seat of the creative process, intuition, the ability to know things in a different way, and ultimately a power greater than yourself.

We may turn to spirituality for comfort, but the process can be more like a trial by ordeal. A spiritual attitude doesn't ease the pain so much as enlist our hurt and suffering in a process that changes and transforms us. Says Dr. Mulready: "I will get through this challenge, and I'll be better because of it."

Somehow, in the end, we emerge more in touch with our own humanity and closer to God. God may have yet more ordeals in store, but we're no longer the spiritual wimps we used to be. We are healing—as individuals, as a people.

The Brain in Love and Lust

On my Web site, Saucy writes: "I fuck like a blender on full speed when I'm in a mania!" Says Bionic Woman: "I got involved with someone at work. He pursued ME. Fourteen years younger. It was just sex. Was I good? Damn I was good. That went on for a year. It was intense. I was a magnet for younger guys. Did I love it? Yes."

It goes on. From Anonymous: "When I was in a relationship, I would wear my poor partner out. To me sex was like potato chips, once you started you couldn't stop until you ate the whole bag. I couldn't stop until the poor guy was begging for mercy, he couldn't perform anymore. Then I would go home and get out the trusty vibrator."

Of course, the depressive side was another story, and Danielle cautions: "I can't say if it's a worthwhile trade to have sizzling sex when you have to take the mania and depression in order to get it."

In a study published in 2002, anthropologist Helen Fisher, PhD, of Rutgers University and a multidisciplinary team of experts recruited forty young people madly in love—half with love returned, the other half with love rejected—and put them into an MRI with a photo of their sweetheart and one of an acquaintance. Each subject looked at the sweetheart's photo for thirty seconds, then—after a diversion task—at the acquaintance photo for another thirty seconds. They switched back and forth for twelve minutes.

The result was a revealing photo album of the brain in love, namely, those areas in the interior of the brain central to reward and motivation fueled by dopamine. In addition, several parts of the prefrontal cortex that are highly wired in the dopamine pathways were mobilized, while the amygdala, associated with fear, was temporarily mothballed.

Just from looking at a sweetheart's photo.

Romantic love, Dr. Fisher explained in a lecture at the 2004 APA annual meeting, is not an emotion. Rather, it's "a motivation system, it's a drive, it's part of the reward system of the brain." It's a need that compels the lover to seek a specific mating partner. Then the brain links this drive to all kinds of specific emotions depending on how the relationship is going. All the while, she went on to say, the prefrontal cortex is assembling data, putting information into patterns, making strategies, and monitoring the progress toward "life's greatest prize."

Love also hurts. Dr. Fisher cited one study in which 40 percent of people who had been dumped by their partner in the previous eight weeks experienced clinical depression and 12 percent severe depression. It is estimated that 50 to 70 percent of female homicides are committed by lovers and spouses. Annually, a million women and four hundred thousand men are stalked.

Dr. Fisher divides love into three categories involving different brain systems: (1) lust (the craving for sexual gratification), driven by androgens and estrogens; (2) attraction (or romantic or passionate love, characterized by euphoria when things are going well, terrible mood swings when they're not; focused attention; obsessive thinking; and intense craving for the individual), driven by high dopamine and norepinephrine levels and low serotonin; and (3) attachment (the sense of calm, peace, and stability one feels with a long-term partner), driven by the hormones oxytocin and vaso-pressin.

"I think the sex drive evolved to get you out there to get looking for anything at all," she told her audience. Romantic love, she thinks, developed to focus one's mating energy on just one individual, while attachment works to tolerate this individual long enough to raise children as a team.

These systems are also connected. "Don't copulate with people you don't want to fall in love with," she half-jokingly tells her students, "because indeed you may do just that."

Romantic love, Dr. Fisher believes, is a stronger craving than sex. People who don't get sex don't kill themselves, she said. On the other hand, it is not adaptive to be romantically in love for twenty years. "First of all," she confided, "we would all die of sexual exhaustion." Not surprisingly, the subjects in her study who had been in love the longest (seventeen months) displayed markers in the brain indicating the beginnings of "the satiation response."

In a related undertaking, Dr. Fisher found evidence that romantic love exists in 150 societies, even though it is discouraged in many of them. But with many women from these countries now entering the workforce and acquiring a sense of independence—together with medical science keeping us relatively younger longer—we can expect to see romantic love on the rise worldwide, she predicted.

Bring it on.

Love and Serotonin

At a different APA forum, "Sex, Sexuality, and Serotonin," Dr. Fisher warned that antidepressants may jeopardize romantic love. As well as high dopamine and norepinephrine, she said, romantic love is characterized by low serotonin. Low serotonin would explain the obsessive thinking attached to romantic love. Serotonin-enhancing antidepressants, she said, blunt the emotions, including the elation of romance, and suppress obsessive thinking, a critical component of romance. "When you inhibit this brain system," she warned, "you can inhibit your patient's well-being and possibly their genetic future."

But there is another point to consider. At the same APA conference, Philip Muskin, MD, of Columbia University, pointed out that untreated depression often causes a lack of interest in sex, and disrupts intimacy.

Transition

Our ability to alternatively fuck like blenders on full speed on one hand or be as responsive as a block of wood on the other can lead to disastrous choices in our relationships. Writes Zia on my Web site: "How's this for a crash and burn story? Middle aged housewife and mother of three divorces husband of 17 years, turns into party animal and has baby at the age of 38 with a 21-year-old man, becomes a single parent, has a manic episode and on a drinking/partying binge picks up a man in a bar that turns into a long-term supportive relationship. Don't try this at home."

We will take a considered look at relationships in Chapter 17.

Inevitably, any discussion of sex raises questions about moral issues. Those of us with bipolar disorder—and to a lesser extent depression—inevitably find ourselves engaging in behavior we will later regret. If we are lucky, a profuse apology or two will get us off the hook. Too often, sadly, we find ourselves hurting others and getting hurt, with our relationships, career, finances, and our very lives in shambles. And too often again, we wind up being caught totally off guard.

Moral Issues

A person in my first support group never saw it coming. In one fell swoop, Hurricane First Episode Mania wiped out what had taken a lifetime to build. A financial officer with a large corporation, he suddenly found he had access to unlimited funds in which to play a modern-day Robin Hood, embezzling some $500,000 and giving most of it to charity. For his efforts, he was prosecuted and convicted and sent to prison.

I am free to divulge these confidential details because they were reported in full in the local paper.

This person's sad experience led me to pose this question on my Web site: "Should people in a state of mania be held legally and morally accountable for their actions? Are there mitigating factors?"

Tasha provides the realist perspective: "We are held accountable, and always will be. Creditors will always want their money back and with interest."

Tina, on the other hand, has this story to tell:

Last September, I was charged with eight counts including one felony count of assault with a deadly weapon (my car, in a police chase). I was in NO way out to hurt anyone. I was completely paranoid and I think in a mixed state. I had been manic for some time, without any prior knowledge of my illness. I have never been in any kind of legal trouble before. I am 22 years old and am in the process of applying to law school. I am so thankful that no one got hurt and that my diagnosis of bipolar was revealed and medicated. I have reacted extremely well to Topamax and am planning on living a wonderful life. I wonder what would have happened had I been held accountable for actions that I had no control over.

Rav is urging revolution:

I think in the end we bipolars are a cultural minority. Society is made by normal people for normal people and ruled as I see it by the biggest assholes among them.

Some of us are natural born heretics. I feel now for many

years a vocation to found an order of people that want an-
other life. St. Francis of Assisi did it. Why shouldn't I?

Nancy provides us with a sobering reminder of the terrible suffering that we can inflict on others:

Recently my husband had an affair with a bipolar woman. . . .
I confronted her and my husband and she burst into tears,
begged me for forgiveness and proceeded to tell both of us
that she was disturbed, that my husband wasn't the first and
she couldn't help it, she was bipolar . . .

I sat there in shock as this very attractive woman (that se-
duces men on a regular basis, I've heard) blamed all her be-
havior on her bipolar condition. Is this crazy? She took no
responsibility or sadness in the fact that she has broken up yet
another home. Our children are broken, I'm broken and now
my STUPID husband is sad to know that HE was just an-
other fling for her! CRAZY! I think we all must take respon-
sibility for our actions. Take the meds—get the treatment!

It works the other way, too. Writes Dotty: "A year ago, two po-
licemen in our area shot and killed a young man who was bipolar.
They considered him a threat to their safety. He had a rubber knife
in his hand and they KNEW he was bipolar, or as they put it, crazy.
Well, I guess they certainly showed him that he was accountable,
didn't they?"
Paula, who has had two full-blown manic episodes, posted this
thoughtful and provocative comment:

Here is my take on it: Though I sometimes have felt quite out
of control, even in serious fog, I find that certain REALLY
important considerations can break through, such as the wel-
fare of my children, basic compassion for my pets, the need to

drive safely to not injure others, the need to not hurt others'
feelings. Therefore, I have concluded that, short of raving psy-
chosis, I must be responsible for my actions. . . .

Short of a frontal lobe injury or a documented psychotic
episode, it would not be wise to count on the justice system
letting anybody off when a bank is robbed or bankruptcy is
declared. The issue of personal responsibility goes to the heart
of who we believe we are—a pile of biochemically charged
synapses, or thinking, soulful being? Don't neglect your soul
while you are trying to find an admixture of pharmaceuticals
that works for you.

There was something about what Paula said that jolted me into
one of those Newton-under-the-apple-tree kind of revelations:
namely, what gets us into trouble much of the time is not doing
wrong in a manic or hypomanic state, but committing an excess of
doing right. We give things away, we give our employers incredible
productivity, we embark on great projects, we light up the lives of
others, and we pursue a spiritual path to its extremes. In these states
of mania, our moral compass gives us a false reading—our actions
and behaviors are in perfect alignment with that inner arrow point-
ing true. Something in our judgment is fundamentally flawed, but
the mind in pure rhapsody over mania's great abundance abdicates
its authority.

Sooner or later, our doing right comes at the expense of someone
else, such as the activities of the corporate financial officer in my
first support group. If we are to accept Paula's view, the sheer im-
mensity of this theft should have intruded a sense of reality into this
person's otherwise delusional state. But what was his moral compass telling him? That he was a modern-day corporate Robin Hood?

Suffice it to say, he would have found no ready takers for an insanity plea. According to the NIMH, the insanity defense is used in
the courts only 1 percent of the time, and is argued successfully only

a quarter of that time. Two states—Montana and Idaho—have abolished the insanity defense entirely. Meanwhile, our chickens come home to roost in the form of wrecked relationships, ruined reputations, unemployability, and impoverishment. As for the person in my first support group, he accepted full responsibility for his actions. He will have served his time by now and, if he is lucky, is reunited with his family and back in the workforce.

Unfortunately, I suspect his job involves saying: "Do you want fries with that?"

Anger

A classic 1983 *Psychology Today* poll asked: "If you could secretly push a button and thereby eliminate any person with no repercussions to yourself, would you press that button?" Yes, said 69 percent of the men and 56 percent of the women, representing tens of millions of would-be dead bosses, coworkers, spouses and lovers and exes, family members, neighbors, politicians, telemarketers, movie stars, news reporters with bad wigs, reality-game-show contestants, and lawyers who appear on *At Large with Geraldo Rivera*.

Another 1980s survey asked college students if the United States could wipe out the Soviet Union with no threat of retaliation, should the government do it? Fifteen percent thought this would be a good idea.

This is pure anger talking, as potentially as deadly as cyanide on a personal level, more powerful than a nuclear weapon on a collective level. Sooner or later, everyone must learn to deal with their anger or face the consequences. For people with mood disorders, the stakes are even higher, as anger is to an episode what a match is to a keg of gunpowder. The process also works in reverse, as our population, including our loved ones, generally have a lot to be angry about.

Anger is "an emotional state that varies in intensity from mild irritation to intense fury and rage," says Charles Spielberger, PhD, in a brochure published by the American Psychological Association.

People prone to anger tend to experience events as more stressful than others. In response to stress, adrenaline and cortisol are pumped into the system, preparing the body for fight or flight, appropriate for caveman daily living and the occasional modern contingency, but not for most situations we find ourselves in. Anger is an adaptive response to threat, arousing powerful aggressive feelings and behaviors.

Depression, goes the old saying, is anger turned inward. Various studies have found anger attacks to be common in 40 to 60 percent of those with unipolar and bipolar depression. The rate is about the same for bipolar mixed states. Surprisingly, no studies appear in the PubMed database documenting anger in mania. Equally surprising, the *DSM* fails to list anger as a symptom for either depression or mania, perhaps because the trait is endemic in the general population as well, and so is regarded as normal (which is a very scary thought).

Make no mistake—any state of mind that can disrupt your work and social relationships and potentially freeze you out of any life worth living should not be regarded as normal. And because our illness amplifies feelings and makes us lose rational control, we need to regard ourselves as skating on very thin ice.

With so little guidance from the psychiatric profession, one could hazard a guess that anger goes unrecognized and untreated. The posts on my Web site unambivalently bear this out. When reviewing what my readers who were patients had to say, only a handful acknowledged their anger, all in passing. Writes Bionic Woman: "There is the road rage. I know a lot of people experience it but in WALMART? It is an awful feeling. I have to keep myself from mowing people down with my cart. Anyone who got in my way. I want to yell and scream get the F out of my way."

If one were put together a bipolar profile based on what family members posted on my Web site, however, anger would be the major symptom. Says Lynne of one or her parents: "This person is getting to the point where mania is rarely seen, and basically all that is seen is anger."

Says Rita of her boyfriend: "I care about him, and want to do the best I can by him, but there are times when I feel I am just a repository for his anger and frustration."

It's not that our population is in denial. The topic is frequently raised in my support group, and we discuss it with the intensity and focus of airline-crash survivors in the Andes debating their menu options. We know what anger does to us and how it hurts those around us. Believe me, we are desperate for answers.

But psychiatry has let us down, leaving us in the dark and disinclined to seek help. Fittingly, it's the other APA—the American Psychological Association—that has made this behavior part of its brief. Its brochure recommends:

- Relaxing techniques such as breathing or visual imagery
- Cognitive restructuring (such as changing exaggerated, overly dramatic thoughts into more rational ones)
- Problem solving (not every problem has a solution, but one can work on a plan to cope)
- Better communication (think before you speak and listen before you respond defensively)
- Using humor
- Changing your environment (such as quiet-time breaks)

Buddhist mindfulness techniques advocate nonattachment to angry thoughts that arise. Basically, one is asked simply to observe one's anger with disinterest and focus on breathing. In a best-case scenario, the anger will dissipate. Thoughts only acquire force, say Buddhist teachers, when we attach ourselves to these thoughts.

Since our inflated egos are our own worst enemies, it pays to think of ourselves as egoless Buddhas full of infinite compassion, even for the people we attribute our anger to.

Modern psychology is heavily derivative of Buddhist mindfulness. Though we may lack an adept's capacity to mindfully dissolve our worst thoughts, we can buy ourselves a few precious seconds before we do something irretrievably stupid. In essence, we can recognize our destructive thoughts as they occur, and then work with them.

Healthy venting can provide a constructive release for anger, but may also add fuel to the fire. Therapists sometimes encourage clients to act out their anger as a form of catharsis, but other experts feel this may only whet the appetite. On the other side of the coin, there is a danger in bottling up your anger, as it can turn inward on yourself, resulting in hypertension, high blood pressure, and depression.

Repressed anger can also wind up surfacing in unexpected situations—often directed at innocent bystanders—a phenomenon known as displacement. Finally, unexpressed anger can result in passive-aggressive behavior, which involves getting back at people indirectly instead of confronting them head-on.

In the movie *Anger Management*, Jack Nicholson plays an unconventional therapist who constantly baits and humiliates the nebbish Adam Sandler to his breaking point. This results in Sandler finally standing up for himself, confronting his boss by smashing a golf club on the office furniture and crashing a game at Yankee Stadium to win back Marisa Tomei (where Rudolph Giuliani, in a cameo, shouts from his box seat, "Slip her a five-second Frenchie!"). Because of his new sense of self-esteem, Sandler has less reason to feel resentful, is far less likely to explode at inappropriate times, and is not afraid to use his anger as a constructive force (though please don't go on a tear with a golf club in your boss's office).

Anger is that pet tiger you take out for a walk. The beast needs occasional air and exercise, but how successful you are at releasing it from its cage depends on your well-honed skill and judgment. If you have any doubt about whether you should sound off or bite your lip, ask yourself if your would-be response is proportionate to your hurt. If you're thinking of mowing down your boss with an Uzi, for instance, it might be better to take a couple of deep breaths and resolve to take up your grievance at a later time.

People who choose the Uzi option may want to consider courses in anger management or seek a therapist. Those who find themselves always putting a lid on it may also find it useful to seek a therapist.

Finally, it pays not to dwell upon *them* versus *us*. It is way too easy to get angry at people we perceive as different from ourselves. The news media play on our worst fears, and unscrupulous politicians, religious figures, and talk-show hosts are quick to find convenient scapegoats to channel public resentment. Because of our illness, we are the ones who find ourselves on the *them* receiving end, subject to opprobrium and ridicule and humiliation. We know from personal experience how destructive *them* versus *us* thinking truly is. Other populations have felt its terrible force in full measure. We need not contribute to this form of madness.

5

Associated Illnesses and Symptoms

Rare is the person who just has depression or just has bipolar disorder. The brain—not to mention the body—simply doesn't work that way. Complicit in both illnesses in particular are the different anxiety disorders and alcohol and substance use, both which arguably should be included as mood symptoms in the next *DSM*. A similar case can be made for pain, though only anxiety is likely to make the cut.

Included in our discussion of anxiety is stress, which is a cotraveler of both mood and anxiety, as well as the prime suspect as a middleman between mood and below-the-neck symptoms, such as the heart and diabetes, a phenomenon I call the perfect mental storm (thank you, Sebastian Junger).

Sleeping too little or too much is both a mood symptom as well as a separate set of illnesses, and requires the patient's and clinician's most urgent attention. (You can find a full discussion on sleep in Chapter 8, "Lifestyle.")

To proceed . . .

Anxiety and Stress

On my Web site, Ben, a stockbroker, writes: "When major depression finally swept over me, it felt like being caught in a huge wave, unable to get my footing any longer, unable to understand which way to the surface, and just helplessly and hopelessly thrown about, powerless to do anything about the hostile world that was coming down around me."

The market was headed south, and his financial situation along with it. He reports:

Every time I have a couple of decent days back to back, I hope that this is the beginning of my recovery. Then something negative confronts me and I get a panic attack and head for the Xanax. I go right down the tubes to hopelessness and constant depression and anxiety. There, even good things are heavily veiled in grey. No shower, no shaving, no energy, no hope. Just scared and remembering back to my childhood diagnosis of "Born Wrong."

Unfortunately, Ben is not alone. So bound up is anxiety to mood that it may be more convenient to think of each as part of the same illness. According to the U.S. National Comorbidity Survey, 51.2 percent of those with major depression also suffer from anxiety; between 31 and 42 percent of bipolar patients also do, according to various studies.

Highly anxious bipolar patients have more suicide attempts, more alcohol use, are less responsive to lithium, and have longer time toward remission.

One's anxiety, however, need not be full-blown to sabotage recovery. The technical term is *subsyndromal comorbidity,* which applies in this context to a mood disorder and under-the-radar anxiety (i.e., some anxiety symptoms, often overlooked but clinically significant).

Think once more of the spectrum phenomenon. Significantly, two studies by one of the Spectrum Project collaborators, Ellen Frank, PhD, and her colleagues at the University of Pittsburgh, found that depressed or bipolar patients with co-occurring panic symptoms experienced significant delays in their weeks toward remission. These patients also had higher levels of residual impairment.

We need to think beyond the *DSM* symptom list, Dr. Frank told the psychiatrists and other mental-health professionals at the 2004 APA's annual meeting. "The *DSM* has made us less sensitive to our clinical intuition."

Both anxiety and mood share the same stress pathway. In an article in the September 2003 *Scientific American,* Robert Sapolsky, PhD, of Stanford, writes on how the fight-or-flight response underpins both anxiety and depression:

The primate stress response, Dr. Sapolsky begins, can be set in motion by the mere anticipation of an event, and when we erroneously believe a stressor is about to happen we "have entered the realm of neurosis, anxiety, and paranoia."

The individual may experience a fight-or-flight response to a voice in a crowd without knowing why, being unable to link the sound of that voice to the similar-sounding voice of a past assailant, resulting in "free-floating" anxiety.

The torpor of depression may appear to be the opposite of anxiety, but—like anxiety—can be related to stress. Moreover, depression is not a passive state. According to Dr. Sapolsky: "The dread is active, twitching, energy-consuming, distracting, exhausting—but internalized. A classic conception of depression is that it represents aggression turned inward . . ." Dr. Sapolsky asks us to imagine a rat trained to press a lever to avoid a mild shock. The anticipation of mastery might activate pleasurable dopamine release to the frontal cortex. If the lever is disconnected, however, so that pressing it no longer prevents shocks, the rat will frantically press the lever repeatedly, attempting to gain control. This, says Dr. Sapolsky, is the essence of anxiety, characterized mainly by adrenaline and norepinephrine secretion and to a lesser extent by cortisol production. As the shocks continue and the rat finds its attempts at coping useless, a transition occurs in which cortisol dominates and key neurotransmitters are depleted. In the words of Dr. Sapolsky: "It has learned to be helpless, passive and involuted. If anxiety is a crackling, menacing brushfire, depression is a suffocating heavy blanket thrown on top of it." With anxiety a virtual trip wire for a mood episode (including mania), successful management of the former is vital to the outcome of the latter. Not surprisingly, depressed or bipolar patients with an anxiety disorder are more difficult to treat.

The *DSM-IV* breaks down anxiety as follows: panic disorder (which can include palpitations and similar physical symptoms); agoraphobia (often manifested as fear of venturing outside); social anxiety disorder or social phobia; specific phobia (such as unreasonable fear of heights); obsessive-compulsive disorder (which may include rituals such as excessive hand-washing); generalized anxiety disorder (excessive unrealistic long-term worry); and post-traumatic stress disorder (often involving reliving a horrifying event).

Stress

A study by Ahmad Hariri, PhD, and others at the NIMH appearing in the July 19, 2002, *Science* divided twenty-eight subjects into two groups: those who had a short form (allele) of the serotonin transporter gene SLC6A4, and those with the long allele. Cells with the long variant express nearly double the serotonin reuptake as those with the short allele (serotonin reuptake is what modern antidepressants target).

The subjects were placed in an MRI machine and completed a simple exercise involving the processing of images of three different faces. The brain scans revealed that those with the short allele displayed a significantly greater response in the right amygdala (governing fear) while engaged in the task. When the subjects were given a thinking task not involving emotions, no variants were seen.

A year later, SLC6A4 featured in a University of Wisconsin–King's College (London) study that analyzed fourteen stressful events (including employment, finances, housing, health, and relationships) in the lives of 847 New Zealanders from ages twenty-one to twenty-six. The study found that 33 percent of those with one or two copies of the short allele and with four or more life stresses developed depression, as opposed to 17 percent with two copies of the long variant. Stressed individuals with the short allele experienced more suicidality (11 versus 4 percent) than those with two copies of the long allele.

Stress is to mood as that iceberg was to the *Titanic,* with therapies increasingly geared toward neutralizing its vast destructive powers. According to the U.S. surgeon general in his landmark 1999 report on mental health: "The compelling impact of past parental neglect, physical and sexual abuse, and other forms of maltreatment on both adult emotional well-being and brain function is now firmly established for depression." At a 2003 APA symposium, Christine Heim, PhD, of Emory University, cited a 1997 Johns Hopkins survey that found that women who reported experiences of childhood abuse had higher depression and anxiety scores, greater drug and alcohol use, and a higher rate of suicide attempts.

Various studies have found higher concentrations of stress hormones in the cerebrospinal fluid of depressed and anxious humans, and a 2002 study found a smaller hippocampus, associated with short-term memory and emotion processing, in depressed patents. Throw in one overworked amygdala and we begin to get a picture of just some of the things that can go wrong under the hood long before depression sets in.

At a symposium at the 2002 APA annual meeting, Charles Nemeroff, MD, PhD, chair of the Department of Psychiatry and

Behavioral Sciences at Emory University, recounted his now-classic study (with Dr. Heim as a lead author) that was published in the August 2, 2000, *Journal of the American Medical Association*. In that study, forty-nine healthy women were recruited into four groups: those with no history of childhood abuse or psychiatric disorder, those with current major depression who had been physically or sexually abused as children, those without current major depression who had been physically or sexually abused as children, and those with current major depression with no history of childhood abuse.

The women were given math tests and made to speak in public. Blood samples and heart readings showed that the women with a history of childhood abuse exhibited increased pituitary and autonomic responses to stress compared with the controls. This was especially true for the women with current depression and anxiety.

"Is the biology of depression the biology of early trauma?" Dr. Nemeroff asked his audience.

A year later, Dr. Nemeroff answered his own question in the form of a secondary analysis of a previous study of 681 women with chronic depression. Of these, about one-third lost their parents before age fifteen, 45 percent experienced childhood physical abuse, 16 percent suffered childhood sexual abuse, and 10 percent endured neglect, representing more than half those in the study. In a classic understatement, Dr. Nemeroff and his coauthors noted that "these findings alone highlight the remarkably high prevalence rate of early life trauma in patients with chronic forms of major depression."

In response to stress, the hypothalamus in the brain secretes CRF (corticotropin-releasing factor), which results in the pituitary gland releasing another hormone, ACTH (adrenocorticotropic hormone; the abused and depressed women in the Heim-Nemeroff study exhibited a sixfold greater ACTH increase over the controls), which activates the adrenal glands that turn loose the stress hormone cortisol. This neuroendocrine feedback loop is referred to as the HPA (hypothalamic-pituitary-adrenal) axis.

Women abused in childhood, Dr. Nemeroff explained, end up with a sensitized brain system, in which CRF receptors are to be found in abundance.

Situational occurrences such as marriage breakup or bereavement also loom large. A study of major depression in twins found that recent stressful events were the most powerful risk factor for an episode of major depression. According to the study, those with the lowest genetic risk of depression had only a 0.5 percent probability of depression that month, but this shot up to 6.2 percent with exposure to severe stress. Those with the highest genetic risk faced a 1.1 percent probability that skyrocketed to 14.6 percent when stress was present.

Two 2000 Centers for Disease Control (CDC) studies examined stress on large populations. The studies looked at the effects of armed conflict on groups of Albanians and Serbians.

In the first study, two-thirds of the Albanians surveyed reported being deprived of food and water, being in a combat situation, and being close to death. More than half had been forced to flee their homes, and nearly 40 percent had experienced at least eight specific traumatic events, from the murder of a family member to rape.

Not surprisingly, the researchers found a high rate of psychiatric disorder among the survivors. What surprised them was how high this figure was—43 percent, twice their expectations. Adopting less-conservative criteria raised the incidence to 83.5 percent.

A study of the Serbian population remaining in Kosovo also surprised researchers, as the findings virtually matched those of the Albanians. Apparently, war in all its terrible horror pays no regard to which group suffers the most. It's simply enough that stress hormones flood into the system like refugees streaming across the border. The stress hormones, of course, are too dumb to know whether the war in Kosovo is the cause of their migration into the bloodstream. Any war will do, as will any situation approximating war. In this regard, we all represent a population at risk.

Those hormones, it seems, have plenty of places to go—the heart, the pancreas, the bones, and so on. Depression has been linked to illnesses from heart disease to diabetes to stroke to bone loss to cancer.

What may be occurring on a cellular level, in response to stress, is that the neurotransmitter glutamate fails to get cleared from the synapse (gap) between the cells, resulting in increased calcium influx through the NMDA (N-methyl-D-asparate) receptors and ion channels into the cell and the activation of certain calcium-dependent enzymes that can result in cell atrophy and death.

Fortunately, our brain circuits are not permanently welded into place. Our thought patterns can be changed, and certain forms of talking therapy are especially useful in restructuring how we perceive and react to stressful and anxiety-inducing situations. With a bit of practice, "It's the end of the world!" can be altered to "Let's find a solution." For those with trauma, coming to terms with past abuse or neglect may be the key to real healing.

Our lifestyle choices play an essential role in nipping stress and anxiety in the bud. A diet of mood-buster foods is simply tempting fate, as is irregular sleep, lack of exercise, and putting off things till the last minute. Ultimately, you may have to lower your expectations—from what you demand of yourself to how clean you want your house to be.

In the meantime, though, it pays to manage your stress and anxiety as if your life depended upon the outcome—which, as we are finding more and more every day, it does.

Dual Diagnosis

On my Web site, Jasmine writes: "I always believed my problem was the alcohol. I drank too much, most of the time. It became very serious—car accidents, drunk driving, jail, suicide threats, etc. Three rehabs didn't seem to work. I did get an education on addiction. I had no denial. What I soon realized was I drank because I didn't know how to feel, and mainly I drank to feel normal."

Eventually, Jasmine was able to figure out that she first needed to manage her bipolar. Now she reports: "I go downhill, real fast. A place I pray I never need to go again. Life is just so good right now. And I'm full of gratitude."

Welcome to the real world, where mental illness rarely is so considerate as to neatly dole out one disorder per person for easy diagnosis and treatment. In Jasmine's case, Mother Nature has dealt her both barrels, a powerful double whammy—a mood disorder coupled with a substance-use problem, commonly referred to as dual diagnosis—where one illness tends to feed off the other.

Without treatment, says the surgeon general, substance use worsens the course of mood disorders.

According to the U.S. Department of Health and Human Services, 51 percent of those with one or more lifetime serious mental disorders have a lifetime history of at least one substance-use disorder. For people with bipolar disorder, the Epidemiological Catchment Survey reports 61 percent with a lifetime substance-use disorder, more than five times the rate of the general population.

In any given year, about 15 percent of those with a serious mental illness experience a substance use problem, according to the U.S. National Comorbidity Survey. For those dealing with current substance use, the picture is far more grim, with 42.7 percent struggling with a mental disorder. Unfortunately, according to NCS findings, of those with co-occurring disorders, only 49 percent are treated for serious mental illness, 29 percent for substance use, and a mere 19 percent for both.

One type of disorder may trigger the other, but 90 percent of the time, according to NCS data, mental illness precedes substance use. On average, mental illness occurs at around age eleven, followed by substance use five to ten years later. On the other side of the coin, drug use can produce psychotic symptoms, result in a relapse of a psychotic illness, or create a need for meds adjustments.

Regardless of which disorder an individual experiences first, the Substance Abuse and Mental Health Services Administration (SAMHSA) emphasizes in a 2002 report that "both disorders must be considered as primary and treated as such."

Self-help

Twelve-step programs are an important component of substance use treatment, and there are dual-diagnosis support groups modeled on AA. (Check out Dual Recovery Anonymous, or DRA, at www.draonline.org.) Others may find it more useful to attend a mood disorders support group one evening and an AA meeting another night.

It pays to keep in mind that AA is not the only model for recovery. *Sober for Good,* by Anne Fletcher, documents the recoveries of 222 men and women, more than half who quit without AA, many on their own, others through the help of therapists, especially those who practice cognitive-behavioral therapy, and others through non-AA groups such as Women for Sobriety and SMART Recovery.

Final Word

With dual diagnosis, it may seem that you are pushing two rocks uphill. Lest you allow yourself to become overwhelmed at the thought, permit me to state that I am familiar with people who successfully manage both their mood disorder and their substance use. They would be the very last to tell you it's a rose garden, but they would also be the first to let you know it's not a reason to abandon hope, either. You have your work more than cut out for you, but keep in mind four simple words: You are worth it.

Pain

In an article published in the May 24, 2002, *New York Times*, Anna Fels, MD, recounted an anecdote told to her by a fellow psychiatrist. He was at a conference about depression in developing countries, where the theme of the lectures was that these people commonly expressed their depression as hard-to-pin-down physical symptoms, or, to use medical jargon, they "somaticized" their depression. Finally, a doctor from India stood to speak. "Distinguished colleagues," he said, "have you ever considered the possibility that it is not that we in the third world somaticize depression, but rather that you in the developed world psychologize it?"

According to Dr. Fels: "His comment, my colleague reported, was met with stunned silence."

Actually, it is the medical profession in the developed world who are guilty of "psychologizing" the illness rather than their patients. According to David Dunner, MD, director of the Center for Anxiety and Depression at the University of Washington, in an article on HealthScout: "Eighty percent of patients with depression come to the doctor with exclusively physical symptoms." But you would never know it by looking at the *DSM-IV,* which makes no reference to pain in its criteria for depression.

John Greist, MD, of the University of Wisconsin, pointed out at the 2002 APA annual meeting that pain is one of the most common physical symptoms. Up to two-thirds of those with unexplained pain meet the criteria for major depression, he went on to say. A 1993 study found that of twenty-six physical symptoms most germane to primary care, nearly one-third were psychiatric or unexplained.

Stress appears complicit in both pain and depression. A 2001 review article cited a large number of studies documenting higher-than-usual stress and anxiety and depression levels in patients seeking health care for migraines, fatigue, and GI symptoms.

Mood and pain are mediated by the same neurotransmitters, serotonin and norepinephrine, both of which have pathways which can be found in the brain, the spinal column, and virtually every organ system in the body. Another key neurotransmitter, substance P, is responsible for sending pain signals up the spinal column into the brain. Substance P, like serotonin and norepinephrine, also plays a role in mood.

Pain in no uncertain terms serves to remind us that our illness is not all in our heads, that our whole physical being is literally held hostage by this debilitating manifestation of mood. Someday, psychiatrists may be advising us to keep pain journals the way we keep mood journals. But first psychiatry needs to stop "psychologizing" depression.

The Perfect Mental Storm

Let's throw away the term *mood* and call it the perfect mental storm instead. Depression and mania aren't just hurricanes in the brain—they're hurricanes plus a Canadian cold front plus a storm at sea, all in disharmonic convergence, each element feeding off the other, generating hundred-mile-an-hour winds and hundred-foot waves that have more than one way of sending their unfortunate victims to the bottom.

We all know that the perfect mental storm is capable of sucking the life force out of even the strongest of individuals, pummeling the victim's brain to antimatter, and reducing one to the level of the living dead, on the brink of total death, as close to actual death without being dead. This is the destructive nature of the storm with which we are most familiar, one that can lead to suicide.

The other killer aspects of the perfect mental storm are just as real, but not readily apparent. Scientists are now beginning to uncover the links between depression and heart disease, depression and diabetes, depression and cancer, and depression and stroke—among others—and what they are finding suggests a cruel illness going to work in a variety of insidious ways, all with the power to kill.

Ken Duckworth, MD, former deputy commissioner of the Massachusetts Department of Mental Health, advised any MDs in the audience at the 2002 NAMI annual convention that "you need to be thinking of [your patients] as if they already had a heart attack."

His epiphany came when, as a young doctor working in a mental-health facility, someone came up to him and said: "Ken, you guys are getting fabulous at doing memorial services." A 1999 unpublished study his department initiated found that the risk for cardiovascular disease for people with serious psychiatric illness in Massachusetts ranged from twice as high to six times higher than normal, depending on age. Respiratory illnesses were four to six times higher and diabetes twice as high. For individuals between the ages of fifteen and sixty-four, the death rate was 1.4 to 3.3 times higher for Department of Mental Health clients than for the general Massachusetts population.

Other studies bear him out.

The Heart

Studies linking depression to the heart seem to roll in by the week. To stick to three of the classics: A 1993 Montreal Heart Institute study found depressed patients with heart attacks were four times more likely to die within six months as their nondepressed counterparts. An editorial in the February 21, 2000, *Journal of Australian Medicine* cited yet another Montreal Heart Institute Study as the basis for the proposition that depression is as great a risk for heart disease as a previous heart attack. A 1995 Johns Hopkins study concluded that those who are depressed are four times more likely to have a heart attack within fourteen years of the onset of depression.

Depressed people are more likely to make bad lifestyle choices that negatively impact their heart. Biologically, depression may set in motion a chain of events leading to atherosclerosis.

Diabetes

A 2004 study by Johns Hopkins and other centers that tracked 11,615 initially nondiabetic adults aged forty-eight to sixty-seven over six years found that "depressive symptoms predicted incident type 2 diabetes." Unfortunately, depressed people tend to eat more and exercise less, which results in weight gain and sabotages efforts at controlling blood-sugar levels.

Cancer

A 1998 National Institute on Aging study found that chronically depressed people were 88 percent more likely to develop cancer. Depression may suppress the body's immune system, which affects the ability to fight rogue cancer cells.

And the Beat Goes On

Commenting on a 2000 study led by Richard Schulz, PhD, of the University of Pittsburgh, that linked even milder forms of depression to increased mortality in the elderly, an editorial in the June 26, 2000, *Archives of Internal Medicine* observed: "Suicide explains only a small proportion of the increase in mortality among the depressed . . ."

The fact that we know nothing about the actual cause and effect of depression and morbidity moved the editorial writer to conclude: "Depression now demands the aggressive level of research in the next quarter of a century that smoking, cancer, and heart disease have received in the past quarter of a century."

Technically, a 1998 World Bank study, *The Global Burden of Disease,* credits depression as the fourth-leading cause of "disease-burden" in 1990 and will be the single-leading cause by 2020. Bipolar disorder is not far behind. But the World Bank fails to account—much less even tries to account—for mood's true kill rate. The Schulz study found that in an elderly population, 17.7 percent who had low baseline depression scores died during six years. This compared to a 23.9 percent death rate among those with high baseline scores.

Doing the math (by dividing the higher figure into the smaller one) indicates that the depressed group had an astounding 26 percent greater death rate than the nondepressed group. This is not to say that depression actually caused these deaths—there is no way to prove that. But it is fair to say that depression represents a great unrecognized health risk for many individuals in this age bracket.

In 2001, according to the Centers for Disease Control, 2,416,425 deaths were reported in the United States, the most by far occurring in the elderly population. By incorporating the Schulz findings into the equation, depression is possibly complicit in some 560,000 of those deaths, dwarfing the yearly figure of 30,000 deaths by suicide in the United States, most which can be attributed to depression.

Please don't read my interpolations to mean that your depressed mother or grandmother has a fatal illness, but do appreciate the potential negative impact of mood on overall health.

A further caveat is that this writer is neither an epidemiologist nor a statistician. A credible finding would require a crack team of experts working for years on the effort. In the meantime, you have my crude figures.

But the perfect mental storm has many more lethal aspects. Because of the sense of hopelessness and isolation depression creates, not to mention sluggish cognition, the illness plays a key role in influencing reckless and destructive behavior. A meta-analysis of twenty-five studies published in the July 24, 2000, *Archives of In-*

ternal Medicine found that depressed patients are three times more likely to be noncompliant with their medical treatment recommendations (all medical treatment, not just depression). Noncompliant behavior includes not taking medication correctly, forgetting or refusing to follow a diet, not engaging in prescribed exercise, canceling or not attending appointments, and persisting in lifestyles that endanger one's health.

We're not finished. A 2000 New Zealand study found that teens with depression are more likely to engage in risky sexual intercourse, contract sexually transmitted diseases, and have sexual intercourse before age sixteen. The fact that depression was linked to these outcomes was of particular concern, according to the authors of the study, as rates of depression are known to escalate from ages fifteen to twenty-one—the period when sexual activity also emerges.

Then there is the whole issue of depression and smoking, depression and alcoholism, and depression and drug use.

So it is that the perfect mental storm cascades upon our inadequate psyches from all points of the compass, threatening us from whichever direction we turn with death by suicide, death by medical complications, death by noncompliance, and death by reckless behavior. Our battered minds, in a state of severe distress, send out Maydays that may never be heard as the animus within us succumbs to forces no one should have to bear.

For those who survive, the feeling can be one of looking up at a pale moonlike sun breaking out from suffocating gray clouds. It is a time of subdued thanksgiving and quiet contemplation. The storm may yet engulf us—if not now, perhaps a few hours from now or a few years from now.

In the meantime, though, we can take comfort in the knowledge of having emerged whole from one of the most destructive and terrifying phenomena in all of nature—the perfect mental storm. Of all things, it is an ordeal that has strengthened us, toughened us, and imbued us with a sense of hope and renewal.

And so we finally reach a safe harbor, where we rededicate ourselves to reclaiming our lives—one day at a time, if it comes to that—with a new respect and profound sense of awe of what we are up against, but also with a new regard for the gift of life.

PART TWO

BRAIN SCIENCE 101

6

Neurotransmitters, Neurons, and Things Your Psychiatrist Doesn't Know

Introduction

The brain, in the words of the surgeon general in his 1999 report on mental health, is "the great synthesizer" of the many biological, psychological, and sociocultural phenomena that make us who we are, the product of our genes and experience working together.

What Woody Allen referred to as his "second-favorite organ" is a three-pound mass containing some 100 billion nerve cells— neurons—thousands of different kinds, each forming more than a thousand synaptic connections with other neurons. In all there may be anywhere between 100 trillion and a quadrillion synapses organized into elaborate networks that account for the brain's vast complexity. Of the twenty-five thousand genes in the human genome, more than half go into the brain's makeup.

So what happens when someone—say, a little man inside—

decides to throw a switch? To start, signals from the neuron travel out a single extension called the axon that may end in several terminals. These signals are picked up by branches—dendrites—extending from other neurons.

Communication between neurons occurs along the countless synapses (gaps) separating axons from dendrites. A structure on the terminal portion of the sending neuron releases specialized messenger molecules called neurotransmitters that cross the synapse and bind to receptors on the receiving neuron. The neurotransmitter's mission is complete when its message is delivered through an opening in the cell membrane to the inside of the neuron.

Neurotransmitters

All told, there are some one hundred neurotransmitters in the brain. The three we are most familiar with—serotonin, norepinephrine, and dopamine—are classified as monoamines according to their chemical makeup. The monoamine hypothesis holds that mood disorders are caused by a depletion of one or more of these neurotransmitters, which makes sense in a flat-earth sort of way, with no reference to recent advances in genomics, neuroscience, and brain imaging.

But neurotransmitters represent the vital first step in linking biology and mood. In a lecture at the 2004 APA annual meeting, Jack Barchas, MD, of Cornell University and a pioneer in the field of how biochemistry and behavior interact, recounted how as a student half a century earlier he proposed investigating neurotransmitters. He was told: "If you want to research biochemistry, study the liver. Nothing is going to happen in the brain for years."

So out of touch was psychiatry with medical science back then that an early mentor actually challenged one of his ideas on these grounds: "How is this justified in the writings of Freud?"

Fortunately, Dr. Barchas paid the man no attention.

Norepinephrine

Norepinephrine (also referred to as noradrenaline) is manufactured in the neuron by enzymes acting on the amino acid tyrosine, which convert it into dopa, then to dopamine (more on dopamine in a minute). Some of the dopamine is then converted to norepinephrine, where it is stored in packages called synaptic vesicles. Just as norepinephrine is created by enzymes, it can also be destroyed by enzymes, such as MAO (or monoamine oxidase, which also destroys serotonin and dopamine). Hence the MAOIs (monoamine oxidase inhibitors) that represent the first family of antidepressants.

When the neuron is working right, it releases norepinephrine through alpha-2 autoreceptors into the synapse—the gap between two neurons—and attaches to alpha-1, alpha-2, and beta-1 receptors on the neuron on the other side of the synapse. From there, a signal is sent into the cell that cues certain genes to switch on proteins governing all manner of activity.

Most of the norepinephrine action takes place in an area of the brain stem known as the locus coeruleus, which monitors external stimuli and our responses (such as fight or flight) and pain. Norepinephrine and the locus coeruleus are also believed to play a role in cognition, mood, emotions, movement, and blood pressure. Difficulty concentrating, fatigue, apathy, and depression are some of the things that can result from norepinephrine going AWOL.

After norepinephrine is released into the synapse and attaches to receptors on the postsynaptic neuron, the presynaptic neuron vacuums some of the remaining neurotransmitters through a reuptake pump (transporter) for future use. The tricyclic class of antidepressants bind to the receptors that act as reuptake pumps, thus keeping norepinephrine in circulation (they also bind in a similar fashion to serotonin receptors). Two of the newer antidepressants that mimic the tricyclics are Effexor and Cymbalta.

Serotonin

Serotonin (5-HT) is synthesized in the neuron from the amino acid tryptophan, which is converted to 5-HTP, then to serotonin. It is released into the synapse in a similar fashion to norepinephrine. Serotonin has some seventeen different types and subtypes of receptors, which underscores its importance as a neurotransmitter.

Serotonin projects from the raphe nucleus in the brain stem to the basal ganglia, frontal cortex, hypothalamus, and limbic system, and down the spinal cord. Serotonin is also found in the GI tract. Not surprisingly, this neurotransmitter mediates a host of functions, from mood to anxiety to sleep to sexual response to food craving and digestion. Unfortunately, SSRIs (selective serotonin reuptake inhibitors) enhance serotonin wholesale, with no regard for the fact that what may be good for mood could be catastrophic for sexuality and other functions. The "selective" in selective serotonin reuptake inhibitors, then, is a complete misnomer.

As in the case of norepinephrine, a presynaptic transporter sucks up excess serotonin from the synapse in preparation for the next release of the neurotransmitter. Both the older tricyclic antidepressants and the newer SSRIs and dual-action meds such as Effexor are believed to work by binding to this reuptake pump, thus keeping more serotonin in circulation. Were this completely true, however, antidepressants would have an immediate effect, instead of taking at least two weeks to start making an impression and another two to six weeks to achieve full clinical benefit.

One explanation is that blocking the transporter desensitizes the neuron in a way that dampens normal firing for four weeks. Another explanation is that antidepressants also work on intracellular processes downstream of the neurotransmitters (more on this in a minute).

Dopamine

Dopamine is to the human brain what nuclear power plants are to the power grid. We need the energy, but we don't want a meltdown. Not surprisingly, several classes of psychiatric and neurological agents target this neurotransmitter, including the antipsychotics, which act as fire extinguishers, and the anti-Parkinson's drugs that give the brain the old zoom-zoom-zoom. The old generation MAOI antidepressants work indirectly to keep dopamine (and serotonin and norepinephrine) in circulation, while Wellbutrin achieves a similar end through a different mechanism.

Dopamine is manufactured by norepinephrine, which in turn is produced from tyrosine. There are several dopamine pathways in the brain. The mesolimbic dopamine pathway, which projects from the midbrain to the nucleus accumbens, is thought to be involved in pleasure as well as delusions, psychosis, and drug abuse.

Cocaine is notorious for enhancing dopamine production, while antipsychotics bind to dopamine D2 receptors and thus inhibit too much of a good thing. Unfortunately, antipsychotics don't just limit themselves to the D2 receptors in the mesolimbic dopamine pathway, leading to what Steven Stahl, MD, in *Essential Psychopharmacology of Antipsychotics and Mood Stabilizers,* calls a "high cost of doing business."

Dopamine agonists (enhancers that mimic the dopamine neurotransmitter) such as the anti-Parkinson's drug Mirapex work on D2 and D3 receptors in the nigrostriatal dopamine pathway (projecting from the substantia nigra of the brain stem to the basal ganglia or striatum). The drug is being tested experimentally on depressed patients. Dopamine agonists are also being enlisted to combat dulled cognition and apathy. A new generation that works on D1 receptors is in development.

Glutamate

Glutamate and GABA (gamma-aminobutyric acid) represent the yin and yang of the neurotransmitters, Darryle Schoepp, PhD, of Eli Lilly explained in a session at the 2003 American Psychiatric Association annual meeting. They are both present in nearly all synaptic function all over the brain, with the former acting in an excitatory capacity and the latter in an inhibitory role. The mood stabilizers are thought to act on one or the other or both.

There are two types of glutamate receptors, ionotropic (iGluR), including NMDA, kainate, and AMPA receptors; and metabotropic (mGluR), which mediate numerous chemical actions. When the NMDA receptor is working right, glutamate and glycine bind to the receptor, which opens up its corresponding ion channel and permits calcium entry into the neuron. This in turn promotes intracellular signaling essential to plasticity and survival. Too much glutamate in the system, however, can be catastrophic. The mood stabilizer Lamictal, with demonstrated efficacy for bipolar depression, is an antiglutamate agent.

GABA

GABA (gamma-amino butyric acid) is formed in the brain from glutamate, glucose, and glutamine, and binds to one of two receptors on the postsynaptic neuron. $GABA_a$-receptors regulate excitability and anxiety, panic, and stress, and are the targets of benzodiazepines such as Ativan, barbiturates, and alcohol. Depressed individuals have decreased GABA in their cerebral spinal fluid and plasma.

Gerard Sanacora, MD, PhD, of Yale has used magnetic resonance spectroscopy to measure GABA in the brain, finding that those with melancholic depression show low GABA concentrations in the occipital cortex, while the depletion is not as pronounced for those with atypical depression, indicating the potential for a far more refined approach to diagnosing depression. Dr. Sanacora has also used before-and-after scans to show that patients treated with anti-depressants or electroconvulsive therapy (ECT) showed significant rises in GABA levels.

Inside the Neuron

Until very recently, it was thought that the brain could not grow new cells. From a mood disorders point of view, this was particularly distressing, as brain scans and postmortem studies have found reductions in the volume of the prefrontal cortex of depressed and bipolar patients, as well as cell atrophy and loss. In a classic 1997 study, Wayne Drevets, MD, chief of neuroimaging of mood and anxiety disorders at the NIMH, found that the subgenual prefrontal cortex of the brain was 38 percent smaller in bipolar patients and 48 percent smaller for those with chronic unipolar depression, irrespective of treatment status or mood state.

In experiments by Robert Sapolsky, PhD, of Stanford University, animals subjected to stress resulted in dead or atrophied neurons in the hippocampus, as well as endangered neurons that were more likely to die when subjected to another stressful event.

One of these casualties is brain-derived neurotropic factor (BDNF). BDNF is a neuropeptide that is crucial to the survival and growth of neurons.

Stress elevates cortisol, which in turn ups the excitatory neurotransmitter glutamate, which increases calcium influx into the neuron and activates certain calcium-dependent "death" enzymes. Cortisol may also reduce the neuron's capacity to take energy-sustaining glucose into the cell, so it doesn't have the strength to deal with a subsequent crisis.

Basically, the cells can't handle the load, Husseini Manji, MD, head of the Mood and Anxiety Disorders Progam at the NIMH, explained in a 2003 UCLA grand rounds lecture. Their atrophy and death tends to isolate neurons, affecting their ability to connect to and communicate with other neurons.

We knew as early as the 1960s that under the right conditions animal brains can grow new cells and shrunken brain cells could grow to normal sizes and make new connections, a process called neurogenesis that takes place mainly in the hippocampus. In 2000, Fred Gage, PhD, of the Salk Institute discovered neurogenesis also takes place in humans.

In 2000, Ron Duman, PhD, and his team at Yale discovered that antidepressants can cause new cells to grow in the hippocampus of rats. A year later, he published a hypothesis that the same effect could take place in humans. Dr. Duman and his colleagues first found that repeated antidepressant treatment "up-regulates" a process known as the cAMP-CREB cascade. The cAMP is a signaling molecule inside the cell that is upstream of the protein CREB, which controls the expression for certain genes, among them BDNF. Significantly, CREB and BDNF play critical roles in neuroplasticity—that is, of the brain's capacity to constantly remap itself by learning and forming memories.

The cAMP-CREB cascade also figures in neurogenesis. Dr. Duman and his team exposed lab rats to repeated foot shocks to induce behavioral helplessness, resulting in a long-lasting "down-regulation" of neurogenesis. But when the animals were treated with antidepressants, the behavior was reversed.

Approximately nine thousand new cells a day grow in the hippocampus of an adult rodent. Of these, about 75 to 80 percent become neurons, and half survive after four weeks. It is estimated that in humans the rate of new cell growth is only 10 to 20 percent of rodents, but this may still be sufficient to influence the function of the hippocampus, Dr. Duman informed this writer.

Meanwhile, a 2000 study led by Dr. Manji found that lithium "significantly increases total gray matter volume in the human brain of people with manic-depressive illness."

Using a gene chip microarray (a process that allows researchers to record the interactions among thousands of genes simultaneously), Dr. Manji and his colleagues started experimenting with lithium and Depakote on brain-cell tissue, and found to their surprise these two completely different medications indirectly affected some of the same cell pathways associated with cell survival and death. One protective protein that utilizes these pathways is Bcl-2, which in one experiment was doubled by lithium and Depakote administration. Subsequent experiments on rats found lithium mitigated the effects of lab-induced stroke and led to the growth of new neurons in the hippocampus. When Dr. Manji asked Dr. Drevets to revisit his study, it was found that those patients on lithium or Depakote did not show brain atrophy.

But producing new brain cells is only part of the picture, and probably not the main part of the picture. What may be even more important is the ability to protect and rescue damaged brain cells and helping them to reestablish connections, Dr. Manji told this writer. To appreciate lithium's possibilities, we need to realize that both depression and bipolar disorder are more than mere mood disorders. The impairments to function and cognition may last far beyond the course of an actual episode, and although not "classic" neurodegenerative diseases such as Parkinson's and Alzheimer's, they are clearly illnesses associated with brain cell loss and shrinkage.

Tellingly, Bcl-2 protects against free radicals that can damage brain cells, as well as Parkinson's and possibly the ravages of mood disorders, Dr. Manji informed a session at the 2002 NAMI annual conference.

Dr. Manji explained how for the last three decades, neurotransmitters have been the focus of mental health research. But recently, he went on to say, we have been learning that mental illness is much more complicated than that. Nerve cells communicate with each other through neurotransmitters, but do not actually go inside the nerve cell. Rather, they are merely the keys that unlock what is going on inside the neuron, "where all the action is."

"You can mess all you want with serotonin and dopamine, etc," Dr. Manji told his audience, this time at UCLA, "but if you don't have the appropriate [cell] circuitry in place it's not going to have any effect."

According to Dr. Manji, there are some ten different potential targets within the nerve cell that we did not even suspect ten years ago that are being investigated.

A potential target inside the nerve cell includes protein kinase C (PKC), a signaling pathway that is implicated in nerve cellular excitability. Dr. Manji's team discovered that lithium and Depakote have very similar effects on the PKC system, taking days or weeks to act. A PKC inhibitor, however, may be more direct. The drug Nolvadex (tamoxifen), used to treat breast cancer, inhibits PKC and has been found to significantly reduce mania scores in one small study. Larger placebo-controlled studies are now under way at the NIMH and at Harvard. If these studies work, he said, we can develop a better PKC inhibitor.

A review article by Dr. Manji and his colleagues at the NIMH in the May 2003 *Biological Psychiatry* concludes that much of the trouble with current antidepressant treatment lies in the faulty assumption that our cell circuitry is intact and will faithfully relay meds-enhanced neurotransmitter activity to their intended targets. In fact, we are discovering just the opposite: that some of our brain cells take the kind of physical beating that necessitates "both tropic and neurochemical support" to restore neuronal connectivity and molecular signaling.

One day, cAMP, Bcl-2, BDNF, and the rest may be as familiar to us as serotonin is today—not as academic curiosities, but as the targets of new drugs that promise to radically improve our lives. Bring on the CREBzac.

The Other Brain Cell

There are essentially two types of brain cells: neurons and glia. Until a short time ago, it was thought that glia were to neurons what bubble wrap is to pottery. "Mind glue," is how German scientists described this lowly second banana, *glia* being derived from glue in Greek. Then researchers started taking a second look, and slowly but surely "the other brain cell" began picking up a bit of respect.

The story begins in the early 1960s, when scientists discovered that the cortices from rat pups living in enriched environments contained more glia per neuron than those from impoverished environments. Apparently, the more active cortical neurons required larger supporting casts. As a general rule, we are stuck with the neurons we are born with, but glia divide and reproduce. Humans have higher glia-to-neuron ratios (about 9 to 1) than lower animals.

Two decades following the rat-pup investigation, four sugar-cube-sized samples of Albert Einstein's brain arrived in the mail of one of that study's researchers, Marian Diamond, PhD, of the University of California, Berkeley. When Dr. Diamond compared a slice of a cortical region associated with higher cognition with similar slices from eleven controls, she found Einstein fairly brimming with glia.

Sophisticated new imaging and listening technology ensured that the glia wouldn't be ignored during the decade of the brain. Our knowledge is far from complete, but what is beginning to emerge is a picture of the glia in continuous dialogue with the neuron.

Astrocytes are a type of glia that surrounds the synapse between neurons. Of particular interest is the neurotransmitter glutamate, which binds to certain receptors on the target neuron and opens up channels in the cell membrane. This permits the passage of calcium ions that essentially announce to the chemical population inside that it's Saturday night. Through a complex set of chemical interactions, astrocytes can strengthen the glutamate signaling by releasing glutamate on its own or weaken it by clearing this neurotransmitter from the synapse.

Glutamate (in concert with GABA) is essential to the regulation of mood, and when something goes wrong, glia can invariably be found at the scene of the crime or else on the lam. Various post-mortem studies on human brains of individuals with major depression or bipolar disorder have detected lower-than-normal levels of glia in certain regions. Without glia, the neuron is essentially left defenseless against glutamate bombardment and its dreaded downstream calcium effects.

In an article in the June 2004 *Neuroscientist*, Bernhard Mitterauer, MD, of the University of Salzburg, proposed a neuronal-glial imbalance hypothesis to explain bipolar disorder. The basis of the hypothesis is a different kind of astrocyte activity involving the release of certain types of proteins into the neuronal synapse. These proteins bind to neurotransmitters, preventing them from reaching their intended targets. When things go according to plan, argues Dr. Mitterauer, a kind of equilibrium is achieved. But over- or under-secretion of proteins may result in not enough or too many neuro-transmitters reaching their targets, with predictable results. This phenomenon (more theory than fact at this stage) may also explain why circadian rhythms (including sleep) are disrupted.

Glial cells service neurons in a host of other ways, making the potential for messing up our minds virtually limitless. We know that glia talk to each other, but we have yet to figure out what they're saying. At least, after all these years, we're starting to listen.

7

DNA, Dollars, and Darwin

Introduction

A wide-eyed first-year medical student eagerly listens to his teacher and faithfully records: "The liver is the most complex organ in the body."

This draws a round of hearty laughter from the audience. The venue is the 2000 DBSA annual conference in Boston, and the speaker is Charles Nemeroff, MD, PhD, of Emory University.

"How gullible was I," he acknowledges. The liver, he goes on to say, has the same composition no matter which way you slice it, while the brain's various parts are as different from each other as the liver is from the kidneys.

"Ninety percent of what we know about the brain," he tells us, "we've discovered in the last ten years."

One can hear some oohs and ahs from the audience, as well as sense a collective feeling of recognition. Of course, five hundred people are thinking at once, this explains everything, doesn't it?

The most exciting stuff is saved for last—the possibility of finding the genes responsible for depression and bipolar disorder and coming up with effective treatments.

In another seminar, Robert Lenox, MD, of the University of Pennsylvania, reels off the locations of the likely bipolar genes: chromosome 18, chromosome 12, chromosome 4, chromosome 22 . . .

Speaking of Chromosome 22

In 2000, John Kelsoe, MD, of the University of California, San Diego, informed this writer: "We have identified a gene on chromosome 22 which we believe plays a role in the susceptibility to both bipolar disorder and schizophrenia."

Before you let your hallelujah ring through the rafters, it pays to recall the false alarm that was raised in 1987 after a study of Amish families supposedly yielded the culprit near the tip of the short arm of chromosome 11. The researchers were forced to concede defeat two years later.

What's so different this time? For one, Dr. Kelsoe and his team have the complete human genome at their disposal. Over the last several years, they have scanned the entire genome in a set of families with bipolar disorder, attempting to identify a chromosomal region consistently associated with the illness.

The approach is called linkage analysis, and it led to "very strong evidence" for the presence of a gene on chromosome 22, identified by two peaks. This region has already been implicated in many studies of schizophrenia.

With the publishing of the entire genome, the team discovered that one of the peaks—at 22q12.1—corresponded to the location of GRK3, whose normal role is to regulate the response and level of sensitivity to several neurotransmitters, including dopamine. It has long been argued that a supersensitivity to dopamine may play a role in bipolar disorder and schizophrenia.

In four human subjects, reduced GRK3 expression corresponded with bipolar I, while the other two subjects not showing a GRK3 decrease had bipolar II.

In parallel with these studies, Dr. Kelsoe and collaborator Alexander Niculescu, MD, PhD, were experimenting with amphetamine administration to rats as an animal model of mania. In Dr. Kelsoe's words:

> We examined the role of 8,000 genes in the response to amphetamine and found that the gene with the biggest response to amphetamine mapped in man to that exact region on chromosome 22 that we identified in our clinical family studies. Since then we have examined this gene in detail and found what we believe are several abnormalities that prevent it from working properly in a portion of people with bipolar disorder.

Together, this set of data implicated the gene both through function and chromosomal position.

Collaborator Thomas Barrett, MD, PhD, then sequenced much of the gene to find six sequential variants—single-nucleotide polymorphisms (SNPs, or "snips")—in the promoter of the gene, that region of the gene that switches it on or off. Dr. Barrett then tested 153 families for association to these mutations and in 2003 found that one of these, P-5, occurs three times more frequently in affected individuals. These findings were replicated the same year at the University of Toronto with a separate set of 237 families.

Thus a picture begins to emerge, albeit still a hypothetical one: a P-5 mutation causing GRK3 to fail, resulting in the brains' receptors' inability to desensitize to dopamine, ending in a situation akin to, in Dr. Kelsoe's words, "being born on cocaine."

Now to the wider scheme of things. The study found that the GRK3 variant occurred in only 3 percent of bipolar families. Since single-gene disorders are a rarity, it is virtually certain this isn't the only gene responsible for illness in this population. For the other 97 percent of those with bipolar disorder, multiple genes are believed to be the rule, as well, leaving researchers with the daunting task of teasing out candidates from some 16,500 genes believed to be expressed in the brain.

Gene Quest

A series of recent Johns Hopkins studies challenges our assumptions about bipolar disorder, namely: (1) psychotic bipolar disorder may be a genetic subtype of bipolar disorder, possibly sharing some of the same chromosomes as schizophrenia, a thought that would have been apostasy until recently; (2) bipolar II may be genetically distinct from bipolar I, with individuals in bipolar II families showing an affinity to chromosome 18q21; and (3) a possible link between bipolar disorder and panic disorder.

What do these findings tell us? Bipolar disorder is a complex illness probably caused by multiple genes, Raymond DePaulo, MD, coauthor of the three Johns Hopkins studies and chair of that university's Department of Psychiatry and Behavioral Sciences, told this writer. It may take any three of ten genes, for instance, to cause bipolar disorder.

But we have to do more than just find the genes. "We have to show biologically what the gene does, what the mutation does, to cause the disease," he explained.

Or, in the words of David Weinberger, MD, chief of the Clinical Brain Disorders Branch at the NIMH, speaking at the 2003 APA annual meeting, we need to find "how we get there from here," from identifying the gene to its cellular function to its role in the systems in the brain to its effect on behavior.

So far, the literature concerning genes and the brain has focused on less than 1 percent of the genome, representing a mere 300 or so genes. Yet our research on mice tells us that roughly 16,500 of our 25,000 genes are expressed in the brain. According to Thomas Insel, MD, and Francis Collins, MD, PhD, directors of the NIMH and Human Genome Project, respectively, in an article in the April 2003 *American Journal of Psychiatry,* part of a feature commemorating the fiftieth anniversary of James Watson and Francis Crick's discovery of the double helix: "We have a treasure trove of new genes to explore, including many that may prove more important than the few neurotransmitters and intracellular signaling molecules that have been studied so intensively these past fifty years."

The hunt for mood genes can be likened to searching for pieces of hay in a haystack. There is no one gene that is likely to stand out. Instead, we're searching for what are probably common and fairly humdrum mutations to what may be more than ten genes, each with a modest effect. The search is further confounded by the fact that unlike, say, diabetes, a mood disorder leaves no discernible biological footprint equivalent to blood glucose. Not surprisingly, our efforts to link social-wallflower genes to phantom footprint symptoms—or "phenotype"—by studying twins and families and isolated populations have been disappointing, yielding at best some possible suspects.

Accordingly, researchers are thinking outside the *DSM* box of phenotype to the underlying biology of "endophenotype," such as sleep and circadian rhythms and appetite regulation. Intriguingly, some of the suspect genes we have identified may be responsible for more than one illness, raising such possibilities as schizophrenia and bipolar patients sharing some of the same psychosis genes.

"The *DSM-IV* was not designed with human gene function in

mind and genes do not encode for psychopathology," Robert Freedman, MD, of the University of Colorado, told a symposium at the 2003 APA annual meeting. Instead, he went on to say, "genes encode simple molecules in cells that alter cell function and brain information processing." His research into schizophrenia provides a model for how researchers are starting to look at mood disorders.

Dr. Freedman has been exploring a link between "sensory gating disturbance" and why people with schizophrenia crave nicotine. A normal person, for instance, can tune out the second of two repetitive sounds. Many people with schizophrenia, however, cannot, and so have great trouble concentrating. Dr. Freedman's team found that auditory gating is modulated by the alpha-7 nicotinic receptor, with linkage to chromosome 15q14. Alpha-7 is reduced in the hippocampi of patients with schizophrenia. In one study, patients on nicotine lost their response to the second sound. Nicotine, Dr. Freedman said, can serve as a model for future treatment, but instead of making a toxin, we can make an agonist.

Should our inquiries down these paths bear fruit, we could eventually redefine mental illness according to "genotype" that would render the *DSM* obsolete.

But we may have to drill down even farther. A 2003 Harvard–McLean Hospital survey of 178 relatives of 64 subjects with major depression and 152 relatives of 58 subjects without major depression found that "affective spectrum disorder" (ASD) clusters in families. ASD at this stage is more an unofficial categorical convenience than a universally recognized phenomenon. Forms of ASD include major depression, ADHD, (attention deficit/hyperactivity disorder), bulimia nervosa, cataplexy, dysthymia, fibromyalgia, generalized anxiety disorder, irritable bowel syndrome, migraine, OCD (obsessive-compulsive disorder), panic disorder, PTSD, premenstrual dysphoric disorder, and social phobia.

The researchers also found that major depression displays a familial affinity with its ASD cotravelers, suggesting that seemingly unrelated illnesses may share the same genetic features. Said one of the study's authors, James Hudson, MD, ScD:

> *Let me give you an analogy. We don't diagnose patients as having "runny nose disease," "sore throat disease" and "cough disease"; they all simply have the common cold. Similarly, the results of our family study suggest that conditions such as major depression, panic attacks, obsessive-compulsive disorder, compulsive binge eating and even certain medical disorders could all be caused by a single underlying disease—the common cold of psychiatry, if you will.*

Is the mystery of the mood spectrum as simple as all that, the quest for the genetic common cold, or do we have to dig even deeper?

Peeling Away the Genetic Onion

The conventional wisdom on genes goes something like this: DNA is transcribed onto RNA, which form proteins, which are responsible for just about every process in the body, from eye color to ability to fight off illness. But even as the finishing touches were being applied to the sequencing of the human genome (completed in April 2003), unaccountable anomalies kept creeping in, strangely reminiscent of the quarks and dark matter and sundry weird forces that keep muddying the waters of theoretical physics.

Enter the science of epigenetics, which attempts to explain the mysterious inner layers of the genetic onion that may account for why identical twins aren't exactly identical and other conundrums, including why some people are predisposed to mental illness while others are not. *Scientific American* devoted a two-part article to the topic in its November and December 2003 issues. To summarize:

Only 2 percent of our DNA—via RNA—codes for proteins. Until very recently, the rest was considered "junk," the by-product of millions of years of evolution. Now scientists are discovering that some of this junk DNA switches on RNA that may do the work of proteins and interact with other genetic material. "Malfunctions in RNA-only genes," explains *Scientific American,* "can inflict serious damage."

Epigenetics delves deeper into the onion, involving "information stored in the proteins and chemicals that surround and stick to DNA."

A December 2004 PubMed search of epigenetics and bipolar disorder revealed but four articles, three by the same author, such is the topic's novelty. Arturas Petronis, MD, PhD, head of the Krembil Family Epigenetics Laboratory at the University of Toronto, in an article in the November 2003 *American Journal of Medical Genetics,* fills in some of the blanks.

We know that there is a high concordance of identical twins with bipolar disorder, but epigenetics, he explains, may account for the 30 to 70 percent of cases where only one twin has the illness. Identical twins share the same DNA, but their epigenetic material may be different. Moreover, whereas DNA variations are permanent, epigenetic changes are in a process of flux and generally accumulate over time. This may explain, Dr. Petronis theorizes, why bipolar disorder tends to manifest at ages twenty to thirty and forty-five to fifty, which coincides with major hormonal changes, which may "substantially affect regulation of genes ... via their epigenetic modifications."

The dynamics of epigenetic changes may also account for the fluctuating course of bipolar disorder, Dr. Petronis speculates, perhaps more so than static DNA variations.

In a pilot study published in 2003, Dr. Petronis and his colleagues investigated the epigenetic gene modification in a section of the dopamine D2 receptor genes in two pairs of identical twins, one pair with both partners having schizophrenia and the other having only one partner with the illness. What they discovered was that the partner with schizophrenia from the mixed pair had more in common, epigenetically, with the other set of twins than his own unaffected twin.

Transition

We've only just scratched the surface. As Insel and Collins conclude: "Students of the history of psychiatry looking back from the Watson and Crick centennial in 2053 may wonder how we could have been so interested in serotonin and dopamine in 2003 when many hundreds of more important factors remained to be found."

Gene Therapy

Meanwhile, back at the DBSA conference, Dr. Nemeroff talked about "antisense technology." Basically, RNA acts as a messenger that is involved in creating disease-causing proteins. Traditional drugs are made to interact with these proteins. By contrast, antisense drugs are designed to inhibit the production of these proteins by wrapping itself around the messenger RNA.

This is possible because the two strands of DNA partly uncoil, with the "sense" strand separating itself from the "antisense" strand. Under normal circumstances, the antisense strand transcribes enzymes that assemble messenger RNA, which leads to the production of proteins.

Antisense drugs are complementary strands of small segments of messenger RNA. Once you know the sequence of messenger RNA, antisense binds to it, gets in the way, and "stops it dead."

Antisense technology, Dr. Nemeroff informs us, is the "ultimate magic bullet."

Ultimate, magic, and *bullet,* I highlight in my notepad, feeling a bit too jaded to take the speaker at his word. There is, after all, a blood-brain barrier (BBB) these new drugs would have to breach. The name conjures up a kind of cross between the Berlin Wall and a coffee filter, but in fact refers to nearly four hundred miles of narrow capillaries throughout the brain, all filled with tightly packed endothelial cells that are exceedingly selective about what gets through. Endothelial cells are also present in capillaries in the body, but the spacing there poses no difficulty.

The BBB is to protecting the brain internally as the skull is to protecting it externally. The problem is the BBB does not differentiate what it keeps out. Lifesaving chemicals, if they happen to be the wrong chemicals, simply won't get through. With very few exceptions, only small molecules soluble in fat clear the barrier. Alcohol, caffeine, and nicotine—all meeting this criterion—have a free pass. So do antidepressants. The problem is, according to William Pardridge, MD, of UCLA, writing in the January 2002 *Archives of Neurology,* "small molecules are largely palliative medicines with often unfavorable safety profiles." There are no chronic diseases, other than infectious diseases, that are cured by small-molecule drug therapy.

Large-molecule drugs have the potential to cure patients with neurological disorders, he notes, but none of them can cross the blood-brain barrier.

The blood-brain barrier makes certain exceptions, allowing passage to large molecules and water-soluble molecules, and exploiting these exceptions is the key to developing new classes of drugs. One binding and transport system in the BBB, for example, permits water-soluble glucose into the brain, and another mediates the bidirectional movement of large molecule peptides. According to Dr. Pardridge: "Based on the knowledge that these endogenous transport systems exist, drugs may be reformulated to enable transport into the brain via the endogenous BBB transporters." A lab-made "chimeric peptide," for example, is half drug (which does not cross the BBB), and half "molecular Trojan Horse" (which does). The Trojan Horses are genetically engineered proteins that have slipped through the BBB in lab animals and could be given to humans now.

The March 20, 2003, *New Scientist* reported that Dr. Pardridge and his team have been working on encasing genes in fatty spheres called liposomes, which are coated with a special polymer, to which certain antibodies are attached. The antibodies trick the brain-capillary receptors into letting the liposomes pass, where they can deliver their payload to brain cells. Dr. Pardridge has produced promising results on rats and monkeys. In one experiment, he doubled the life spans of rats with the successful delivery of antisense RNA to its target.

Lo and behold! The antisense RNA got through after all. But don't hold your breath waiting. First the bad news. Gene therapy is unlikely to have a clinical application in psychiatry for some time to come. The good news is we're working on it. An article by Robert Sapolsky, PhD, of Stanford University, in the February 2003 *American Journal of Psychiatry* tells us how far we've come and where we need to go. Dr. Sapolsky, the recipient of a McArthur "genius" grant and other awards, uses gene technology to import modified genes into the damaged hippocampi of lab animals, and studies baboons in the wild to see how their social behavior affects stress-induced illnesses.

According to Dr. Sapolsky: "The biology of psychiatric disorders is not about inevitability but is instead about vulnerability and propensity. It is only in certain environments that the disease is likely to emerge." Many psychiatric disorders, he writes, are based on "if-then" logic; for example, "*if* you are exposed to a stressful life event, *then* your risk of depression increases" and the more complex "*if* you are exposed to a stressful life event and you have a low sense of self-efficacy, *then* your risk of depression increases." The genome, Dr. Sapolsky states, "represents an informational system of if-then clauses."

The intermediary between the *if* of stress and the *then* of depression appears to be the stress hormone cortisol, which is secreted as part of the caveman fight-or-flight response to a perceived threat. Cortisol, however, has a way of going on a caveman rampage of its own when modern man fails to respond as anticipated. For example, stress can awaken dormant herpes viruses and cause them to replicate. The viral genes responsible for setting this process in motion are controlled by a promoter (gene activator) that contains an element that responds to cortisol. Prompted by these findings, researchers have developed vector (gene-material) systems that exploit these promoters. Dr. Sapolsky and his colleagues have constructed a family of herpes virus vectors responsive to cortisol introduced into the hippocampi of the brains of lab animals. Their aim is to alter normal hippocampal function during stress so that any number of protective transgenes are switched on—say, one that floods tryptophan hydroxylase (which leads to serotonin production) into the brain.

Dr. Sapolsky and his team are also working on anxiety and conditioned fear, centering on the amygdala of the brain.

What is especially intriguing about Dr. Sapolsky and his fellow researchers' application of if-then logic is that we do not have to identify specific mood genes in order to take advantage of gene technology. Still, gene therapy is more about potential than progress. Disappointments and dead ends tend to be par for the course, and a host of thorny technical issues remain to be resolved. Nevertheless, Dr. Sapolsky envisions a day when a few deceptively simple tweaks to our genes are likely to serve as the brain's own internal 911 system, dispatching an array of crisis-intervention chemicals to neurons in distress, in response to all those clear-and-present dangers that have a way of rendering us helpless. Never say never.

Bad News

The NIMH funds about $80 million a year in bipolar disorder research compared to $280 million for schizophrenia, and that same ratio is reflected in the published literature. According to a 2003 report by the Treatment Advocacy Center and Public Citizen, the NIH in 1999 spent $2,240.88 per AIDS/HIV patient in researching AIDS/HIV and $476.26 per lung-cancer patient in researching lung cancer. For schizophrenia, the per patient figure was $74.95; for bipolar disorder, it was $25.95, and for depression, $18.60.

Mental illness has no equivalent of a Framingham study, and all the classes of psychiatric meds were discovered serendipitously rather than grounded in scientific research, Edward Scolnick, MD, president emeritus of Merck Research, pointed out at the 2003 NAMI annual convention.

Because we have such little understanding of mental illness and have yet to identify a suitable range of molecular targets, Dr. Scolnick went on to say, "no one really knows how to make a better version of Clozaril."

The Clozaril class of drugs works on about a dozen targets at once, with predictably multiple side effects. By contrast, the drugs for hardening of the arteries and other illnesses work on a single target and are well tolerated.

The advent of lithium in the seventies and its promise as a magic bullet resulted in a considerable loss of interest in bipolar disorder, Thomas Insel, MD, head of the NIMH, explained to this writer. Unfortunately, catching up is problematical, owing to the fact that there is considerable debate about study designs, which leads to peer-review committees turning down grant requests, resulting in frustrated researchers leaving the field. "We eat our young," Dr. Insel confessed.

If only we had the budget the AIDS and cancer researchers have.

The Great Darwinian Challenge

The late Caltech geneticist Theodosius Dobzhansky once wrote: "Nothing in biology makes sense except in the light of evolution."

Welcome to evolutionary biology, or Darwinian medicine, which theorizes that many diseases or their symptoms may be trade-offs that nature has built into our survival gear. A high fever, for instance, may aid in the destruction of deadly pathogens, and without the inconvenience of coughing, we would all likely die from pneumonia. The sickle-cell gene, in turn, is protection against malaria.

So what about mental illness? Ask the evolutionary psychiatrists (or psychologists). Randolph Nesse, MD, of the University of Michigan, writes: "Psychiatrists still act as if all anxiety, sadness, and jealousy is abnormal and they don't yet look for the selective advantages of genes that predispose to schizophrenia and bipolar disorder."

Our behaviors and emotions, according to evolutionary psychiatry, are adaptations the mind has made to recurring problems. You want to know why we get depressed? Well, maybe it had something to do with ensuring that the inevitable losers in those prehistory tribal power struggles accepted their lot and didn't do something that would get them expelled from the group or worse. Even the winners probably needed some discouragement against getting too big for their breechcloths. There's even a theory for postpartum depression, if you're prepared to believe that Mother Nature at her most brutal was willing to step in and sacrifice the newest born for the sake of the other members of the family.

Mild depression can amount to a "failure of denial." In this state of mind, the rose-colored glasses come off, allowing its wearer to see things as they really are. In this context, depression represents the unclouded mind that results in making realistic choices, from giving Mr. Wrong the mammoth-hide boot to calling off that wild dodo bird chase.

Depression may have also constituted a form of social extortion, a cry for help that enlisted the support of the other members of the group.

The fight-or-flight response, the bane of our stress-filled modern lives, clearly had an adaptive purpose. Those lacking the necessary genes became the animal kingdom's next value meal.

According to the late David Horrobin, MD, PhD, in his 2001 book *The Madness of Adam and Eve*, the diet of the hunter-gatherer would have predisposed our ancestors to better mental health, with mental illness restricted to whatever the evolutionary traffic could bear.

In *Touched with Fire*, Kay Jamison suggests that bipolar disorder may be the price nature is willing to pay for allowing artistic, imaginative, leadership, and entrepreneurial traits to be passed down from generation to generation.

Jim Phelps, MD, an Oregon psychiatrist specializing in bipolar II, argues that the severe form of the illness in the gene pool may be a fair exchange for the advantages of its milder side.

Or it could be a lot more elemental. Several writers have theorized that bipolar disorder could be an adaptation to the changes in the seasons. Think of those fur-clad hunter-gatherers shivering in their caves. For whatever reasons, our genetic codes got hewn, shaped, and sanded and polished there. "Human biology," says Dr. Nesse, "is designed for stone-age conditions." Or, as Leda Cosmides, PhD, and John Tooby, PhD, of the University of California at Santa Barbara put it, "our modern skulls house a stone-age mind."

In other words, we are the beneficiaries of a group of genes that did not anticipate credit cards, artificial light, processed foods, digital timepieces, rush-hour traffic, and rap music blaring from twelve-inch subwoofers mounted in oversized SUVs. Still, despite a world that seems booby-trapped to make us fail, many of us rise to the occasion to lead full and productive lives. Call it the twenty-first-

century Darwinian challenge. Our ability to feel on levels deeper
and higher than the rest of the population, crippling as it may be,
has also given wings to our thoughts, ones that motivated us to
climb out of our cozy rock condos in the first place and now seem
destined to have us reach for the stars.

PART THREE

ROADS TO RECOVERY

8

Lifestyle

Sequentially, this is the stage in this book when we should be talking about medications, talking therapy, and other so-called mainstream treatments. But when I came back from the 2004 American Psychiatric Association's annual meeting, I changed my mind. As usual, the pharmaceutical industry was out in force, with circuslike displays dominating the exhibition hall of Great Plains dimensions at New York's Jacob K. Javits Center. Literally, one could not see end to end. The poster sessions featured mostly studies initiated and backed by the drug companies, and nearly half of the sessions I attended were industry sponsored, virtually all which managed to get in a plug for their featured medication disguised as scientific research.

As the sessions wore on, I began getting the impression that despite listening to some of the most brilliant practitioners in the profession, I would not like to get treated by them. Yes, some of the speakers referred to talking therapies, but most of them seemed intent on demonstrating their complete lack of ability to think outside the medicine cabinet. None of them suggested, for instance, that when the standard meds options fail it would be a good idea to make enquiries about the patient's nutrition (better late than never). As for long-term treatment, only one speaker talked about the value of a support group.

So how to decide which gets top billing? Medical treatment or lifestyle management? Ultimately, it came down to the fact that although meds can be real lifesavers, bad lifestyle habits severely limit their effectiveness.

Simply put, meds work much better when people take care of themselves. A 2002 Harvard study of 322 depressed patients on Prozac found that those with high cholesterol levels were "significantly more likely" not to respond to the drug than patients with low cholesterol.

Once the drug companies get with the program, we will see more findings of this sort, along with high-profile academic psychiatrists getting out the word.

Lest I convey a misleading impression that all psychiatrists have a professional blind spot for lifestyle choices, I must point out that most of the information presented here comes from mainstream psychiatrists, therapists, medical doctors, and biological researchers, a good deal of it presented at psychiatric conferences and published in reputable journals.

So here's in anticipation of the day that all of psychiatry is attuned to lifestyle.

Food and Mood

A 2003 issue of *Time International* reports on forty-one-year-old Amanda Jodhpuria, who had bad luck with lithium, and sought out a nutritionist who diagnosed a B-vitamin and fatty-acids deficiency, which prompted her to change her diet—no coffee, sugar, or salt, and more fish. She told *Time:* "My mood has leveled out, and the depressions are much shorter." The same article reports a survey from the British mental-health charitable organization Mind, which found that 80 percent of those who followed a diet low in sugar, caffeine, chocolate, and alcohol and high in water, vegetables, fruit, and oil-rich fish reported improved moods, with 26 percent citing major improvements.

Scientists are coming up with new findings all the time now, from folates to fish. Eating right should not be regarded as a cure for a mood disorder, but common sense dictates that what works for the heart and other organs also applies to the brain. Some people may experience extreme reactions to certain foods or classes of foods, but all of us need to worry about sugar and bad fats, which are the focus of the next several pages.

Sugar and Carbs

The average American eats more than 125 pounds of white sugar a year, comprising 25 percent of our daily calorie intake. According to Rita Elkins, MH, in *Solving the Depression Puzzle*: "We have become obsessed with sugar, not fully recognizing what excessive sugar consumption not only does to the body, but also the mind."

Cutting down on your sugar consumption, the author recommends, can be one of the best things you do for your health. It can also be one of the hardest.

The author cites studies by Richard Wurtman, MD, and Judith Wurtman, PhD, of MIT (Richard Wurtman is coauthor of *The Serotonin Solution*), who found that sugar and starch in carbohydrates temporarily boosts serotonin levels, which would account for the carbohydrate cravings in people prone to depression. Additionally, depressed people are drawn to sugar and fat combinations such as those found in cookies and chocolate.

A 2002 University of Texas Southwestern Medical Center survey of six countries found those populations with higher per capita refined sugar consumption corresponded with higher rates of depression (the depression data was based on a landmark 1996 epidemiologic study). At the bottom was Korea, with less than a hundred sugar calories a day and an annual depression rate greater than 2 percent. Topping the list was New Zealand, at almost 500 calories and a nearly 6 percent annual depression rate. In between were the United States (300 calories/3 percent depression rate), and France, Germany, and Canada (300 to 400 calories/4.5 to 5-plus percent depression rate).

Arthur Westover, MD, coauthor of the study, cautioned that it is premature to jump to any conclusions, though "eating healthy is a good idea whether there is any relation to mood disorders or not," he told this writer.

According to a number of experts, excess consumption results in a crash and worse. Soon after a carb or sugar binge, even though the stomach is full, the brain is signaling for more. Foodwise, you have enough in your tank to see you through a parched sub-Saharan summer, but craving-wise your brain is telling you you're in the middle of winter in the Donner Pass. Now we have a problem, for speed-dialing Domino's or whatever 911 equivalents you have for rushing carbohydrates to the scene can stimulate insulin overproduction, which can paradoxically lower blood sugar and result in further cravings.

Women are in double jeopardy, for the sugar cravings that many experience during PMS, pregnancy, or menopause could be a response to the ebbs and flows of estrogen. Estrogen may have an impact on serotonin levels.

In *The Antidepressant Survival Guide,* Robert Hedaya, MD, of Georgetown University, says the quick energy rush of sugar and carbohydrates is followed by an inevitable crash, leaving one sluggish and drained of energy, and further depressed.

Rita Elkins recommends that you avoid eating when you are anxious, bored, depressed, lonely, or frustrated; avoid nibbling when the meal is over; don't use food as a reward; drink when you have the urge to eat (and then eat if you are still hungry); and join a support group.

Dr. Hedaya's program starts with tossing out that bagel and coffee in the morning, then bidding a tender farewell to that Cherry Garcia ice cream, followed by saying hello to more protein, folates, unrefined foods, and omega-3 fatty acids. Each meal of the day is based on roughly one third protein to two-thirds carbohydrates (with fruit and vegetables counting as carbohydrates). A typical dinner might be four ounces of chicken or fish with brown rice and vegetables topped off by fruit and cheese. Breakfast might be based around an egg, and lunch some tuna fish.

If you think you can cheat by going to a sugar substitute, think again. Many people are particularly sensitive to aspartame, and Ralph Walton, MD, of Northeastern Ohio Universities College of Medicine, argues that people with mood disorders are at special risk. In 1993, Dr. Walton conducted a small study that was called to a halt "because of the severity of reactions within the group of patients with a history of depression."

Many readers who contacted me confessed to drinking virtual reservoirs daily of Diet Coke (which contains aspartame). It's probably fair to say that they would get equally sick drinking the same amount of something that was healthy for them. Moderation is the watchword, here.

Messing with the Food Chain

A review article in the September 2003 *International Journal of Circumpolar Health* by biologist Abel Bult-Ito and associates, of the University of Alaska Fairbanks, offers an excellent case study on what happens when various populations change from their traditional means of procuring and consuming food to steak and Crisco and a lot of junk.

Though the traditional diets of circumpolar people vary from region to region, the menu generally draws from marine mammals, fish, hoofed animals, fur-bearing animals, birds and their eggs, plants, and berries. These foods are rich in nutrients, with high levels of protein, omega-3 fatty acids, and antioxidants, while low in carbohydrates. Until contact with Westerners, obesity, diabetes, and cardiovascular disease were virtually unknown to the frozen North. That changed with the introduction of a Western diet, which is high in carbs and saturated fats and low in essential nutrients such as omega-3. Bad physical and dental health followed like six-month night after six-month day. Mental health also headed south as a result, contend the authors of the article.

Studies have found that rates of depression, seasonal affective disorder, seasonality, anxiety, and other mental illnesses are on the rise in circumpolar regions, especially among nonisolated populations. Suicide rates have increased sevenfold in many northern populations over the past several decades. The suicide rate for the Canadian Inuit from 1987 to 1991 was 3.9 times higher than that of the general Canadian population.

The authors of the article acknowledge that the mental distress of the Inuit and their brethren can be attributed to social, cultural, and lifestyle upheaval, as well as increases in chronic physical diseases, but they argue that "the combined decline in mental health and the disappearance of traditional diets in circumpolar peoples makes a direct connection between diet and mental health in these people a very real possibility."

Carnivores may want to consider switching to grass-fed beef, which is much higher in omega-3 and lower in saturated fats than the grain-fed hormone-injected marbled slabs that end up on our tables. Grain-fed beef has a 20 to 1 ratio of omega-6 to omega-3, while grass-fed beef is about 3 to 1. The ideal diet is considered to comprise equal parts of omega-3 and omega-6. Where grass-fed beef is not available, opt for the leaner cuts and moderate-sized portions.

Diet and Obesity

In the 2004 documentary movie *Super Size Me*, filmmaker Morgan Spurlock made himself a human guinea pig by eating nothing but McDonald's fare for one month and reducing his normal exercise. He was thirty-two, six foot two, and 185 pounds, with an enviable cholesterol count, triglyceride levels to die for, and certified by three doctors and a workout coach as being in excellent health. The three doctors concurred that the worst that could happen was his triglycerides would rise a little and perhaps a little weight gain. Famous last words.

By the end of the experiment, Spurlock gained twenty-five pounds, raised his cholesterol by 60, dropped his libido, and to the utter astonishment of his doctors began to turn his liver into goose pâté. Such was the state of his liver, along with chest pains, that his doctors strongly advised he end his affair with Mickey D's well before scheduled and to prepare for immediate admission to a hospital. That wasn't all. By day nine, Spurlock was experiencing depression, and soon after was developing wild mood swings from all the sugars and other McPoisons. And the unkindest cut of all— he eventually became addicted to the stuff, literally craving Big Mac highs.

Spurlock may have taken things to an extreme, but he was quick to show in his film how we have become a fast-food nation with alarming numbers of supersized citizens.

In 2001, the U.S. surgeon general declared an obesity epidemic, reporting that approximately three hundred thousand U.S. deaths a year are associated with obesity and an overweight condition as compared to more than four hundred thousand deaths a year from cigarette smoking. In 2002, the World Health Organization reported that "[u]nhealthy diets and physical inactivity are . . . the leading causes of the major noncommunicable diseases. . . ."

"Obesity hits every organ system in the body," endocrinologist

Judith Korner, MD, PhD, of Columbia University, told a session at the 2004 APA annual meeting. This includes the heart, sleep, diabetes, cancer, and psychosocial ills. Ten years from now, she said, obesity will exceed lung cancer as a cause of death.

Eating the wrong food can result in the weight piling on fairly quickly. Dr. Korner cited an example: One New York City muffin, she said, contains about 600 calories, and a twenty-ounce cola 250. Assuming this little snack begins as a temptation that turns into a daily habit, in addition to normal regular food intake, it takes just four days to cross the 3,500 calories/one pound threshold and one month to put on seven pounds.

How easy is it to take off weight and keep it off? Unfortunately, we run into a wall when we lose 10 percent of our body weight, Dr. Korner reported. Adipose tissue shrinks, which results in less leptin, which puts the hypothalamus on red alert. The body goes into survival mode, increasing hunger pangs and lowering metabolism. Within three to five years, she said, almost all dieters are back up to original body weight.

All this comes as cold comfort to those of us caught in the pincers of our illness and our meds. Depression sends many of us into the warm embrace of ice cream and chocolate, while our meds can amount to hot fudge sundaes in pill form with none of the pleasures. Weight management obviously needs to be regarded as a lifetime task—eating the right foods and getting plenty of exercise, while setting realistic goals.

Setting these goals may mean that aiming for a Rubenesque ideal is okay for now. Trying to accomplish too much too soon is counterproductive and will only lead to disappointment.

Watching What We Eat

Unfortunately, the fast-food restaurants we find ourselves eating out at offer us little choice but the notorious fat-sugar duo. A McDonald's meal of a Quarter Pounder with cheese, medium fries, and a chocolate shake well exceeds the daily saturated fat limit. Substituting a medium Coke yields the same sugar as the shake, the equivalent of fifteen teaspoons. Imagine emptying fifteen packets of sugar into a large Starbucks coffee and you get the picture.

McDonald's advertises on its Web site that "McDonald's wide range of high quality foods can fit into a balanced diet." Its entry nutrition page shows über-athlete Serena Williams happily nibbling on a salad (significantly, not gorging on fries).

But the salads can be worse than the traditional fare. A fully loaded McDonald's Fiesta Salad contains more saturated fat than a Quarter Pounder.

No section on fast foods would be complete without mentioning pizza. According to the pizza industry, Americans eat a hundred acres of pizza each day, or about 350 slices per second, adding up to 46 slices a pizza a year for every man, woman, and child. Two slices of a Pizza Hut twelve-inch pizza with pepperoni (America's favorite topping) add up to about the same total fat as a Quarter Pounder. Amazingly, Pizza Hut has this to say on its entry nutrition page on its Web site: "Pizza can be a part of a well-balanced meal."

WHO Recommendations

In May 2004, the World Health Organization issued the final draft of its Global Strategy on Diet, Physical Activity, and Health. Its main recommendations concerning diet include:

- Achieve energy balance and a healthy weight.
- Limit energy intake from total fats and shift fat consumption away from saturated fats to unsaturated fats and toward the elimination of trans-fatty acids.
- Increase consumption of fruits and vegetables, and legumes, whole grains, and nuts.
- Limit the intake of free sugars. Limit salt (sodium) consumption from all sources and ensure that salt is iodized.

The WHO also recommended at least thirty minutes of regular, moderate-intensity physical activity on most days.

My Weight-Gain Experience

In January 1999, when I first sought help for my bipolar disorder, I was first put on a notorious weight-gaining mood stabilizer and equally notorious antidepressant by a crisis-intervention psychiatrist who only saw me twice and failed to warn me about their side effects (why is this no surprise?). Within a few weeks, I had ballooned from 156 pounds to 187, an alarming gain of 20 percent of my original body weight. Since I am six-one, the meds ironically filled out my beanpole frame and made me look better than I ever looked in my life, bald head and all.

Had I started out at a more normal 200 pounds for my height, a 20 percent weight gain would have represented 240 pounds, well on my way to looking like the "Before" Jared Fogle of Subway diet fame. Any temporary gain from stabilizing my mood, I am convinced, would have been lost by the long-term depression from weight-induced sluggishness and the mood swings of extra sugar and other poisons in my diet. My meds would have been engaged in a losing battle with my runaway metabolism, which would have turned me into one of those cases psychiatry calls treatment-resistant, which implicitly lays the blame on the patient. I would be a prime candidate for diabetes, which runs in my family, and considering my current cholesterol count my heart probably would have stopped beating by now. As it was, with my base metabolism so skewed toward being skinny, the meds worked like a charm.

If Calvin Klein calls asking me to appear in an underwear ad, tell him I'm busy . . .

Meds and Weight

Thoroughly discuss the weight implications of any new drug your psychiatrist may recommend and hold him or her fully accountable. Psychiatrists and especially primary-care physicians are notorious for not bringing up weight side effects. Moreover, many of them mistakenly regard the extra weight as a fair trade-off for stabilized mood, failing to consider how putting on pounds effects one's mental well-being in the long term. Accordingly, consider switching to no-fat or low-fat food alternatives from the very beginning of treatment on the general principle that an ounce of prevention is worth twenty or more pounds of a diet cure. Stop paying your cable bill, if you have to, and think about seeing a nutritionist.

Everyone responds differently to meds, and the weight side effects are no exception. Some patients may actually lose weight on their meds. Among the antidepressants, Effexor and Wellbutrin are considered weight-friendly while Remeron is such a notorious weight gainer that some doctors use it for treating anorexia. Originally, SSRIs were thought to reduce weight, but that misconception was based on short-term studies, usually eight weeks or less.

Among the mood stabilizers, both lithium and Depakote are weight gainers. The other mood stabilizers are considered weight-neutral, while Topamax (not effective for mania) is often used as a diet pill.

As for the new-generation antipsychotics, all represent a potential weight risk, with Zyprexa and Clozaril the most notorious.

The three meds (or more) combinations most bipolar patients find themselves on can add up to recipes for dietary disaster. In 2003, for instance, the FDA approved Zyprexa as combination therapy with lithium or Depakote for treating initial-phase mania. Anyone taking Zyprexa with either of these drugs, however, is simply begging for an audition as the next Macy's Santa. Adding drug number three or four virtually clinches the deal.

But as bad as these meds are together, one must always bear in mind that absolutely none of them should be taken with a Big Mac. Or a shake. Or fries. Or a Coke. Or a loaded salad. Or a pizza. We may have no choice with our meds—especially if the weight-friendly ones fail us—but we can choose to eat smart and exercise right and use every sensible weight-management technique to our full advantage.

Calvin Klein is calling . . .

Exercise

Make no mistake, exercise may be as effective as any antidepressant, plus you don't gain weight. The only catch is you have to go out and do it.

A 1999 Duke University study divided 150 participants with depression who were age fifty or more into three groups. One was put on an exercise regimen, another administered the antidepressant Zoloft, and a third given a combination of the two. Those in the exercise group worked out on a treadmill or stationary bicycle at 70 to 85 percent of their maximum heart rate for thirty minutes, three times a week.

At the end of four months, all three groups showed significantly lower rates of depression.

The big surprise came from a follow-up conducted six months later when it was discovered that those in the exercise group experienced significantly less relapse than those in the Zoloft or combination groups. Only 8 percent of the exercise group had their depression return, compared to 38 percent of the Zoloft group and 31 percent of the combination group.

As to why the combination group should fare worse than the exercise alone group, lead researcher James Blumenthal, PhD, speculated in a press release: "Simply taking a pill is very passive. Patients who exercised may have felt a greater sense of mastery over their condition and gained a greater sense of accomplishment."

A 2001 University of Bristol meta-analysis of fourteen studies concluded that the short-term effect of exercise equated to the benefits of cognitive therapy, but cautioned that owing to the poor quality of these studies, it is premature to make sweeping generalizations.

Experts speculate that exercise works against depression in a number of ways, including reducing the stress hormone cortisol, which is linked to depression; restoring one's sleep and eating patterns, and raising energy levels, all critically important to feeling alive; releasing endorphins, which are associated with good mood; raising serotonin levels; increasing brain cells or slowing brain deterioration; and raising body temperature, which may induce relaxation.

Finally, getting in shape improves self-esteem.

In a 2001 study, researchers at the University of Nottingham measured phenylethylamine (PEA) levels in twenty men before and after exercise and discovered all but two had increased levels twenty-four hours later. The researchers speculated that PEA may be responsible for the euphoria of "runner's high." Significantly, PEA is a key ingredient in chocolate, which along with fat and sugar is thought to account for the treat's temporary feel-good effect. One can easily imagine humankind divided along two poles, all based on how we seek our PEA fix.

When considering an exercise regime, it pays to keep realistic goals in mind. If your body is not accustomed to activity, it is going to fight back and enlist your mind in an elaborate campaign of rationalizations. Don't expect to run a marathon your first week. Walking for thirty minutes (even for just five or ten minutes to start) is perfectly acceptable, and represents a giant step forward for those who have been inactive. Don't expect your depression to begin lifting until at least a few weeks, and don't look forward to slacking off when you start feeling better. Working out should be a lifelong commitment.

Older people need to be especially mindful, for they tend to engage in less physical activity as they age.

Of course, the last thing any of us want to do when caught up in a killer depression is crawl out of the covers and try to win three gold medals. You will probably have to wait until the worst of your symptoms abate before you take the plunge. Even then, the prospect of taking one's body for a quick spin around the block seems daunting. One step at a time . . .

Sleep

I was going to bed at around eleven or twelve in the evening and getting up at eight or nine the next morning. There was only one problem: These were West Coast hours and I was living on the East Coast. My inability to establish a regular sleeping pattern was directly related to my state of depression, which seemed to have me in a permanent headlock. Only half-jokingly, I told my psychiatrist that perhaps a move to California would solve the problem.

Ever since college, I preferred working at night, even when required to keep daytime hours. Not uncoincidentally, that's when my bipolar features began to manifest in full measure, with devastating results. Still, I lived for the night, when the world had shut down with no distractions, and it was just me and my manic-fueled creative surges. But now I was faced with undoing thirty years of conditioning or having to submit to a force that had staked a claim to my brain. I had fought back hard, but make no mistake about it: I was still in the battle of my life, for my life.

Sleep and mood are virtually joined at the hip. A 2004 DBSA survey found sleep disturbance to be "one of the most common problems associated with mental illness." According to Thomas Roth,

PhD, chief of sleep medicine at Henry Ford Hospital in Detroit, sleep is one of the few things in medicine that is both a disorder and a symptom. Dr. Roth was addressing a symposium, "Sleep Disorders and Psychiatric Illnesses: Scientific Foundations," at the 2002 APA annual meeting.

The *DSM-IV* catalog of sleep disorders includes primary insomnia, narcolepsy, and circadian-rhythm sleep disorder, to name a few. Meanwhile, "insomnia or hypersomnia" and "fatigue or loss of energy" are listed as symptoms for both major and mild depression, and "decreased need for sleep" is a symptom of mania and hypomania.

According to Dr. Roth: "As many as 60 percent of psychiatric outpatients complain of disturbed sleep. Studies of depressives indicate that as many as 85 percent will at some point experience insomnia." Research has linked persistent insomnia with the onset of another major depressive episode within one year, and sleep complaints are a reliable predictor of future relapses.

In bipolar disorder, the loss of a single night's sleep can place the patient at severe risk. Says the British Association for Psychopharmacology, "Sleep disturbance is perhaps the most commonly described final common pathway to mania . . ." A 1998 study by Ellen Frank, PhD, of the University of Pittsburgh, and others found an association between disrupted social routines (including sleep) and onset of mania.

Modern times work against us. Back before electric lights, most people slept about ten hours. Now it's down to seven, with one-third of us below six. Throw in shift work, jet travel, and the demands of having to be in two places at once, and one can see why many more of us—children included—fall victim to mood disorders.

Sleep Hygiene

Sleep hygiene may be as important to fighting your depression or mania as any medication or talking therapy, if not more so. Maintaining a regular sleep schedule, with eight or so hours of consolidated sleep, is considered paramount. It need not conform to the schedule of someone who must be at work at 8:00 or 9:00 AM, but it needs to be consistent. Excessive sleep is counterproductive, and napping should be resorted to only sparingly (as this can throw off one's sleep schedule).

In a 2004 interview with this writer, Dr. Frank said "there's something about the sleep-wake cycle—it's telling us something." At the 2001 Fourth International Conference on Bipolar Disorder, Dr. Frank reported on her use of interpersonal and social rhythm therapy. IPSRT evolved out of interpersonal therapy for depression developed in the sixties.

Part of her therapy (which complements meds) is getting patients to compile a life chart. This helps patients make the connection between many of their bipolar episodes and major life events that lead to marked changes in routine, such as the birth of a child. The therapist will work with the patient in finding the most unstable life-time rhythms and setting goals (with reasonable expectations) for change, meanwhile searching for triggers likely to cause any disruptions. Rotating shift work for people with mood disorders, Dr. Frank told this writer, is like "working with asbestos without a mask." Patients in this position, she advised, may want to disclose their diagnosis to their human resources department (but not necessarily their boss) and ask for special consideration.

Dr. Frank acknowledges that those with bipolar disorder seem to be phase-delayed, preferring to rise later. At first, she tried to get her patients to conform to the rest of the population. Now she doesn't unless it's essential to the job. Nevertheless, of all the goals that need setting, "getting out of bed seems to be the most important one."

Create an association between the bed and sleep, Dr. Frank advises. Bed is "not where you read your book, not where you watch television." A lot of Americans have established the habit of doing maybe fifteen things in their bed, she went on to say. "What we want is the Pavlovian response to being in the bed and putting your head down that will initiate sleep." (Sex is allowed.)

Many people find it useful to have a one- or two-hour winding-down period prior to turning out the lights. This can involve various relaxing routines, including yoga, visualizations, breathing, and meditation. There is no shortage of tapes and CDs to assist. Those requiring further aural support can go to the bed to the sound of gurgling brooks and fountains and distant oceans (make sure your bladder is completely empty).

Reading (including audiobooks) and TV and radio are two standbys. Be mindful of books that are gripping page-turners you can't put down, however, and stay away from programs that are bound to set off a strong emotional response.

Caffeine is to sleep as Attila the Hun was to a nice quiet day in the Roman Empire, though it may not be as simple as cutting out the stuff altogether. The Rip Van Winkles among us may legitimately need a pick-me-up, as well as those who find themselves waking up groggy from a meds hangover. *Sparingly* is the watchword. That morning caffeine is still in the system in the evening. Evening caffeine should be considered taboo (unless you work nights). Note that caffeine is often loaded in other foods and medicines, various cola products being the most obvious example. Two tablets of Excedrin contain 130 milligrams (mg) of caffeine, about the same as a cup of brewed coffee, while 12 ounces of Mountain Dew contain 55.5, about the same as a cup of tea and 20 mg more than the same amount of Coke.

Alcohol is good for initiating sleep, but it destroys deep sleep. Establishing regular mealtimes and exercise routines are also part of good sleep hygiene. Exercise early in the day rather than late in the day, as exercise stimulates rather than settles.

Bear in mind that light at night is the enemy. A flick of the switch does more than turn on the lights. It throws out your body's biological rhythms, as well. If you must go to the bathroom in the middle of the night, learn how to negotiate your mission with the lights out, and with the toilet seat where you would expect to find it.

In the meantime, many of you may be faced with making some tough choices: If you are a shift worker, you may have to find a job with regular hours. If your work involves travel, you may have to find employment that keeps you close to home. You may have to change from a fast career track to one not so demanding.

Students who burn the midnight oil are particularly susceptible. All-nighters are a necessary fact of academic life, but many of them can be avoided by staying on top of course loads.

Personal Note

For me, my Herculean struggle to bring my system to within a time zone or two of the one I was in was compounded by the spring changeover into daylight saving time. I literally felt like poor Sisyphus, forced to push a rock uphill for eternity, only to have it roll down to the bottom just as he neared the summit. For a while, I achieved a reasonable level of success by sticking to a strict lights-out policy no matter how wide awake I felt at the time.

Then I made the fatal mistake of loading the video game *Civilization III* into my computer. For those of you unfamiliar with *Civilization,* it takes a good week of dedicated playing to go from fending off Stone Age marauders to triumphantly rolling your armored vehicles into the capital city of your last rival superpower. You guessed it—it was impossible for me to go to bed in the middle of a life-or-death struggle between my Persians and those sneaky Iroquois (who had built the Sistine Chapel and the Pyramids and had a fleet of aircraft carriers off my shore), with the nuclear-capable Babylonians ready to enter the fray on the side of the Iroquois and seal my doom, unless I could convince the French to come to my aid, which depended on them not holding a grudge against me just because I leveled their stupid little Great Wall of China six centuries ago.

Just fifteen or twenty minutes, I would say at 11:00 PM. Then all sense of time would disappear, and next thing I knew it would be three in the morning. An hour later, I would still be awake under the covers, plotting my revenge on those no-good Babylonian bastards.

It took me many long months before I came out of denial and faced up to the fact that this was an addiction I couldn't control. I'm proud to say I've been *Civilization*-free for better than three years. My sleep is still far from perfect. There are nights when my racing thoughts threaten to keep me awake into the next millennium. There are mornings when my brain has gone missing and I realize it's going to be one of those days. There are afternoons when the power goes down like a plug being pulled from an appliance and the only option is to lie down.

I may not be 100 percent in control, but I'm not entirely helpless. I'm grateful that I work from home, where I can still manage to cobble together fifty or so productive hours a week without the stress of being on my game for a full working day, five or six days a week. I do the best I can with what I've got. It's kind of a working arrangement, an uneasy truce between my ideals and my limitations. So far it's working, with no manic episodes since my diagnosis in early 1999. My occasional hypomanias are nothing serious to worry about, while my chronic low-grade depression, though a concern, is not incapacitating. In short, I have my life back, but I can never take this state of affairs for granted. I constantly need to remind myself that I'm one night's missed sleep or a morning or afternoon of oversleeping from possibly destroying everything I've worked to so hard to build.

If there's a sword of Damocles suspended by a thread in my brain, sleep is it. I've learned the hard way to respect this fact. Please don't repeat my follies. Resolve right now to treat sleep as if your life depended on it. It does.

Staying Well

If you want to learn what patients do to stay well, the obvious source are the people who live with our illness. Only one researcher, Sarah Russell, PhD, of the Melbourne-based Research Matters, has figured this out, which makes me an enthusiastic fan of hers.

In an article in the March 2005, *Australian and New Zealand Journal of Psychiatry,* Dr. Russell reports how she recruited a hundred bipolar patients who had stayed well for the past two years or longer. Staying well to some patients meant being symptom-free and behaving normally. For others, it meant a sense of control over their illness. Seventy-six percent of the participants were in paid employment, 38 percent were parents.

Dr. Russell discovered that successful patients needed to be mindful of their diagnosis and "how they were responding to their mental, emotional, social, and physical environment." Rather than simply taking their meds and forgetting about their illness (an impression created by their doctors), patients would "move swiftly to intercept a mood swing." Moving swiftly often meant a decent night's sleep and other strategic stop-and-smell-the-roses moments.

The study patients were adept at identifying their mood triggers, which needed to be picked up much earlier, they reported, than what their doctors recommended. By the time the sex, productivity, and spending of hypomania started to roll around, they said, it was already way too late. Instead, they were microscopically attuned to subtle changes in sleep, mood, thoughts, and energy levels.

Most participants were fanatic about maintaining their sleep. When disruptions to their routines did happen, they did not hesitate to take a sleep medication. In addition, participants did what they could to minimize stress in their lives. Smart lifestyle choices (diet, exercise, etc.) were a must, and this included drastic career changes, if push came to shove. Self-education was vital, and support also mattered, but more in a social and community sense rather than seeking out fellow patients.

The patients in the study tended to shop around until they found a psychiatrist who suited them. Eighty-five percent were on meds. Adjusting doses was par for the course, but meds changes were seen as minor compared to the life and lifestyle changes the participants were willing to make. Many combined meds with complementary treatments that included cognitive therapy, nutritional supplements, naturopathy, psychotherapy, Chinese medicine, massage, tai chi, meditation, and yoga (often over the objections of their psychiatrists). Ten participants stayed well on talking therapy without meds.

Dr. Russell was particularly impressed by the "stay well plans" of the patients, which ranged from verbal understandings with family members and others to informal written documents. It wasn't that the patients were obsessed with their illness. Rather, she writes: "When participants were feeling well, the illness was in the back of their minds. It did not play a large role in their lives, but they knew it was there. On the other hand, when participants encountered triggers and felt 'early warning signals,' it was necessary to become more vigilant."

No doubt many of you are doing exactly what the patients in this study are doing, and are still struggling. Nevertheless, it is highly significant that when you ask a hundred reasonably healthy patients a simple question, you turn up a fairly uniform set of answers. Nearly as significant, one researcher felt the question was important enough to ask.

Suicide Prevention

For many of us, our illness at its worst is like a spike driven through the skull. Suicide is often not a question of life and death, but simply escaping the pain. As Violet describes it: "Even though I really don't want to die due to fear of going to Hell, I want my pain to stop. I feel like if something doesn't happen soon I could relapse and do something drastic again."

More people survive depression than die from it, but the prospect of finding ourselves in the lucky majority brings us only small relief. The experience has exposed us to our worst vulnerabilities, and deep inside we no longer trust what tomorrow may bring. We may still be walking and breathing, but we have been as close inside death as this side of life permits, and our minds will never let us forget it.

We ponder the fates of the unlucky minority, and sometimes we say a prayer. We contemplate the tortures their brains exposed them to, and know for a fact that no God would ever hold judgment against them. For the time being we are the lucky ones, but tomorrow that may change.

Nevertheless, you can plan for tomorrow. You can start by watching your thoughts and feelings very carefully. You may be able to pick up subtle signals in your mind before a full-scale crisis overwhelms you.

In the meantime, cultivate friends or family members you can call on. If you have no friends or family you can trust, then seek out a support group. Your friends or loved ones should be the ones making the decisions in an actual crisis, including escorting you to the emergency room.

Hope is a nonstarter in the throes of a crisis. The best you can do is promise yourself another twenty-four hours, and to try to hold on to the thought that your state of mind is only temporary. According to a 1978 study by Richard Seiden, PhD, who tracked 515 people who had been prevented from jumping from the Golden Gate Bridge, 94 percent were still alive twenty-five years after their attempt or had died of natural causes, while only 6 percent had killed themselves. Said Dr. Seiden in an ABC News piece: "The whole linchpin of suicide prevention is that a person's not suicidal their entire life. It's related to crisis. And if we can get them through that crisis, there's a good chance they can have a decent life."

Coping with Work

In an earlier chapter, we discussed how stress is biologically linked to mood. Unfortunately, the demands of working life tend to reinforce that fusion.

A 2000 Gallup Poll found that 80 percent of U.S. workers felt stress on the job, and nearly half said they needed help in coping with it. Twenty-five percent have felt like screaming or shouting due to job stress, 14 percent felt like striking a coworker, and 10 percent worried about a colleague becoming violent. Stress accounts for some $300 billion a year lost by U.S. business in the form of absenteeism and other costs, and is often a prelude to depression.

At Bank One, in 1989, psychiatric disabilities (mostly depression) were the seventh-leading cause of short-term disability (STD) and fourth in STD days. By 2000, the figures were number two in both categories (number one is pregnancy and childbirth). "We're not an anomaly," Daniel Conti, PhD, director of the employee assistance program at Bank One, told a session at the 2002 DBSA annual conference.

Part of the reason is that depression tends to strike people in their productive years, as opposed to, say, heart disease, which takes its major toll in late life. But public enemy number one appears to be today's work environment, with no end of potential stressors. Stress is now accepted as the most commonly endorsed health risk. The jobs that are most toxic are those with high responsibility and low control.

Vast numbers of us now working in information technology or customer service have more to fear from depression—which affects our ability to think and relate to people—than many types of physical injuries. An ad for a teller, for instance, reads: "Superior inter-personal skills . . . handle delicate issues . . . create enthusiasm."

"What would depressive illness do to that?" Dr. Conti asked.

For bipolar disorder, the figures are positively distressing, with numerous surveys finding high rates of unemployment.

But should we just give up on the idea of ever leading a productive and rewarding life? In 1999, a past president of the American Psychological Association and Stanford University professor, Albert Bandura, PhD, attacked his own peers. "The field of psychology is plagued by a chronic condition of negativity regarding human development and functioning," he said in a speech to the APA. "People have the power to influence what they do and to make things happen," he went on to say.

That he felt compelled to state the obvious speaks volumes for the misperceptions that pass for wisdom in the mental-health profession. Marsha Langer Ellison, PhD, and Zlatka Russinova, PhD, of the Center for Psychiatric Rehabilitation at Boston University, had this to say about their professional brethren:

> *Professionals in the mental health system, employers, and the general public often cast a dispirited and pessimistic eye to those who have a severe mental illness and yet aspire to careers as professionals or managers. People with psychiatric conditions often talk about how they have heard that they will "never work again," or that they must resign themselves to the simplest, least rewarding, and lowest paying work.*

Ellison and Russinova's comments were part of a 1999 study that surveyed five hundred professionals and managers, all with serious mental illness. They found that 73 percent were able to achieve full-time employment in occupations that ranged from nurses to lawyers and CEOs. An additional 6 percent were self-employed.

Sixty-nine percent increased their responsibilities since starting their jobs, and more than 20 percent earned more than $50,000 a year.

Unfortunately, says Dr. Conti, "we teach people to become disabled." Once an employee has left his or her job, returning to work is very difficult. "Run like hell [from disability], if you can," Dr. Conti told the DBSA conference. "Leave the job only if you have to, if you can no longer perform the job."

Once a person is away from the workplace, motivation for activity drops, with predictable results. To that we can add the destructive isolation of staying at home.

The Americans with Disabilities Act (ADA) mandates that employers must provide reasonable accommodation to employees with disabilities, which includes people with mental illness. There are exceptions (workplaces with fewer than fifteen employees are exempt, for example), and the U.S. Supreme Court keeps looking for new ways to undermine the will of the other two branches of the federal government. In practice, there is probably little you can do to prevent your employer from acting like a bastard, but a good many companies have found it in their best interests to act according to the spirit of the ADA and other federal and state laws.

Your key dilemma is whether you should disclose your illness to your employer and risk the type of harassment that leaves you no choice but to resign. The upside is that an enlightened employer may allow you to work a number of days from home and make other arrangements.

Should you decide to disclose, it is advisable to go through your employer's human resources department, if your employer has one, rather than your boss. Legally, human resources is required to maintain confidentiality, and in theory will run interference for you.

Not all of us, of course, are able to return to work. Sometimes, the only criterion of success we have is our own self-knowledge of what we are up against and our own heroic efforts in fighting back.

Mentally ill? Perhaps. Mentally tough? The rest of the world can't even begin to imagine.

Support

In an article in the December 2002 *American Journal of Psychiatry*, researchers from Johns Hopkins reported their survey of 103 participants in several Internet forums. Overall, 33.8 percent had resolved their depression symptoms, though "a causal relationship," the authors cautioned, "cannot be determined."

Among frequent users (more than five hours a week), the success rate was 42.9 percent compared to 20.7 percent for infrequent users.

One of the groups surveyed was Walkers in Darkness (www.walkers.org). Walkers is run by Mark Oberg, who twelve years prior to the study went from being vice president of a high-tech firm to sleeping in a shelter. Mark had been struggling with severe depression, and the outpouring of goodwill from total strangers made a profound impact. "You have no idea how [Walkers] changed my life," he confided to this writer. A year or two later, in 1996, when founder David Harmon decided to step down, Mark assumed full-time responsibility "as a way of repaying the debt which gave my life back." Since then, Walkers has become his "life's work and passion."

"It was like all of a sudden I am not alone," says Merfox, a Walkers regular. "Others out there know how I am feeling."

Walkers is not an isolated phenomenon. Entering "depression support" or "bipolar support" on Google turns up hundreds of choices, though most of these are outdoor stalls compared to Walkers' Wal-Mart.

My experience with online support was very briefly recounted as part of a June 25, 2001, *Newsweek* cover story, "The New Patient Power," on health and the Internet. Following my diagnosis of bipolar disorder in early 1999 after a series of crushing depressions, I dragged myself to the computer to find out what I could. I checked out several message boards and gravitated to one in particular, run by Colleen Sullivan at Bipolar World (www.bipolarworld.net). Colleen encouraged me to write on depression for a Web site, which led me to my newsletter and my own Web site. These days, my e-mails back and forth from readers have replaced my participation on message boards, but the principle and the practice remain the same—we are all part of a community helping each other and we are not alone.

The major advantage of Internet support over live support is the convenience and anonymity of not having to leave home, but staying inside at the expense of face-to-face contact is the Internet's biggest downside. Social isolation—which is arguably the most destructive behavior of our illness, be it depression or bipolar disorder—is the very last thing we need to encourage. The Internet needs to be regarded as a gateway into the wider world rather than a substitute for it.

Getting out of the house is generally a battle for anyone with a mood disorder, but the rewards are well worth the effort. DBSA likes to emphasize the educational advantages of fellow patients sharing their experiences, but the biggest advantage that I see as the cofacilitator of a DBSA support group in Princeton, New Jersey, is the fact that members start perking up soon after they walk in the door.

Since we are the only ones who truly understand each other, no one looks at you funny when you tell them how you ordered 437 books from Amazon.com last night or what you felt like doing to yourself when you lost custody of your children.

A support group is not a pity party, nor is it group therapy (ours can be more like open-mike night at a comedy club). It is about fellow patients intelligently discussing how they can manage their illness and cope with some of the heavy burdens in life their illness imposes on them. There is no secret formula for success. Most of the time just showing up can work wonders.

The DBSA has a list of more than a thousand support groups with contact info on its Web site (www.dbsalliance.org). Your state or local NAMI or mental-health association and the info line 211 can also assist you in finding a nearby group.

In lieu of formal support, try to develop an informal network. In a 2003 interview with this writer, Kay Jamison said: "I have a lot of friends who have depression or bipolar illness, and we've had sort of an informal support line, the manic mafia. People keep informal tabs on how everyone else is doing."

There are millions of us out there. Try linking up with at least a few.

Using Your Bag of Tricks

Support groups are an invaluable source for learning to recognize the ebbs and flows of your illness—including potential triggers and other dangers—and for picking up a personal bag of tricks to navigate your way through each day, from managing anger to dealing with stress to not having a meltdown when your family starts pushing your buttons. Over time, what once left you helpless begins to become manageable.

Because of our tendency to isolate ourselves—which can result in our illness feeding upon itself—getting out of the house is critical, even if it is just to go to the mailbox to get the mail. Meeting a friend for coffee (preferably decaf) may work better than an antidepressant, or help your antidepressant achieve better results. Those who are unable to work are strongly encouraged to do a day or two a week of volunteer work.

One of my most indispensable coping techniques is the Seinfeld Gambit. My mind has a million things going on at once, but paradoxically I can only focus on one of them at a time. Thus, when I'm laughing, I'm not thinking the dark thoughts that feed on my depression. The simplest way to banish these thoughts and put a smile on my face is by my recalling anything from a *Seinfeld* episode—astronaut pen, master of my domain, the Moops, the marble rye—and suddenly my mental TiVo is replaying the scene and I'm rolling in the aisles, in a manner of speaking. This is a strictly short-term fix, mind you, but it is singularly effective for its limited purpose.

Emily, one of my newsletter readers, offered her own variation: "I found that the pure joy of tickling my children and hearing them shriek with laughter, helped me when I was kicking myself for being a depressed parent. You can't help but smile! The kids go to sleep peaceful, relaxed and feeling loved."

KJ, who is an animal lover and volunteers at an animal farm, writes:

> When I am having a particularly bad time I try to transport myself mentally to the farm and I go from pen to pen visiting Dottie the pig, Nashville the Tennessee Fainting goat, Raisin the llama, plus many more. It is very soothing and really helps rachet down the negative feelings I may have been experiencing up to that point. I have many, many fond, warm and loving feelings for these animals so "visiting" them in my mind has a powerful positive effect.

Ed offers this take: "I try to be positive and associate with people who are positive. I avoid negative thinking and negative people. It doesn't take much for me to be depressed."

Tom's technique of "giving up" takes his mind off his obsessing about settling old scores and allows him some peace of mind.

Several readers suggested activities they enjoy: taking walks, watching funny movies, watching a TV cooking show, reading, and so on. I literally wrote my way out of my last depression, and it keeps me from future ones. And don't underestimate the serotonin value of a pet. This is my cue to mention our cat Holly, whom I endearingly refer to as Monkey Pants.

Just Start Anywhere

I love this advice. It comes from Kathleen Crowley's *The Power of Procovery*. Kathleen was driven to madness by intense and unrelenting chronic pain. As she explains on her Web site: "The fundamental focus of procovery is one of moving forward when you can no longer move back, of letting go of what was and rebuilding new dreams."

Part of the process involves the recognition that big problems don't necessarily require big solutions. "Small changes," she says, "can have big impact." "Where do we start?" is a proposition that tends to immobilize us. "Whether it's number one or number five or number 30 on the task list," she advises, "whether it's getting a goldfish or getting a job, just start anywhere."

The inertia of depression, however, can turn even small tasks into huge ones. Nowhere is this more evident than in our own homes, where laundry defiantly refuses to wash itself, the plates do not obediently march off to the kitchen, and clothes and other objects materialize out of closets and their storage spaces in the middle of the night and dump themselves unceremoniously onto every square inch of floor.

The solution? Just start anywhere.

Meditation and Yoga

Meditation is a highly personal affair, and it will probably take a process of trial and error to find what works for you. My mind, for one, is like a Circuit City showroom, with TVs and VCRs and home sound systems blaring all at once from all sides, and Kmart bluelight specials and beepers and police radios going off against a truckload of gongs clattering down marble steps. Filtering out even the top layer of all this racket would have been an exercise in extreme futility, so I hit upon a preliminary yoga warm-up routine, much like an athlete limbering up before attempting some really heavy lifting.

Gradually, a few of the TVs and VCRs in my mind click off and go silent.

Now, for the first time, the seat of my pants meets the seat of my floor cushion. I bend my legs into a semi-lotus position, but my back sags under the strain. But then come my breathers, which lift me ramrod straight.

I have now achieved the benefits of an excellent workout, a sure stress buster, and a positive deterrent to depression and mania. But I am not about to miss the big payoff, especially so close to my goal. Who knows? Just around the corner could be nothing less than the big E—enlightenment, the Boddhi tree spectacular, the Fourth of July in my head I keep hoping for, when all those TVs and VCRs and blue-light specials resolve into one glorious chord that puts me in harmony with Christ and Buddha and all creation.

But I am willing to settle for much less.

Now comes what is simultaneously the simplest and most difficult activity ever devised by a living being: I attempt to shut out all other thoughts as I follow my breath in and out my nose. The ideal, according to the Buddhist monks, is to concentrate all thinking on the tip of the nose, but I am quite content to keep my thoughts confined to the immediate planet.

Fortunately, the monks have come up with a fallback meditation known as "mindfulness meditation." As you sit quietly, you simply watch your thoughts in a detached manner, refusing to be drawn into any dialogue your mind's many TVs and VCRs may want to engage you in. When you find yourself "thinking," you simply let the thought go and resume your meditation.

Like *Seinfeld,* we are talking about a show about nothing. But there is far more to nothing than meets the eye. No self, no other. Who can truly say what lies beyond?

What you take away from the experience is for you and you alone. You may be content with five minutes in a chair, or you may set aside a whole hour. It could be ten minutes of torture or the first time you may find yourself experiencing real peace of mind.

A 2003 University of Wisconsin study found that mindfulness meditation produces "lasting positive changes" in the brain and the immune system. The meditators recorded increased electrical activity in the left frontal region of the brain—found in earlier research in people who are positive and optimistic—when compared to the controls. The meditators also produced more antibodies after receiving a flu vaccine.

Amy Weintraub, author of *Yoga for Depression: A Compassionate Guide to Relieve Suffering Through Yoga* and a senior yoga instructor trained at Kripalu (a leading yoga center in Western Massachusetts) who has used yoga to battle her own depression, offers these insights.

" 'Living in this mortal body,' " she quotes the Buddha, " 'is like living in a house on fire.' " We suffer. "Depression," says psychologist and yogi Stephen Cope in Weintraub's book, "is the common cold of the deluded human being." Don't take this personally— we're all deluded, including your psychiatrist and therapist. But we're also all divine, or at least we're connected to the divine. Yoga is about establishing this sense of oneness. It is probably fair to say a good many people take up yoga simply as a proven stress buster or alternative to Richard Simmons, but they may also find themselves reaping unexpected rewards, such as beatific inner calm or heightened awareness. Some also find it helps their depression.

In a 2004 UCLA study, twenty-eight mildly depressed young adults attended two one-hour yoga classes twice a week for five weeks. Midway into the course, subjects "demonstrated significant decreases in self-reported symptoms of depression and trait anxiety," which they maintained to the end. Subjects also reported decreased negative mood and fatigue following class.

What is going on in the body, says Amy, is muscular relaxation, restored natural diaphragmatic breathing, improved oxygen absorption and carbon monoxide elimination, and increased alpha-wave activity.

Yoga is an eight-limbed path that uses postures, breathing, and meditation as both a means and an end. Back bends, which open up the chest and increase lung capacity, are especially useful for depression. So are inversions such as headstands and shoulder stands, which stimulate the brain (but which should not be attempted without the guidance of a qualified yoga instructor). Some positions are meant to be calming and others energizing. Anxious types are advised to employ calming positions, while energetic positions are de rigueur for those who find it hard to get out of bed.

Breathing exercises follow the same energizing-calming dichotomy. One reason so much emphasis is placed on the breath is that most of us have forgotten how to breathe. Instead of using the diaphragm, we use the chest, which is not as efficient since the lower portions of the lungs are not exposed to air. The yogis imbue the air we breathe with a spiritual quality called Prana (with a capital P).

Amy's breakthrough came in a yoga class while holding the bridge pose, supine with pelvis and chest thrust upward. She released the posture ten minutes later to a flood of sensations and a "time-out for the rational mind, a few moments of deep rest, a glimpse of samadhi [cosmic consciousness]."

What if, she asks, that intelligent awareness of bliss is not an altered state but your natural state? "Eventually, through practice," she informs us, "those moments of samadhi expand until they are firmly established in your mind and you are living with your eyes wide open."

Now, if you don't like the Eastern flavor of meditation, you can change its focus to reflect your own cultural beliefs. But the beauty of yoga and meditation is that you can practice it without any of its religious trappings whatsoever. We are talking about a show about nothing, remember? No self, no other . . .

. . . and, perhaps, no depression or mania.

God Power

Some three hundred years ago, the Age of Faith gave way to the Age of Reason. Out the window went the power of prayer, to be replaced by the belief that the key to physical and mental recovery resided in the hands of medical science, even if the doctors of the era happened to kill far more people than they saved.

Now science has done a complete 180. To date, there have been about twelve hundred studies on the healing power of faith and the health effects of spirituality, according to Harold Koenig, MD, founder of the Center for the Study of Spirituality Theology, and Health at Duke University. Among them, he has been involved in the following:

- A 1998 study of eighty-seven depressed older adults, which found that the rate with which those who recovered from depression the fastest corresponded to the extent of their religious belief.
- A 1998 study of 542 patients aged sixty or older admitted to Duke University Medical Center, which found that those who attended religious services weekly or more often reduced hospital stays by more than half.
- A 2002 study of 116 depressed geriatric patients, who were given standard medications treatment over twelve weeks. The recovered patients in the study reported "significantly more frequent public and private religious practices, greater positive reli-

gious coping, and less negative religious coping" than those who remained depressed.

In 2001, Dr. Koenig, along with the late David Larson, MD, MSPH, a fellow Duke scientist, and Michael McCullough, PhD, of Southern Methodist University, published *Handbook of Religion and Health*. In preparing the book for publication, the authors reviewed more than a hundred studies on the relationship of religion to depression. Two-thirds of those studies found religious persons have less depression than those who are nonreligious, and if they become depressed, they recover more quickly.

Skeptics cite the placebo effect as a likely cause of the benefits of spiritual belief, together with the fact that religious communities offer the kind of support networks that reduce stress and ease mental anguish. Additionally, those who attend religious services have better health habits, such as drinking and smoking less. Finally, religions encourage marriage, which is a reliable predictor of longer life.

Dr. Koenig does not dispute this, saying in numerous interviews (including a January 23, 2005, ABC News piece) that religion gives people hope and optimism and helps them better overcome a negative life experience. Some religious people may think God is punishing them or become overburdened with guilt, but religion can also relieve guilt and grant forgiveness.

Even though no one is certain how spiritual practice aids in recovery, it is apparent that a number of processes in the body are being enlisted in the cause, from the brain's relaxation response to the release of hormones to the strengthening of the body's immune system.

Clearly, something is going on, and psychiatrists are stupid not to open up a dialogue with their patients. A 1997 Gallup Poll found 97 percent of those in the United States believe in God or a universal spirit. In addition, 88 percent of Americans consider religion "very important" or "fairly important" in their lives. At the 2002 APA annual meeting, Dr. Koenig cited a 1997 survey that found 80 percent of psychiatric inpatients consider themselves spiritual or religious persons, with 68 percent relying on religion as a source of strength "a great deal."

Yet, according to a 1996 USA Today poll, even though 63 percent of patients believed it was a good idea for doctors to talk to patients about spiritual faith, only 10 percent said their doctor has discussed the matter.

That may change. Most medical schools in the United States now require spirituality and healing classes for graduation, while many include body-mind as a component of a required class. In 1994, only four medical schools offered these classes. This is a far cry from the legacy of Freud, who described religious beliefs as a mass delusion and the Catholic faith as the enemy. As recently as the 1990s, the *DSM-III-R* used religious behavior in 23 percent of its examples of psychopathology.

According to Herbert Benson, MD, president of the Mind/Body Medical Institute of Boston's Beth Israel Deaconess Hospital and Harvard Medical School, quoted in a June 24, 1996, *Time* cover story: "Anywhere from 60 percent to 90 percent of visits to doctors are in the mind-body, stress-related realm."

In his book *Timeless Healing,* Dr. Benson contends that humans are actually engineered for religious faith: "Our genetic blueprint has made believing in an Infinite Absolute part of our nature."

Before you say religious or spiritual practice is not for you, think again. That Gospel choir music you heard blaring out of a building you walked past didn't add a spring to your step? Those yoga postures you practice don't help you clear your mind and give you a head start on the day?

Sometimes all you need to do is close your eyes and chant, "Peace."

Whether you are an atheist or deeply religious, a good daily practice is recommended. This can range from a short Bible reading to a long meditation. It is helpful to abide by a strict schedule and set aside a certain part of the house, lighting candles or incense, if necessary, to set the mood. If you have bipolar disorder, bear in mind you are capable of inspiring yourself into a state of mania, and that retreats that have an all-night component should raise the yellow caution flag with you.

Finally, remember that spiritual and religious practice should be regarded as a complement rather than a substitute for proper medical care. A 1998 University of California study reviewed the medical records of 172 children who died after their parents relied on faith healing instead of standard medicine. The majority of these children would have survived if had they received normal medical care.

9

Seeking Help

Facing Facts

The toughest challenge on the road to recovery is probably the first—that of admitting you need help. If you're depressed, the guilt that may be a part of your illness may tell you that you don't want to burden your loved ones, or that you don't have a real illness worthy of medical attention. Something like that was going through my mind when my family took me to the local emergency room. Notwithstanding the fact that my suicidal depression was every bit as life-threatening as a heart attack and just as serious a medical concern, I somehow felt I had no right to burden the attending physician with my problem, whose time was better spent sending a real patient to get his wrist x-rayed. By contrast, a couple of years later, when I turned up in the same place in absolute misery from a

gastrointestinal complaint, I felt my physical distress was suffi-
ciently serious to warrant jumping the queue.

While a depressed individual may be too guilt-ridden to seek
help, someone in a state of mania or psychosis by definition is beyond reason. The intoxication of hypomania can deceive one into
thinking life is finally going right, while those in irritable or angry
moods are likely to shift the blame to their loved ones and others.

Finally, there's the old denial factor. Who, after all, wants to admit they're crazy? Who wants to own up to the stigma and the
shame? Typically, it is only when we run out of options (and ex-
cuses) that we seek help. The best authorities on this are my own
readers.

"What caused me to seek help?" writes George on my Web site.
"Almost losing my job and my wife."

Julie reports:

> Recently, I was forced to get help after experiencing two ma-
> nia episodes. The first one I reasoned away that I was not ill.
> The second one I could not reason away and I had to look in
> the mirror and accept that I was bipolar and would be on
> medications for the rest of my life. Because of my resistance to
> deal with my illness, I lost a job and my apartment. I have also
> learned a tremendous lesson—things can always be worse and
> they can also be better. My illness is now something I live with
> in a healthy way. I am no longer hiding from my shadow self.
> Me and my shadow are working on becoming one.

Says Anonymous:

> I was always told I was an out of control teenager who was
> too immature to handle certain situations (ie anger, peer pres-
> sure). I never got help because I was always told by my par-

ents that I was making these thoughts up. Another reason why I waited so long to seek help was because there were several periods of time when I felt on top of the world or even just "normal," whatever that is. These periods supported my parents' notion that there was nothing wrong with me.

Says Marg: "When my depression started two years ago, I blamed it on everything around me: work, being a single mother with three kids, being lonely, although I was in a relationship with a man recovering from alcoholism." It took her at least a year to be correctly diagnosed for bipolar disorder and put on the right meds. She concludes: "I ended up losing my job, my boyfriend, making my kids feel confused and afraid. I am still trying to recover all of it and unsure about the future. I only hope the road of my life will have less curves from now on."

William, age nineteen, has this to say: "I have been battling severe depression my entire life, but even when I was old enough (around 17) to realize that maybe wanting to kill myself everyday wasn't entirely 'normal,' pride and the notion that I was weak from not being able to pull myself out of it kept me from getting help."

Finally, this observation from Gayle, following several suicide attempts: "Probably the bravest thing I'll ever do—I GOT HELP!!!"

Your Next Step

For most people, their default first port of call is their primary-care physician. By far, more prescriptions for antidepressants are written by this branch of the medical profession than by psychiatrists, often for people who insist on going to specialists and getting expert lab work done for every other aspect of their health. Unfortunately, in a routine physical exam, there is no time for more than a few cursory questions.

A 2001 UCLA study found that only 19 percent of a sample of depressed or anxious people they surveyed received appropriate treatment from their primary-care physician. By contrast, 90 percent of those who saw a mental-health specialist got proper care.

Unfortunately, for suicidally depressed patients and floridly manic or psychotic patients, one's first contact with a psychiatrist is usually via the emergency room and a locked ward. Don't be frightened by the prospect of being a "prisoner." In all U.S. jurisdictions, there are strict limits on involuntary commitment (generally, only if you pose a risk to yourself or others), and it's frightening how fast you're no longer considered a danger when your insurance runs out after two days.

Those with premium health coverage are often encouraged to remain as inpatients for thirty days before they, too, find themselves miraculously recovered and sent out the door.

Hospital day programs may take up the slack, but again patients receive a clean bill of health the day their insurance runs out. Thereafter, psychiatric and talking-therapy treatment is on an outpatient basis—that is, until the next life-threatening crisis occurs.

Those who suspect that they may have a mental illness are encouraged to make an appointment with a psychiatrist or talking therapist. A psychiatrist is an MD who has completed a three- or four-year psychiatric residency. Most specialize in medications treatment.

Psychologists are PhDs or PsyDs who have completed six or seven years in a doctoral program, comprising both a formal curriculum and supervised clinical work. They specialize in any of the hundreds of forms of talking therapy and (except in the states of New Mexico and Louisiana after taking additional training) are not licensed to prescribe meds.

Counselors, therapists, and specialized social workers are generally people with master's degrees (MA, MS, or MSW) and two or more years of clinical experience. Licensing varies from state to state.

I will use the term *talking therapist* to encompass psychologists, counselors, therapists, social workers, and some psychiatrists.

Even the most meds-oriented psychiatrist needs to be a skilled talker and listener, as his or her knowledge of your illness is only as good as what you tell him or her. Because neither depression nor bipolar disorder leave a readily identifiable biological marker that can be spotted in a lab test, blood sample, or brain scan, a psychiatrist is largely dependent on what you say. Under ideal conditions, an insightful practitioner can elicit all the necessary information from you to make a precise diagnosis and initiate the type of treatment most likely to work for you. But in practice, for patients with bipolar disorder, it takes many years and a succession of doctors to figure out what is wrong. The onus, then, is very much on you to get your story right, which is not always the easiest thing to do while in the throes of a killer depression or out-of-control mania.

On my Web site, Anonymous describes her frustration: "For years I had been going to doctors and they would tell me that I just needed to slow down in my everyday work, try to get me to listen to soothing music, when I would visit the doctor I would try and try to tell him that wasn't the problem. Finally one doctor put me on Valium so I could sleep. That was the first time in years that I felt decent and could function and sleep."

Unfortunately, she became addicted to the Valium, then to Xanax, from two different doctors. By this time, her mania manifested full strength, which involved going through her and her husband's savings. Only after a suicide attempt was she finally correctly diagnosed: "It just sends knives in me knowing that for approximately ten years I had been going through all this with the doctors. It ended up I quit my job, and there are jobs that I will not be able to get because I got in trouble with the law over credit card fraud, so now I have a criminal record on top of everything else. It isn't fun to be mentally ill."

I find myself suggesting to readers who have contacted me to put their concerns in writing before their initial or next visit to the psychiatrist, for, if nothing else, this is a good way to organize your thoughts.

Think of those times you felt depressed and write down what it felt like. Did something bring it on—say, a relationship breakup—or did it seem to occur out of the blue? Did you feel like you couldn't go on living? Did you entertain thoughts of suicide? Did you feel like you couldn't get out of bed? Or, just the opposite, maybe you couldn't get to sleep. Are you eating more or less? Not feeling your usual self? What's different? Are you doing a great acting job hiding your distress from your friends and family and colleagues, or do they think you're acting a bit out of character, too? Are your work and family and personal relationships feeling the strain? Provide details. Are you less patient with people lately? Short-tempered, angry, aggressive? Or perhaps the very opposite: submissive, guilt-ridden, and ready to give up without a fight? How long has this been going on? Have you felt like this at other times in your life?

A good psychiatrist will be asking these questions, but you can save both of you a lot of time and effort if you have your answers ready. Your psychiatrist will also probe for personal and family history, looking for more clues. Now is hardly the time to talk at length about past trauma and abuse, as this may destabilize some patients at their most vulnerable. It is essential, however, to inform your psychiatrist whether you are a survivor of trauma or abuse, as this can have a bearing on your treatment. Later on, in talking therapy, you can try to resolve trauma and abuse issues.

You will also want to write down what it feels like to be normal. If normal for you is feeling constantly depressed, that's a very good clue. Also try to recall what it's like feeling happy. Some people may have felt a little too happy in the past, which may be the only way your psychiatrist may suspect you have bipolar disorder.

Many people suspect they have bipolar disorder long before they see a psychiatrist. But even people who merely think they have depression need to focus on all those times they didn't feel their normal selves or felt too much like their normal selves. You might want to go back over those times in your life you would rather forget—such as embarrassing yourself in public or attacking your spouse or walking off your job or getting arrested—or where you were unusually productive—working twenty-hour days, cleaning the house in the middle of the night, writing a term paper in three hours—and try to remember what you were feeling during those times and the times that led up to these events. If you felt you were smarter than the rest of the world, describe it. If you were in a raging white heat, fill in the details.

Admitting that there may be something wrong with you is one of the most difficult tasks there is. Add to that fear and ignorance of others and the stigma, and you begin to appreciate why so few people seek help or get a correct diagnosis.

As I wrote earlier, my psychiatrist didn't pick up on my bipolar disorder during my first visit, such was the state of my depression. It was only after the antidepressant he prescribed sent me into a state of mania (which, ironically, pulled me out of my depression and may have saved my life) that my diagnosis became a no-brainer. Two visits to a crisis intervention team followed. When I went back to my original psychiatrist, this time I had a written opus ready for him. Amazingly, I recalled a full-blown manic episode from some twelve years earlier that I had somehow written off as a stressful time in my life. Imagine dismissing a heart attack in a similar fashion, and you can begin to appreciate the power of denial when it comes to confronting one's own madness.

When I ask psychiatrists what they find works best in treating patients, many reply that establishing a trusting relationship with the patient is essential. These are the psychiatrists I would hire.

Without this trust, those degrees on the wall aren't worth the paper they're printed on. Your end of the bargain is to keep your psychiatrist fully informed and to stay on your meds and other treatments. His or her end of the bargain is to be there for you in a crisis, day or night, and work with you in getting well and staying well. If your meds aren't working or you are experiencing bad side effects, inform your psychiatrist rather than simply quit the drugs on your own. Together, the two of you can work on new doses and/or new meds. If he or she suggests adding a new med to your cocktail, by the same token, you should expect to be informed of the risks and side effects as well as the benefits. If you object to that med, he or she should respect your judgment. And on and on it goes—mutual trust and respect.

Sometimes, though, achieving a good working relationship may involve auditioning more than one psychiatrist. Writes Linda: "I went through ten psychiatrists in one year until I found one able to call down to rock bottom and tell me the footholds up. That was luck. Otherwise I'd be sitting in front of television waiting for the next meal, the sound of doors locking behind me."

Sunny, who replaced a psychiatrist with whom she had a bad experience with another "who was very good, nice, knowledgeable, and didn't pry into things that weren't his business," advises, "Don't be afraid to fire a bad doc."

Or, another way of saying it: Put the same care into finding a good psychiatrist that you would into finding into a good hairdresser. It's amazing how people regard the inside of the skull as less important than the outside. Don't be one of them.

10

Antidepressants and Controversial Meds Issues

You've been diagnosed with depression or bipolar disorder, plus maybe co-occurring anxiety or alcohol or substance use. Now what? Do you risk taking very imperfect medications with all their side effects, or do you feel you can manage your illness by other means? There is no pat answer that applies to everyone, but as a general rule it is safe to say that better outcomes are achieved by combining different treatments, which also includes integrating smart lifestyle choices into various psychiatric and talking therapies. The intent of the next several chapters is not to recommend one type of treatment over another, but to help you make informed choices.

We will first take an extended look at medications treatment, then move on to talking therapy, and finally to electroconvulsive therapy (ECT, also known as shock treatment) and related experimental therapies.

Antidepressants for Depression

Antidepressants are used for treating depression and anxiety. The American Psychiatric Association advises its members to avoid treating bipolar patients with just an antidepressant. This is owing to the strong potential for an antidepressant to switch a bipolar patient into mania or rapid-cycling. Even the use of an antidepressant with other medications in treating bipolar disorder is a highly controversial issue (more on this in Chapter 11).

Using antidepressants to treat kids is also controversial, a topic we will discuss in depth in Part Four, "Special Populations."

Let's start with the bad news. Antidepressants are not magic bullets. Success is measured in terms of a 50 percent response (i.e., at least 50 percent of the test subjects getting at least 50 percent better), which would be unacceptable for any other illness. Fewer still actually achieve remission (i.e., become nearly symptom-free). In addition, Prozac and its cousins poop out on as many as 50 percent of their users, bringing on perhaps their second major depressive episode in the space of a year—a situation about as acceptable as two bypass operations in twelve months. Consequently, you should regard antidepressants as but one small part of your wellness program.

You may find antidepressants do their job better if you lower your expectations. Don't expect an antidepressant to make your miserable life bearable. If the underlying cause of your depression is a toxic relationship or abusive working situation or something similar, at best an antidepressant will perk you up enough to help you resolve it. Doing nothing invites depression back in.

Antidepressants will not replace your bad memories with good ones, nor will they take over the heavy lifting in changing sad thoughts to happy ones. But they may get you back on your feet again, and that certainly is a start.

The Players

The fine points of the biochemistry of antidepressants have already been discussed in the "Brain Science" portion of this book. For the purposes of this chapter, we simply need to know there are four broad classes of antidepressants that all target one or more of three neurotransmitters, namely:

MAOIs—These date back to the fifties, but are still in service as a last resort or as an early option for treating atypical depression. Side effects are as subtle as an 800-pound gorilla (including the risk of stroke in reaction to tyramine in foods such as bananas). MAOIs operate by blocking out the enzyme, monoamine oxidase, which gives the neurotransmitters serotonin, norepinephrine, and dopamine a chance to do their work.

Nardil (phenelzine) and Parnate (tranylcypromine) are the best known. A supposedly kinder and gentler MAOI, EMSAM (selegeline), is applied as a transdermal patch. RIMAs, another more benign branch of the MAOI family, are available in Canada, but can be obtained by U.S. patients via special FDA consent through one's doctor or psychiatrist.

Tricyclics—Another oldie but goodie from the 1950s. The side effects gorilla is slightly lighter than MAOIs, but still packs a wallop. Overdoses can be fatal. Tricyclics work by keeping serotonin and norepinephrine in play. Tofranil (imipramine, Norpramin [desipramine] and Pamelor or Aventyl (nortriptyline) are the best known.

SSRIs—The hype that surrounded the introduction of Prozac (fluoxetine) in the late 1980s motivated millions to get their depression treated for the first time, though this class of antidepressant is no more effective than its predecessors and still carries a pretty heavy side-effects gorilla. They work by keeping serotonin in circulation.

Other companies were quick to follow up with their own versions, including Paxil (paroxetine), Celexa (citalopram), Lexapro (escitalopram), Luvox (fluvoxamine), and Zoloft (sertraline). Though technically "me-too" drugs in relation to Prozac, trying the "Pepsi" after the "Coke" has failed (or vice-versa) may make all the difference in the world.

Other New-Generation Meds—Same old neurotransmitters, all working on dual targets, some primary, some secondary. These include Effexor (venlafaxine), Cymbalta (duloxetine), Wellbutrin (bupropion), and Remeron (mirtazapine). Serzone (nefazodone) was recently taken off the market due to a remote risk of liver damage or liver failure, but it is available in generic form.

Efficacy

Published studies indicate that antidepressants result in a response (i.e., a 50 percent reduction in depression scores) in two-thirds of subjects over the course of a usual four to eight week trial. The FDA database, however, which includes studies not published, reveals the success rate is more like 50 percent. Factor in the high rate of dropouts in these studies and the true success rate is spectacularly dismal.

Less than fifty percent of patients getting only fifty percent well is not exactly encouraging. Add to that the phenomenon of Prozac poop-out and the prospect of a high rate of relapse, and one is entitled to question whether the side effects are worth trying an antidepressant in the first place.

Indeed, a good case can be made that depression remits naturally rather than through the intervention of an antidepressant. Critical analysis of antidepressant trials indicates that the drug companies have essentially failed to prove their products' worth (much more on this later).

But one can also look at the matter far more charitably. For one, it's irrational to give up after your first failure, especially if you still have a 50 percent chance of success on your next try. (If the same people who trash antidepressants for failing half the time dropped out of the dating game after their first rejection, few of them would ever get laid.) Treatment guidelines, in fact, anticipate initial failure. The American Psychiatric Association in its 2000 *Practice Guideline for the Treatment of Patients with Major Depressive Disorder* recommends switching to another antidepressant if the first one does not work and to a different class of antidepressant if the second one fails.

Several open-label studies published in the *Journal of Clinical Psychiatry* over the years have demonstrated the value of switching to a second SSRI after the first one has failed, with response rates ranging from 42 to 71 percent. In one study, many of those who had failed on Zoloft had much better results on Prozac. Conversely, in another, many of those who failed on Prozac got lucky with Zoloft. Likewise, a multicenter double-blind study published in the March 2002 *Archives of General Psychiatry* illustrated the benefit of switching to a different class of antidepressant. In that study, of 117 chronically depressed patients who failed to respond to Zoloft after twelve weeks and 51 patients with similar bad luck on the tricyclic imipramine, more than half from each group benefited from switching to the other.

Other strategies include combining your antidepressant with another antidepressant or augmenting your antidepressant with a different class of drug such as a thyroid drug or lithium (more on this shortly).

You can also improve your chances by not quitting on your medication. A 2003 multicenter open trial of 840 patients on Prozac found that of the 607 who completed the study, 424 achieved remission at week 12. Thirty-one to 41 percent of patients who were unimproved at week six achieved remission at week 12. Twenty-three percent of unimproved patients at week eight had remissions by week 12. At week 10, however, patients reached the point of diminishing returns. Concluded the study's authors: "Nonresponse to [Prozac] should not be declared until eight weeks of treatment have elapsed."

Still, even the most persevering can be frustrated by a long and drawn-out game of pill roulette that can take months or even years to resolve—that is if they don't give up in despair first.

But even the lucky ones are in for a difficult initial several weeks, for antidepressants have a perverse way of making their side effects known almost at once, weeks before their healing power kicks in, when the depression is raging at its fiercest. The side effects tend to diminish over time, but too late for many distressed patients who have given up long before then. Here—and this is tough—you must have faith. Barring some extreme side effect or medical emergency, you need to give your prescription a full eight weeks to work—and if that one fails, another eight weeks with a second antidepressant.

Why Antidepressants Aren't Magic Bullets

The pharmaceutical industry, like the film industry, has a blockbuster mentality. Despite the fact that no two depressions are the same, drug companies treat them as if they are, according to Gordon Parker, MD, PhD, of the University of New South Wales in an article in the June 2004 issue of *Australian and New Zealand Journal of Psychiatry*.

When drug companies test an antidepressant, they lump all depressed subjects (except kids) together and view the illness as a single entity, with no regard to subtype, gender, cause, and other considerations. The pay-off, should the trials succeed, is an FDA license to print money: the right to exclusively market to mass populations.

If shoe manufacturers had this one-size-fits-all mentality, they

would be out of business. Some people obviously do well on antidepressants, others do not, but we have no way of knowing in advance
which ones and why. Drug companies have no incentive to investigate further and independent academic researchers lack the means.
To be fair, the FDA is not exactly encouraging drug companies to
find niche markets.

The little evidence we have suggests these limited treatment options:

▌ The APA's 2000 *Practice Guideline* states: "MAOIs may be
particularly effective in treating subgroups of patients . . .
with atypical features." A 1993 study found a response rate of
72 percent for patients with atypical depression on the MAOI
Nardil compared to 44 percent on imipramine.

▌ The American Psychological [not Psychiatric] Association's
2002 *Summit on Women and Depression* notes that women
respond preferentially to SSRIs and men to tricyclics. Women
in postmenopause, however, respond less well to SSRIs, but
there is evidence that hormone replacement therapy restores
this preferential response.

▌ Because SSRI manufacturers have invested huge sums in tapping into a lucrative market for patients with anxiety—with
clinical trials to back them up—we can infer from these findings that these drugs work reasonably well for depression with
anxiety features.

▌ For bipolar depression, we have a handful of conflicting studies to go on (more on this later).

Not surprisingly, no drug company is about to sign up my Web
site readers for glowing testimonials. Writes Anonymous: "I have
tried Serzone, Neurontin, Paxil, Ativan, and Effexor. None of these
have worked. In actuality, no antidepressants will ever work for
me. The most important thing is to decide to get up every morning,

go for a walk or exercise every day and to look for the positive things in life, and not dwell on the negative things that can/do happen to us."

Says Dynamo:

I have been on Buspar, Ativan, Wellbutrin, Zoloft, Paxil, and Effexor throughout various parts of my life. I have gone off every single one of them. The best was Effexor, but I was in the lucky .00000001 percent of the population that experiences heart problems while taking the drug. I am now medicine-free, and unless something miraculous occurs, I will stay that way the rest of my life.

Josquin, however, contends that people doing well on meds are less inclined to write than those not doing well. He reports: "For two years I have experienced complete relief on 50 mg Zoloft (after having experienced depression all my life). The side effects are fine with me. I feel more tired than before, but I like taking naps, so it's no problem. I have 'delayed orgasm,' but I like having sex longer so it's no problem. I feel comfortable and am happy. End of story."

Experimental Antidepressants

Researchers are looking at alternative targets to the three neurotransmitters we know best. One major neurotransmitter is glutamate, which has an excitatory effect. The Amyotrophic Lateral Sclerosis (ALS) drug Rilutek (riluzole), a glutamate inhibitor, acts as an antidepressant. Based on this knowledge, it may be possible to develop a similar compound.

Valdoxan (agomelatine) targets melatonin, which is how serotonin winds up. Melatonin is essential to sleep and regulation of circadian rhythms. The drug is in Phase III clinical trials (the major testing phase).

Other potential treatments focus on the neuroendocrine pathway—the HPA axis—where stress can trigger depression. Several companies have in development a "CRF antagonist" that would inhibit the release of the stress hormone CRF. The pregnancy termination pill, Mifepristone, (RU-486) prevents the synthesis of another stress horomone, cortisol, and may be effective in treating psychotic depression.

Researchers are also looking at the molecular pathways inside the neuron responsible for cell function and maintenance. The Parkinson's drug, Mirapex (pramipexole), is known to boost a protective chemical—bcl-2—in one of these pathways. Preliminary studies indicate it may work as an antidepressant.

Aiming for Remission

Considering how imperfect antidepressants are, using them to achieve remission may seem like a pipe dream. Yet, said Michael Thase, MD, of the University of Pittsburgh at a symposium at 2002 APA conference, "This is the outcome that should be targeted." This means "no symptoms" and a "return to functional self," corresponding to a Hamilton-17 Depression score of 7 or lower.

Even the presence of residual symptoms can pose a risk. A 1998 Cambridge University study found that these symptoms were "strong predictors" of subsequent relapse.

Dr. Thase observed that depression needs to be vigorously treated at high doses for adequate duration. Doctors need to ensure patient adherence, as two-thirds to three-quarters of patients do not take their antidepressants, he said. Doctors also have to measure patient outcomes, as "a simple finding of a symptom or two determines if a patient is in the response zone or the remission zone."

Significantly, Dr. Thase said that remission needs to be the goal of the acute (initial) phase of treatment.

Dr. Thase's point about high doses was seconded by Maurizio Fava, MD, of Harvard, at the same APA meeting. Paxil on 40 mg/day runs the risk of a 23 percent recurrence to depression, while 20 mg/day of the same drug puts patients at more than double the risk at 51 percent, he said.

High doses, nevertheless, need to be weighed against side effects, where lowering the dose may be the only way of staying on a medication (more on this in a few pages).

Augmentation and Combination Strategies

Augmenting an antidepressant with another drug is an important option in helping achieve remission, a number of speakers pointed out at the 2002 APA annual meeting. Augmenting carries forward a partial response from an antidepressant and buys time, Andrew Nierenberg, MD, of Harvard, noted in one symposium. It also helps avoid discontinuation, may achieve a more rapid response, and can be used to treat breakthrough symptoms. Holly Swartz, MD, of the University of Pittsburgh, observed in addition that augmentation may result in synergy, while Richard Shelton, MD, of Vanderbilt, mentioned the possibility of lowering doses and expanding therapeutic effect.

On the minus side are cost issues, the uncertainties of dosing, and the possibility of drug-drug interactions. Unfortunately, most of what we know is based on a small number of open studies and anecdotal reports. "There is not enough data," Dr. Swartz cautioned. Dr. Nierenberg alluded to the phenomenon of the "augmentation of the month club" where once you have a study involving five patients, "everyone does it."

Augmentation strategies include adding lithium, thyroid (T3),

Buspar (a novel antianxiety med that may speed up response and improve sexual dysfunction), pindolol (a blood pressure med that may speed up response of an SSRI), Viagra (which may counter SSRI sexual dysfunction side effect), stimulant and dopamine agonists (such as the Parkinson's med Mirapex), anticonvulsants (for bipolar depression), Provigil (for fatigue), Ritalin (for a short-term energizing effect at a low dose), atypical antipsychotics (at low doses), estrogen, inositol, and metyrapone (which stops production of cortisol).

As opposed to augmentation, in which a different type of drug is used to boost an antidepressant, combinations involve mixing two or more antidepressants. Typically, combinations involve two different classes of antidepressants—say, an SSRI with an antidepressant that works on norepinephrine (such as Effexor, with a dual serotonin-norepinephrine action, plus a weaker dopamine action).

Unfortunately, virtually no data on combinations exist. Confessed Dr. Nierenberg at the APA meeting: "A lot of time I make my patients better by getting rid of the drugs [the pharmaceutical companies] give out."

Long-Term Treatment

According to Dr. Thase at the 2002 APA annual meeting, between 50 and 70 percent of those who have experienced one episode of major depression will experience another at some later stage. The risk of subsequent episodes or recurrent depression increases from 50 to 70 to 90 percent across the first-three depressive episodes. Chronic minor depressive disorders similarly place the individual at risk of major depression.

The odds, however, can be much improved by staying on your antidepressant. A 2003 Oxford University, Nagoya City University (Japan), and Western Psychiatric Institute (affiliated with the University of Pittsburgh) meta-analysis of thirty-one placebo-controlled antidepressant trials comprising 4,410 participants found an 18 percent average rate of relapse for those remaining on their antidepressant, compared to 41 percent on a placebo. According to the authors of the study, this means that continuing with antidepressants reduces the risk of relapse by 70 percent, a figure that held fairly steady in their review across all classes of antidepressants, condition of patient, and length of time on an antidepressant prior to a particular study.

This study and others represent perhaps the most convincing proof of the efficacy of an antidepressant. Whereas it is difficult to demonstrate that these pills actually get you better, researchers have made a fairly strong case that sticking with these meds offers a far better chance of keeping you well than not taking them.

The APA's *Practice Guideline for the Treatment of Patients with Major Depressive Disorder* (2000) recommends four to five months of "continuation" treatment on an antidepressant following satisfactory resolution of symptoms, but has nothing to say concerning the subsequent "maintenance" phase, other than the treating physician should have regard to the risk of recurrence, the severity of symptoms, side effects, and patient preferences.

The British Association for Psychopharmacology's *Evidence-Based Guidelines for Treating Depressive Disorders with Antidepressants* (2000) is far more specific, recommending that patients remain on their antidepressant at the same dose beyond six months and for as long as five years or indefinitely if they have had more than three major depressive episodes in the past five years or more than five episodes altogether, or if social or personality or other factors make a relapse or recurrence likely. The BAP also recommends twelve months of antidepressant therapy for elderly patients.

Unfortunately, by week ten, 50 percent of patients stop taking antidepressants, according to Dr. Fava at the 2002 APA annual meeting, either because of the side effects, or they feel they don't need the medication, or they feel better, or they feel the meds aren't working, or they forget to take them.

If it's working, an antidepressant needs to be regarded as the equivalent of insulin to a diabetic. You can't just stop taking them as soon as you start to feel better, however much you would like to. It was four years before my psychiatrist gave me the okay to stop taking my antidepressant. I still have the bottle in the medicine cabinet as a keepsake (I lie; I'm way too much of a slob to actually use the medicine cabinet). If I need to be cheered up, I simply look at the bottle rather than take the pills inside. It's a right I earned by being a model patient.

Side Effects

A 2001 DBSA survey found that 40 percent of patients believe they have to tolerate avoidable medications side effects. Nearly half the patients in the study reported side effects, a finding that would have been much higher had the survey queried patients who had dropped out of treatment. (A DBSA survey from two years earlier reported 80 percent having experienced side effects.) Of those reporting side effects, more than half expressed their dissatisfaction with their antidepressant.

One psychiatrist finally came clean on the issue. In the February 29, 2000, *Washington Post,* Robert Hedaya, MD, of Georgetown University, wrote: "Sadly, some doctors do not appreciate, or may even dismiss, their patients' complaints about side effects. . . . This all-too-common response by physicians not only lacks compassion, it's also bad medicine. By dismissing antidepressants' side effects as something patients must learn to live with, doctors are forfeiting their patients' chances for full recovery."

Since serotonin mediates so many processes in the brain and body, any interference in the serotonin traffic pattern can result in a range of unwanted side effects.

Agitation/Mental Restlessness

Potentially the most dangerous side effects include anxiety, agitation, emotional instability, and mental restlessness. The labeling on Prozac warns that 12 to 16 percent of the Prozac patients in clinical trials reported anxiety, nervousness, or insomnia, compared to 7 percent on a placebo. The labeling also cites as "frequent" adverse events emotional lability (mood swings) and agitation. "Infrequent" events include akathisia (mental restlessness), hallucinations, hostility, and psychosis, among others.

We will look at these issues in far greater depth further down under "The Crazy Factor." What you need to know for the time being is that agitation and anxiety tend to be transient effects and generally subside as your body adjusts to the drug. Nevertheless, should you find yourself feeling unusually agitated or hyper or anxious, you should notify your physician at once.

Mania

Physicians frequently fail to recognize bipolar disorder and diagnose patients instead as having clinical depression. Then they prescribe an antidepressant, which can cause the patient to switch into mania or rapid-cycling. In rare cases, patients with clinical depression can have a similar reaction. Please notify your physician at once if you experience mania while on an antidepressant.

Drowsiness and Fatigue

The flip side of agitation is the torpor and inertia many patients experience, particularly in the early phases of taking the drug, when the body has not yet adjusted. All antidepressants come with the warning to be careful about operating heavy machinery, and this includes your car.

Sexual Dysfunction

The most notorious side effect of the SSRIs is sexual dysfunction, which also affects women. The worst antidepressants in terms of sexual dysfunction, according to a 2002 survey of more than six thousand men and women on antidepressants, were Paxil, at 43 percent; Remeron, at 41 percent; and Prozac, at 37 percent. The lowest were Wellbutrin (22 percent) and Serzone (28 percent). Falling in between were Zoloft, Effexor, and Celexa.

For those not predisposed to sexual dysfunction, the same study found a reduced effect ranging from 7 to 30 percent.

The Remeron finding should not be regarded as conclusive, as a 2002 review of previous studies found the drug at the lower end of the scale.

Weight Gain

Weight gain is also worrisome. Effexor and Wellbutrin are considered weight-friendly, while Remeron is such a notorious weight gainer that some doctors use it for treating anorexia. A 2000 Massachusetts General Hospital study of 284 patients on either Paxil, Prozac, or Zoloft found Paxil patients experienced a significant weight increase over twenty-six to thirty-two weeks compared to modest gains for Prozac and Zoloft. The older antidepressants are even greater weight gainers.

Other Side Effects

Other side effects can include sleep problems, GI complaints/nausea/diarrhea, and fatigue or low mental alertness. The product labeling on the newer antidepressants reports clinical trials dropout rates due to adverse events ranging from 12 to 20 percent.

Working with Side Effects

Side effects can be reduced by lowering the dose, though this may increase risk of a relapse. Jay Cohen, MD, of the University of California, San Diego, and the author of *Over Dose: The Case Against Drug Companies: Prescription Drugs, Side Effects, and Your Health,* argues that the starting dose for antidepressants is too strong for many patients.

Do not underestimate smart lifestyle choices. The labeling on all antidepressants advises informing your physician if you take alcohol (who is sure to tell you that this isn't such a great idea). Equally relevant warnings would advise against mixing antidepressants with pizza, cheeseburgers, Starbucks, and Entenmann's.

In the meantime, we simply do not know the long-term effects of many of these drugs. Trials are typically conducted among rather small populations for periods that tend to range from six to eight weeks. Yearlong trials are an extreme rarity, and ten-year data regarding the newer antidepressants are simply not available.

The 2001 DBSA survey strongly hinted that better outcomes can be achieved through clear communication between you and clinician. This may necessitate that you keep badgering your psychiatrist to the effect that burdensome side effects and diminished quality of life are not the prices you should be paying for resolving your depression. For one, having to deal with physical and emotional fallout of side effects sets you up for another depression. For another, the object of medical treatment is to restore you to where you were before you got sick and send you back to full functioning.

It may take several attempts before your earth-to-psychiatrist messages finally get through. If your psychiatrist is still lost in space, don't be afraid to fire him or her.

Meds Management

Your psychiatrist should know all the drugs you are taking, including those prescribed by another physician, as some drugs affect the metabolism of others. These include over-the-counter meds (especially those that used to be prescription meds, such as Sudafed) and herbal supplements (especially Saint John's wort). Please keep both psychiatrist and other physicians informed of any meds changes.

It pays to be mindful of the practice that drug companies are now employing in the use of different names for the same drug for marketing purposes. Sarafem, which is prescribed for premenstrual dysphoric disorder, is a new trade name for Prozac. One psychiatrist referred to it as Prozac with Barbie colors.

More worrying is the fact that the FDA has allowed Glaxo-SmithKline (GSK) to market its antidepressant drug Wellbutrin as an antismoking drug under the name Zyban. Wellbutrin should not be prescribed for people who are at risk of having seizures. An unwitting Wellbutrin patient innocently slapping on an antismoking patch may find his family dialing 911.

Then there is Symbyax, which is Prozac and Zyprexa combined in one pill for treating bipolar depression.

Your physician and psychiatrist and pharmacist could be charged for malpractice for not keeping track of your prescriptions, but mistakes can happen. A simple rule to go by: When it comes to managing your meds, there is only one safety net—you.

Pregnancy and Breast-feeding

In its *Practice Guideline,* the American Psychiatric Association advises:

> *There is no evidence that tricyclic antidepressants, [Prozac], or newer SSRIs cause either intrauterine death or major birth defects. However, in one large study, three or more minor physical anomalies occurred more commonly in infants exposed to [Prozac] than in a comparison group. This study also demonstrated that fetuses exposed to [Prozac] after 25*

weeks' gestation had lower birth weights, which were associated with lower maternal weight gain.

In June 2004, the FDA mandated labeling changes on new-generation antidepressants, which now include this warning: "Neonates exposed to Effexor, other SNRIs (Serotonin and Norepinephrine Reuptake Inhibitors), or SSRIs (Selective Serotonin Reuptake Inhibitors), late in the third trimester of pregnancy have developed complications requiring prolonged hospitalization, respiratory support, and tube feeding. Such complications can arise immediately upon delivery."

The APA advises that going off an antidepressant, however, carries its own risks, including low birth weight (associated with the mother not looking after herself), suicidality, marital discord, the inability to engage in appropriate obstetrical care, and difficulty caring for other children.

There are no right or wrong choices, only informed and uninformed ones. Please consult your physician before making any final decisions.

Drug Metabolism

Not having luck with your antidepressant? It could have to do with the way your body metabolizes drugs. Cytochrome P450s, in the words of an article in the April 8, 2000, *British Medical Journal (BMJ)*, are "a multigene family of enzymes found predominantly in the liver that are responsible for the elimination of most of the drugs currently used in medicine."

Not everyone has the same cytochrome P450s, which explains why different people react so differently to the same drug. Of particular interest is the cytochrome P450 CYP2D6, which breaks down a large number of psychiatric drugs—including Prozac, Paxil,

Zoloft, Effexor, the tricyclic antidepressants, and the antipsychotics Haldol and Risperdal—in the liver. According to the article, this enzyme is "highly polymorphic" (i.e., prone to mutation) and is inactive in 6 percent of white people.

Poor metabolizers are at risk for drug accumulation and toxicity. Those taking antipsychotic drugs risk exacerbated side effects such as postural hypotension and oversedation.

Then there are complications from drug interactions. Enzyme *inhibition* involves competition with another drug for the enzyme binding site. For example, Serzone, Luvox, Zoloft, Paxil, and Prozac can interfere with P450 enzymes responsible for the metabolism of a patient's other medications. But these are fairly weak compared to the cardiac drug quinidine.

Enzyme *induction* drugs, on the other hand, enhance the enzyme's metabolizing capacity on other drugs, which is an opportune moment to introduce yet another P450 enzyme, this time CYP3A. For example, Tegretol (a bipolar drug) induces CYP3A, requiring higher levels of Depakote and Lamictal (both bipolar drugs), antipsychotics, and the benzodiazepines, and makes birth control problematic.

Drugs metabolized through CYP3A include Elavil, Tofranil, Serzone, Zoloft, Effexor, and the benzodiazepines. Grapefruit is a strong inducer of CYP3A, with known dangerous interactions to the tricyclics and benzodiazepines (for treating anxiety and insomnia), as well as calcium channel blockers experimentally used to treat bipolar disorder. Further study may yield further interactions. Please ask your doctor about grapefruit before being put on a new med. You may want to avoid the fruit altogether.

Modern DNA testing requires only a small tissue sample—blood from a finger prick, cells from a mouth wash, or hair follicle cells—to provide a rapid and reliable patient genotype. In January 2005, Roche entered the U.S. market with an AmpliChip CYP450 test costing about $350 to $400 per test.

In the meantime, much of the information your doctor needs is right at his or her fingertips, in the drug-product labeling found in the *Physicians' Desk Reference*. In the words of the *BMJ*: "This may allow the choice and doses of specific drugs, particularly those for treating psychiatric disorders, to be used more appropriately."

Other Things You Should Know

Even if all goes well with your treatment, there are bound to be adjustments along the way. For example, soon after your system has adapted to its medications, your doctor is likely to increase your dose to maintenance levels, and should you need to switch medications or go off them entirely, the doctor will "taper" your doses rather than having you go cold turkey.

Lack of disposable income should not prevent you from seeking antidepressant therapy. True, each pill retails in the neighborhood of two dollars in the United States, but few individuals wind up paying the full price. Private health plans and state welfare usually pick up the tab or most of the tab, and for those who otherwise do not qualify, the best-kept secret in America is that pharmaceutical companies have patient-assistance programs that give away drugs to those in need.

You need to work through your prescribing physician to take advantage of these programs. The drug companies have 800 phone numbers for your physician's office manager to call. Once the paperwork is completed, you will be able to pick up your medications at your doctor's office. The Pharmaceutical Research and Manufacturers of America (PhRMA) has information on its Web site (www .phrma.org).

Be sure to shop around if you are paying out of pocket for generic drugs. When a drug goes generic, the pharmacist purchases it wholesale from new manufacturers at a fraction of the price of the brand-name drug. The pharmacist then marks up the retail price of the drug to that almost approaching that of the brand-name drug and pockets the difference.

Take-Home Message

A reader survey of depressed patients published in the October 2004 *Consumer Reports* found that more than 80 percent said that treatment helped. Meds had a quicker impact than talk therapy, but it often took trial and error to find the right med. More than half the antidepressant users had tried two or more drugs; 10 percent, five or more. For people with severe problems, treatment by mental health specialists yielded significantly better results than primary-care physicians.

The take-home message: Consider your brain an organ every bit as important as your heart, together with a quality of life free from permanent side effects, and find a doctor or psychiatrist who feels the same way.

The Crazy Factor

In 2001, a Wyoming jury returned a verdict against GlaxoSmith-Kline (formerly SmithKline Beecham), makers of Paxil, with damages amounting to $6.4 million. On February 13, 1998, Donald Schell, age sixty, took two Paxil tablets, then shot to death his wife, daughter, and granddaughter before killing himself. Unpublished data from SKB revealed that its own investigators had attributed a variety of side effects to the drug, including akathisia (mental agitation), mania, psychosis, aggression, and attempted suicides.

Eli Lilly had better luck in an earlier wrongful-death suit involving Bill Forsyth, a retiree living in Hawaii, who unaccountably stabbed to death his wife of thirty-seven years, then impaled himself on a kitchen knife soon after taking Prozac.

Eli Lilly won the case, but possibly lost a long-term war, for the company was obliged to make public incriminating internal documents that showed prior knowledge of psychosis, akathisia, and restlessness in some patients.

The database of FDA antidepressant trials supports contradictory conclusions. A 2003 analysis by Arif Khan, MD, and his colleagues at the Northwest Clinical Research Center (Washington State) found an insignificant difference in suicide rates between those taking newer antidepressants and those on placebos—less than 1 percent in both groups. Seventy-seven patients committed suicide during the trials.

But a reanalysis of the same data by David Healy, MD, of the University of Wales, indicates that the odds are much higher between the antidepressant and placebo groups, both for suicides and suicidal acts. Still, we are talking about a tiny percentage of people taking antidepressants: 1.28 percent for the new antidepressants and 1.53 percent for SSRIs, according to Dr. Healy's figures. But the numbers conceivably could have been higher had the drug companies specifically measured for suicidal behavior.

Please do not chuck your antidepressants out the window. Population data indicates that untreated depression runs a far greater suicide risk than the bad effects of taking antidepressants. John Mann, MD, of Columbia University, representing the American Foundation for Suicide Prevention, told an FDA panel in 2204 that since 1987, after a steady three-decade rise, suicide rates in the United States began dropping. Women, who were prescribed twice the number of SSRIs as men, experienced proportionately lower drops in suicide rates. Areas in the United States with the highest SSRI prescription rates had the biggest decline in suicides. According to Dr. Mann, for every 10 percent increase in prescription rates, the U.S. suicide rate declined 3 percent.

What is not in dispute is that these meds can induce an unwanted state of mind in some patients, openly acknowledged in the product labeling. A 2001 Yale University retrospective review of hospital admissions found that 8.1 percent of patients admitted to a psychiatric unit over fourteen months were the result of antidepressant-induced mania or psychosis.

If you start feeling uncharacteristically hyper soon after beginning antidepressant treatment, call your doctor at once and stop taking the medication while you still have your wits about you. Your doctor may adjust your dose or switch medications to get you on something that works for you. If you are experiencing anxiety or agitation in the early going, the effect is usually temporary, but it is strongly advised that you keep your doctor informed.

Paxil Withdrawal

According to the BBC current-affairs program *Panorama,* aired in October 2002: "The Maudsley Hospital in London runs a national information service for people taking psychiatric medicines. Trouble coming off Seroxat [Paxil] is the number one complaint from callers. Doctors too report far more withdrawal problems from patients on Seroxat than on any other drug."

Said David Taylor, chief pharmacist at the Maudsley Hospital: "If a patient is to stop taking Seroxat suddenly, then usually they would quite soon become quite anxious. They may feel very dizzy and unsteady on their feet. Often people experience electric shock sensations. They may also have a fever and feel generally unwell and they also may experience mood changes or very vivid nightmares for example."

According to the World Health Organization, as reported in the July 21, 2002, issue of the *Guardian,* Paxil topped the list for drugs in terms of difficulty to quit, followed by Effexor at number two,

Zoloft at number four, and Prozac at number seven. The benzodi-azepines Ativan and Valium came in eleventh and thirteenth.

If you are on Paxil, please do not panic. Should you no longer need to stay on the drug, GlaxoSmithKline advises physicians to recommend "a gradual reduction in the dose rather than abrupt cessation." Paxil washes out of the system more quickly than other SSRIs when stopped. In recent clinical trials, GSK decreased the daily dose by 10 mg a week (doses can range from 10 to 60 mg a day), then stopped treatment after reducing the dose to 20 mg. The August 27, 2002, *Washington Post* reports Frederick Goodwin, MD, former head of the NIMH, as in favor of an even more gradual taper, "dropping the dose every four or five days by as little as possible, even if that means cutting pills in half."

The Placebo Factor

Invariably, a new drug's efficacy is compared to that mysterious entity known as the "placebo group." In a typical clinical drug trial, one group of patients, unknown to them, receives the experimental drug while another group unknowingly is given an inert compound having no medical benefit. Those assigned to hand out the real and dummy pills are not told which is which, thus ensuring a "double blind."

With antidepressant drug trials, the placebo effect is high enough to cause a full half of these studies to end in failure, which has set off fierce debate over whether an antidepressant is little more than a placebo with side effects. The focal point of the controversy are two studies by Irving Kirsch, PhD, of the University of Connecticut.

The first, a 1998 meta-analysis of nineteen double-blind anti-depressant trials, found that the placebo effect accounted for a mind-boggling 75 percent of an antidepressant's result—any anti-depressant, you name it.

Four years later, the July 2002 *Prevention and Treatment* published another study by Dr. Kirsch that analyzed the FDA database of forty-seven placebo-controlled short-term clinical trials involving the six most widely prescribed antidepressants approved between 1987 and 1999. These included "file-drawer" studies; that is, trials that failed but were never published.

What Dr. Kirsch found was that 80 percent of the medication response in the combined drug groups was duplicated in the placebo groups, and that the mean difference between the drug and the placebo was a "clinically insignificant" two points on both the seventeen-item and the twenty-one-item Hamilton Depression Rating Scale, regardless of the size of the drug dose. The placebo factor ranged from a high of 89 percent for the Prozac response, according to the study, and a low of 69 percent for the Paxil response. In four trials, the placebo equaled or achieved marginally better results than the drug.

Three commentators responding to the study briefly alluded to the fact that some patients may be more responsive to certain medications than others, but none of them drove home what many of us know from personal experience—that if our initial antidepressant doesn't work, it is good practice to try another one.

One of my newsletter readers, Ned, made this exact point after I first reported on the Kirsch study in my newsletter:

> *It is so frustrating and unfair to see those studies are misinterpreted to mean that "antidepressants are just placebos with side effects." I mean, if they are placebos, then how come so often the seventh one or the ninth one works? In 1984–5 I was tried on maybe six tricyclics, all failures, and then one MAO inhibitor, a fairly rapid and extremely impressive success. There is NO WAY that was a placebo effect.*

In the meantime, there is clinical consensus that antidepressants do work. It's just that we have no fail-safe method of proving it.

11

Bipolar Meds

The Meds

The story begins in an Australian lab in 1949 when John Cade, MD, senior medical officer in the Mental Hygiene Department of Victoria, had a hunch that urea would be effective in the treatment of bipolar disorder. He needed an agent to help the substance dissolve in water, which turned out to be the common salt lithium. He quickly found the solution had a calming affect on guinea pigs, but further experimentation showed that it was the lithium and not the urea that was the active ingredient. He then tried lithium on human subjects, with eye-popping results.

Lithium can be considered the first of the mood stabilizers—an agent that reduces the severe mood swings characteristic of bipolar disorder—and today it still remains a first-option treatment. It was approved by the FDA in 1970 for the treatment of mania.

Two drugs for treating epilepsy (commonly called anticonvulsants), Tegretol (carbamazepine) and Depakote (divalproex sodium), experienced similarly bizarre accidental discoveries. (Valproic acid, the compound on which Depakote is based, was the result of a search for a butter substitute by the Germans in World War II.) Depakote and a generic version of Tegretol are FDA-approved for treating mania.

Newer anticonvulsants include Lamictal (lamotrigine) for bipolar depression, Trileptal (oxcarbazepine) for mania, and Neurontin (gabapentin) and Topamax (topiramate) in various adjunctive capacities. Only Lamictal among these has an FDA bipolar indication.

Atypical (new generation) antipsychotics were developed for treating schizophrenia, but are now employed as first options for treating mania. Like the mood stabilizers, their discovery (of the first-generation meds) was accidental. Thorazine, an old-generation antipsychotic, debuted in the 1940s as a TB med.

Zyprexa (olanzapine), Risperdal (risperidone), Geodon (ziprasidone), Seroquel (quetiapine), and Abilify (aripiprazole) have been approved by the FDA for treatment of mania. Clozaril (clozapine) is used off-label as a last choice.

No Magic Bullet

Unfortunately, fewer than half of those who take mood stabilizers or antipsychotics achieve a satisfactory result without experiencing troublesome side effects. These can range from hair loss to rash to drowsiness to dulled cognition to weight gain to Parkinson's-like tremors to involuntary spasms. Not surprisingly, people with bipolar disorder have trouble remaining compliant with their medications.

Barring some intolerable side effect, however, you need to give your meds at least several weeks to work. We are all unique, but often the side effects are merely transient.

The other danger stems from the opposite pole, when the success of these medications leads some to mistakenly believe they are cured. Kay Jamison—one of the leading authorities on bipolar disorder, as well as a patient—admits this happened to her. Her inevitable relapse and attempt at suicide forced her to learn her lesson the hard way.

The intoxicating high of mania or hypomania also works against patients taking their meds. On my Web site, Kris, age seventeen, inquires: "When I'm manic, I love it. I feel great. I think to myself, 'why take meds, I don't need them.' When I'm depressed, I feel that the meds do nothing for me. Can someone please give me some advice on how to manage?"

To which I responded:

Hi, Kris. Your desire to not take meds is natural. That's the nature of this illness. You might want to do a cost-benefit analysis. In one column write down all the great things about being manic. Also note how many quality manic moments you have a month and how long they last. In another column, write down all your bad mania moments—the times you flew into rages, alienated your friends, couldn't do your schoolwork, couldn't concentrate, spent too much money, nearly killed yourself doing something stupid, and on and on and on, plus any hospitalizations or run-ins with the law. Add to that all your depression bummers. I'm sure that you will discover that you are paying one hell of a price for those few and relatively brief "quality" manic moments. Now ask yourself: Is it worth it? I'm sure you will make the right choice.

I should be so smart. Kris at least had the brains and the courage to seek help when she realized something was wrong with her. It took me till age forty-nine, after a lifetime of denial. At the time, I felt like an animal caught in a steel trap, forced to chew off its leg in order to free itself. There goes my creativity, I lamented, as I took my first pill.

Fortunately, my worst fear did not materialize, and I never had to put life on three legs to the test. My creativity emerged intact, and so I remain a model of compliance.

Lest one get me wrong, loss of mental acuity and quality of life should not be the price one has to pay for getting stabilized on meds. A universal complaint is that once on meds, one can wave good-bye to thinking with the preternatural clarity one has grown accustomed to. So fearful was I of this happening to me that soon after I was put on my meds, I went online and started taking every IQ test I could find.

Call it an identity crisis. Was my old "normal" really normal, or was it merely the artificial intelligence of hypomania, even when I wasn't demonstrably hypomanic? And heaven help this "new normal." If this is what true normal is, I hear from many, then I want no part of it.

It may take you some time to figure out your "real normal," but once you get a true read, you have the right to insist that your psychiatrist work with you in achieving it and maintaining it, or at least in getting you to within very close proximity. This includes your right to work with your psychiatrist in maintaining a mild hypomania, if that is your true baseline.

Nevertheless, so frightening is mania to the psychiatric profession that it is my belief that they tend to err on the side of over-sedating. When I put this to Kay Jamison in a 2003 interview, she replied:

"I think that's sometimes true, often true, maybe, but I think that's where people really need to go in and badger, really go in and say, look, is there any possibility of a different medication that might work or if I can take it in a lower amount? Are there any things that I can do that might mean I don't

*have to take as much medication? And that these are debili-
tating side effects. I think sometimes doctors have to hear it a
lot, and sometimes even put it in writing."*

The catch is how to properly badger your psychiatrist without
raising every professional alarm bell in his or her office. If your
complaint is something along the lines of "I can't think like I used
to," they are conditioned to react with something like "You're not
supposed to," though they will be far too polite to be so blunt. And
if you carry on about how nimble-witted and sociable and productive you used to be, their inclination is to reply, "But at what price?"

(Heaven help us, don't walk into their office happy—they are
likely to raise all your doses. Just joking, but not quite.)

What you need to do is frame your request in terms a psychiatrist
can relate to. First, put your psychiatrist at ease by acknowledging
how grateful you are to be stabilized on your meds and that you in-
tend remaining a model patient for life. Then carefully explain any
problems in cognitive function you may be experiencing. Use precisely that term, *cognitive function,* then itemize exactly how these
"cognitive deficits" are affecting you, with reference to objective
criteria, if you're able, such as not being able to meet work deadlines
or problems reading a book. At all costs, avoid the temptation to
brag about the Oscar Wilde/Noël Coward/Dorothy Parker you were
in your life before meds.

A competent psychiatrist will work with you in good faith, but
the responsibility of constructive engagement lies with you.

Be prepared to accept that there may be an old part of you that
you may have to let go of. I miss the mental fifth gear I used to have,
but many car wrecks along the way have forced me to acknowledge
the devastating liability of having a high-performance brain. I am
much better off in four gears, with some slippage in my ability to
play Jeopardy, but in firm possession of peace of mind rather than
bewailing the loss of pieces of mind.

Be advised that our meds may be our best insurance against further cognitive deterioration. As we discussed in an earlier chapter, bipolar disorder is more than just a mood disease—it attacks our ability to think and function, even in states of wellness. Left untreated, our illness is likely to render our brains to mush on its own accord. Please keep this in mind before you decide to quit on your meds.

Also keep in mind that a mood episode can be a traumatizing experience, with lingering effects, and that it takes time to heal. Over time, as nature takes its course, you may find your meds far more effective and less burdensome.

Even compliant patients face a high rate of relapse, and the reality is that full recovery without further episodes is rare. Nevertheless, when compared to the alternatives—a life of madness and institutionalization or worse—bipolar meds represent deliverance from one of the cruelest illnesses on the planet. The drugs may not work perfectly, there may be a lot of heartbreak in finding the right treatment followed by yet more heartbreak when a future episode breaks out, but the mood stabilizers and antipsychotics do hold out the prospect of leading a full and rewarding life, and for that we have a lot to be thankful.

Caveat

Before we engage in a detailed discussion of bipolar meds, it needs to be pointed out that the science that is supposed to be guiding us can mislead us as well as inform us. Compared with other illnesses, bipolar disorder is notoriously understudied and research unconscionably underfunded, resulting in a paucity of reliable study data. Much of the evidence for treatment is tentative at best and often contradicts other evidence, leading to disagreements among experts on matters that should have been laid to rest years ago. Accordingly, the most important thing you need to know is that you are unique and that what is said below may or may not apply to you.

The Mood Stabilizers

Lithium

According to a review of the literature by Mark Bauer, MD, and Landis Mitchner, MD, of Brown University, lithium is the only true mood stabilizer, with published studies proving its efficacy in all phases of bipolar treatment, including acute (initial phase) mania and mania prevention, and acute depression and depression prevention. This ability to be all things at once holds out the promise of a simplified one-drug treatment for those fortunate enough to respond.

On the flip side, as an augmenter, the drug can boost the performance of another drug.

These days, due to the lack of drug companies promoting the drug and the extra care doctors must use in treating patients with it, other medications have become more popular, though lithium still remains a first-choice option on all the treatment guidelines.

The evidence strongly suggests that lithium works well for uncomplicated euphoric mania but is considered problematic for rapid-cycling, mixed states, and co-occurring illnesses such as anxiety or substance use. Lithium also tends to work better in patients who have few mood episodes.

For suicide prevention, lithium users experienced one-third to one-half the suicidality compared to Depakote users.

Because of lithium's toxicity, regular blood levels are required. The modern therapeutic window for lithium is 0.6 to 1.0 milliequivalent per liter (mEq/l), lower than the recommended 0.8 to 1.2 mEq/l of the past.

Dehydration resulting from, say, a fever may raise lithium levels, while sodium and caffeine may lower levels. To avoid dehydration, it is advisable to maintain an adequate daily fluid intake. Since lithium is a salt, you will almost certainly find yourself craving fluids anyway. Dasani is to a lithium user as Tang is to an astronaut.

The drug carries a risk of renal failure over the long term, as well as hypothyroidism (the latter can be corrected by a thyroid supplement).

In its *Practice Guideline for the Treatment of Patients with Bipolar Disorder* (2002), the APA says that up to 75 percent of patients treated with lithium experience side effects, usually of a minor nature that can be reduced or eliminated by reducing the dose or changing the dosing schedule. Slow-release preparations that smooth out lithium concentrations in the blood are advised.

The most visible side effect is tremors, sometimes of Parkinson's dimensions. As well as making dose adjustments, tremor can be ameliorated by reducing caffeine or adding a beta-blocker. Other common complaints are gastrointestinal (nausea, diarrhea, increased urine output), cognitive impairment, weight gain (13.9 pounds in one study), hair loss, and skin problems.

Depakote (divalproex sodium)

Because of lithium's shortcomings in treating rapid-cycling, mixed episodes, and mania complicated by co-occurring disorders, Depakote is the treatment of choice here. It is also as effective as lithium for treatment in the acute (initial) stage and maintenance stages of mania, and is also favored for use in patients with co-occurring substance use.

A 1994 study found the drug successful for patients with ten or more episodes, while lithium failed at this threshold.

Depakote is not regarded as a drug for treating bipolar depression. Some small studies have found there may be a use, but strong evidence is lacking.

The drug takes at least three weeks to achieve its full effect. A 2003 Abbott Laboratories pooled analysis of 348 manic patients found those on high doses of Depakote from the outset did better at days five, seven, eight, and ten than those on the standard gradual dose, and fared the same as those on Zyprexa, with better tolerability than Zyprexa.

Because of its toxicity, regular blood tests are required. The drug's packaging carries black-box warnings about the risk of damage to the liver, neural-tube defects to the fetus (3 to 8 percent during the first trimester), and pancreatitis (very remote). The labeling also advises that Tegretol can double the clearance of Depakote, which means raising its dose accordingly if you are taking both drugs together. The labeling additionally advises that doses of Lamictal need to be lowered if taken with Depakote.

Depakote is a notorious weight gainer (fourteen pounds in one study). Those who are put on the drug are advised to immediately replace their Ben & Jerry's with nonfat frozen yogurt and find other low-fat or nonfat alternatives at once, and cut down on sugar.

The drug poses certain risks for young females, and the following warning posted on the Web site of the NIMH bears quoting:

Valproate may increase testosterone levels in teenage girls and produce polycystic ovary syndrome in women who began taking the medication before age 20. Increased testosterone can lead to polycystic ovary syndrome with irregular or absent menses, obesity, and abnormal growth of hair. Therefore, young female patients taking valproate should be monitored carefully by a physician.

The antidote to this is folate.

Tegretol, Equetro (carbamazepine)

Because the drug's manufacturer, Novartis, did not pursue an FDA indication for mania, no large studies have been done until recently, even though its efficacy was widely recognized. That changed when Shire Pharmaceuticals recompounded the formula, funded successful trials, and was granted an FDA indication. The drug contains a black-box warning about risk of agranulocytosis (affecting white blood cells), but that risk is extremely remote.

Tegretol induces the enzyme cytochrome P450 34A, which can affect the metabolism of other drugs and reduce their efficacy, including other psychiatric drugs and oral contraceptives. Accordingly, those taking concomitant Depakote, Lamictal, Topamax, antipsychotics, benzodiazepines such as Xanax, and tricyclic antidepressants need to consider raising the doses.

The drug's labeling warns that dual administration of Tegretol and lithium may increase the risk of neurotoxic side effects.

On the reverse side of the coin, the following psychiatric drugs can raise Tegretol levels: Depakote, Luvox, Prozac, and Serzone.

Trileptal (oxcarbazepine)

Trileptal is what is known as an analog of Tegretol, a structural derivative of the older drug. In theory, all the data about the efficacy of Tegretol should apply to Trileptal, but this hasn't been tested.

The drug is generating a good deal of buzz because it apparently has the benefits of Tegretol without causing the type of drug-drug interactions of its chemical cousin.

Lamictal (lamotrigine)

Lamictal is being touted as the one mood stabilizer singularly effective for bipolar depression, even though the drug does not have an FDA indication for this purpose. Instead, in June 2003, the FDA approved Lamictal for the long-term maintenance of bipolar I to delay the time to occurrence of mood episodes.

The manufacturer, GlaxoSmithKline (GSK), sold the FDA on the strength of two studies involving 1,305 bipolar I patients who were stabilized, then put on either lithium, Lamictal, or a placebo for eighteen months. Lamictal was found to be superior to lithium at delaying time to relapse into a depressive episode, while lithium was superior to Lamictal at delaying time to relapse into mania.

In granting its indication, the FDA did allow GSK to put on the product package labeling that the findings for Lamictal maintenance treatment were "more robust for depression."

The reason why GSK did not go the usual route in seeking an indication for the acute (initial) phase of treatment probably has to do with the fact that the drug requires very slow gradual loading over six weeks before patients are finally put on a clinical dose. Nevertheless, a 1999 study involving 195 patients did find that even doses in the lower range (50 mg/day) produced a benefit over seven weeks.

The drug has the advantage of low incidence of weight gain, but contains a black-box warning about risk of serious rash, which was found in 0.08 percent of adults receiving Lamictal as initial therapy for bipolar disorder and 0.13 percent for those receiving the drug as adjunctive therapy. The risk of rash is greater in children and adolescents, and is only approved for this group in treating a certain form of epilepsy. The labeling recommends that the drug be discontinued at the first sign of rash and not be restarted unless the potential benefits clearly outweigh the risks.

Owing to risk of serious rash (Stevens-Johnson syndrome in its most extreme form), GSK recommends gradual increases to a full dose, starting at 25 mg/day for the first two weeks, 50 mg/day for weeks three and four, 100 mg/day for week five, and 200 mg/day for week six.

If also on Depakote, GSK recommends 25 mg every other day for the first week, 25 mg/day for weeks three and four, 50 mg/day for week five, and 100 mg/day for week six.

If also on Tegretol or other enzyme-inducing drugs, the recommended schedule is 50 mg/day for weeks one and two, 100 mg/day in divided doses for weeks three and four, 200 mg/day in divided doses for week five, 300 mg/day in divided doses for week six, and 400 mg/day in divided doses for week seven.

If you are discontinuing the drug, GSK recommends a gradual taper over two weeks, unless safety concerns require a more rapid withdrawal.

Neurontin (gabapentin)

For treating mania, studies have found it is better to use a placebo. The drug is reputed to be effective, however, as an add-on for anxiety, which frequently co-occurs with bipolar disorder.

Topamax (topiramate)

Topamax is receiving notice for its appetite-diminishing and weight-reducing properties (in one study, patients experienced a mean weight loss of thirteen pounds at the end of one year). It has few interactions with other mood stabilizers, which facilitates its use as adjunctive therapy. Unfortunately, it is not the antimania agent its manufacturer, Ortho-McNeil, was hoping it would be.

As an add-on, the drug may have a benefit. A 2004 study of fifty-six patients with various types of bipolar disorder who were not responsive to lithium, Depakote, or Tegretol found that fifty-three reacted well when the drug was added.

The drug's greatest benefit may lie in treating behaviors and effects that go with bipolar disorder and bipolar meds, including impulsivity, bulimia, binge eating, substance use, post-traumatic stress disorder (PTSD), and obesity. As Susan McElroy, MD, of the University of Cincinnati, put it during a 2003 grand rounds lecture at UCLA: "I use it in bipolar when managing some of the shmutz that goes with the illness."

For some people, the drug noticeably dulls cognition, which is why it is unofficially known as "Dopamax."

Antipsychotics

Recent studies have challenged the claim that the newer atypicals are more efficacious and have a better side-effects profile than the older antipsychotics. The main point of contention is that first generation antipsychotics such as Haldol (haloperidol) may be getting a bad rap because patients in old studies received extremely high doses. Indeed, in the old days, it was standard practice when starting treatment to raise the dose until the patient exhibited muscular twitching and involuntary spasms collectively known as EPS (extrapyramidal symptoms). Then the dose was adjusted slightly downward.

Tardive dyskinesia refers to chronic EPS symptoms, generally setting in after six months or more.

The atypicals also pose their own risk of EPS and tardive dyskinesia. The drugs also run the risk of sedation, cognitive dulling, weight gain, diabetes, sexual dysfunction and raised prolactin, and heart-rhythm irregularity. Some of these effects involve just one drug, others more than one.

Before proceeding further, it is important to note that risk does not equate with certainty. Risk is obviously something that needs to be discussed with your psychiatrist. On the other hand, a psychiatrist who prescribes Zyprexa to a borderline diabetic before trying other meds is probably guilty of malpractice.

EPS

According to Zyprexa's labeling, 46 percent of patients report at least one EPS effect at approximately 15 mg a day, 34 percent at approximately 10 mg a day, and 23 percent at approximately 5 mg a day. Risperdal has a 13 to 31 percent risk of EPS, depending on dose, and Geodon has an 11 percent risk. Seroquel and Clozaril run slight risks, while Abilify—other than the possibility of initial akathisia (a type of mental restlessness)—has virtually none.

Dosing recommendations when the atypicals first hit the market were either too high or too low or too vague, but it is now generally accepted that the following doses equate to 8 mg of the old-generation Haldol: Zyprexa (15 mg), Seroquel (500 mg), Risperdal (3 mg), Geodon (100 mg), and Abilify (15 mg).

Tardive Dyskinesia

The labeling on the atypicals all warn of potentially permanent "dyskinetic" movements (such as involuntary spasms). As opposed to EPS, which is immediate and usually transitory, tardive dyskinesia manifests over time, in all likelihood as the result of cumulative doses. Accordingly, the labeling advises to continue with long-term treatment only if other treatments are not effective. The labeling also advises the smallest dose for the shortest duration.

For tardive dyskinesia, says the APA's *Practice Guideline for the Treatment of Patients with Schizophrenia* (2004), the risk that atypicals pose is about one-tenth that of the older-generation antipsychotics.

Sedation

Nearly all of the atypicals are potential horse tranquilizers, often merely in the initial phase of treatment before the body has a chance to adjust, but severe enough to be worrying, especially in these days of hit-and-run psychiatry, when patients are sent out onto the streets disoriented and confused after maybe one or two nights in the hospital. In clinical trials, 39 percent of patients on Clozaril reported sedation, followed by Zyprexa at 29 percent, Seroquel at 18 percent, Geodon at 14 percent, and Abilify at 12 percent. Only Risperdal caused no apparent sedation.

Seroquel's sedating effect is paradoxically most potent in the lower dose range (100 to 200 mg), which makes it a favored sleep aid by psychiatrists (generally on an "as-needed" basis, often at doses as low as 25 mg).

Sexual Dysfunction

A 2003 Spanish study of 636 outpatients over four weeks or more found that frequency of sexual dysfunction was high with Haldol, Zyprexa, and Risperdal (38.1 percent, 35.3 percent, and 43.2 percent, respectively). Seroquel users experienced sexual dysfunction at a rate of 18.2 percent.

A 2000 FDA briefing document reported that Risperdal elevated blood prolactin to more than 90, well above Haldol (at less than 30) and Zyprexa (at a borderline less than 20). The other atypicals did not result in significantly high prolactin levels. Hyperprolactinemia turns off ovaries and testes function, increasing risk of breast lactation and breast enlargement, leading to disrupted menstrual function and impaired sexual function in women and impotence and loss of libido in men. The APA's schizophrenia *Practice Guideline* reports that women suffer these effects more than men.

Weight Gain

A 1999 study found that Clozaril resulted in a mean weight gain of 9.8 pounds in ten weeks, 9.1 for Zyprexa, 6.4 for Risperdal, and negligible for Geodon. Seroquel wasn't evaluated, and Abilify was unavailable at the time. A 1997 study found patients on Zyprexa gained twenty-seven pounds over one year. Product labeling shows nearly 30 percent of Zyprexa users added 7 percent or more body weight over six weeks and 56 percent over one year. Twenty percent of Seroquel users, more than 15 percent of Risperdal users, around 10 percent of Geodon users, and less than 10 percent of Abilify users crossed this "clinically significant" threshold over the short term.

Diabetes

With weight gain and change of metabolism comes the risk of diabetes. In 2003, Eli Lilly and the other manufacturers added a diabetes warning to their product labeling.

In 2004, a joint panel of the American Diabetes Association, the American Psychiatric Association, the American Association of Clinical Endocrinologists, and the North American Association for the Study of Obesity issued a consensus statement recommending that doctors screen and monitor their patients on atypical antipsychotics for (1) personal and family history of obesity, diabetes, high cholesterol, hypertension, or cardiovascular disease; (2) weight and height; (3) waist circumference; (4) blood pressure; (5) fasting blood glucose; and (6) fasting blood cholesterol.

The panel also advised doctors to refer their patients to specialists, if necessary.

The Drugs

Zyprexa (olanzapine)
In addition to Zyprexa's antimanic effect, recent studies have found a modest but significant antidepressive effect, possibly enough to qualify for an FDA indication for this phase of the illness. Instead, Eli Lilly went to the FDA with a Zyprexa-Prozac combo, found to be more potent than Zyprexa alone, according to clinical trials.

Symbyax
In 2003, the FDA approved Lilly's combination Zyprexa-Prozac pill, Symbyax, to treat bipolar depression, the first med indicated expressly for such a use.

The same worries about diabetes and hyperglycemia, drowsiness, weight gain, EPS, and other concerns in Zyprexa also apply to Symbyax.

Clozaril (clozapine)

Clozaril is the first of the atypicals, but because weekly blood work is required due to risk of damage to white blood cells (agranulocytosis), the drug is regarded as a last treatment option. The black box on the product labeling also carries warnings of the risk of seizures, fatal myocarditis, and other cardiovascular and respiratory effects.

Treatment guidelines recommend its use as a last option for treatment-refractory patients.

Risperdal (risperidone)

In 2003, the drug's manufacturer, Janssen, received FDA approval to market Risperdal for acute mania and for mixed episodes.

Seroquel (quetiapine)

In 2004, the FDA approved Seroquel for the treatment of acute mania, either as monotherapy or as an adjunct to lithium or Depakote. A major 2005 study found the drug also has a significant and fast-acting antidepressant effect.

Geodon (ziprasidone)

In 2004, the FDA approved Geodon for treating acute mania and mixed episodes.

The FDA delayed approving the drug for several years due to worries over heart rhythms (lengthening of the so-called QTC interval of the heartbeat). The drug's labeling contains warnings about QTC prolongation and the possible risk of sudden death, but does not include the dreaded black-box warning. As of 2005, with 2 million patients treated on Geodon and no QTC-related deaths, psychiatrists are regarding the QTC issue as behind them.

Abilify (aripiprazole)

The drug is being touted as having a relatively benign side-effects profile.

Combination Therapy

At the 2001 DBSA annual conference, Joseph Calabrese, MD, of Case Western Reserve University, observed: "The main thing I have learned over the last decade is there is no one medicine that does the job." Combination therapy is now standard, with three or more drugs considered normal, and the emphasis is on using meds that have complementary efficacy, such as Lamictal (which is strong against depression) and Zyprexa (which works from the opposite pole on mania).

At the 2003 APA annual meeting, Frederick Goodwin, MD, cited several rationale for using combined therapy to treat bipolar disorder, including:

▐ Targeting different symptom clusters, such as those mentioned by Dr. Calabrese.
▐ Different mechanisms of action. Lithium and Depakote have multiple targets in the signal transduction pathways inside the neuron that may complement one another.
▐ Nonresponse or partial response. For example, one study of adding Zyprexa to lithium or Depakote found the combination kept patients well longer than either mood stabilizer alone.
▐ Side effects. Adding two meds together at lower doses may keep each drug below its side-effects profile. One study of 140 bipolar I patients found 59 percent compliance with Depakote monotherapy, 48 percent compliance with lithium monotherapy, but 100 percent compliance with combined therapy at less than full doses.

On the downside, combination therapy raises the potential danger of toxic drug interactions, which can be minimized by adding new medication in modest amounts and raising the dose slowly.

Unfortunately, the main message from combination treatment is that our meds leave much to be desired. As Bruce Cohen, MD, PhD, psychiatrist in chief of McLean Hospital in Belmont, Massachusetts, explained at the 2004 APA annual meeting, "putting people on mixed cocktails indicates to me that we don't have the right medications."

It is not uncommon to include benzodiazepines such as Valium (diazepam), Klonopin (clonazepam), and Ativan (lorazepam) as part of the mix, especially in situations where stabilization and the need to establish sleep is a top priority. But because of their depressant effects and dangers of addiction, these agents are generally regarded as a short-term solution. Many psychiatrists, however, feel the addiction potential is overstated.

Combination therapy with an antipsychotic and a mood stabilizer is now recommended as a first choice in most treatment guidelines. A large 2002 Harvard University study found that either Risperdal or Haldol with a mood stabilizer outperformed a mood stabilizer alone. Other studies have found that Zyprexa or Seroquel combined with a mood stabilizer was more effective than a mood stabilizer alone.

Short-Term Treatment for Mania

Psychiatry breaks down treating patients into two phases: (1) the acute (or initial) phase, with the goal of stabilizing patients, hopefully to remission; and (2) the maintenance (or continuation) phase, following remission, which can go on for several years to life, with the goal of preventing relapses and maintaining full functioning.

Essentially, it boils down to getting well and staying well.

In its *Practice Guideline,* the APA suggests that an atypical antipsychotic combined with either lithium or Depakote may be more effective than either of these agents alone. For patients who are less ill, monotherapy with one of these drugs may be sufficient.

The first option if patients continue to experience episodes is to optimize doses. When first-line medications fail, the APA recommends changing drugs.

The Texas Implentation of Medication Algorithms (TIMA) *Bipolar Algorithms*, put out by the state of Texas and, the British Association for Psychopharmocology's (BAP) *Guidelines*, by contrast, recommend a one-drug first approach, and then moving to combination therapy if the results are less than optimal.

Treating Hypomania

Owing to a complete lack of data, the guidelines are silent on treating hypomania. Since hypomania can represent a legitimate baseline for many, on the one hand, or a precursor to full-blown mania for others, this is a matter of grave concern. In an interview, John Gartner, PhD, author of *The Hypomanic Edge,* informed this writer, "the most common form of this disorder is being treated as if it were a rare weird variation."

When psychiatrists become aware of hypomania in their patients, he went on to say: "I think their tendency is to overreact, react as if it is the same as mania." Dr. Gartner likens a patient with hypomania to the pitcher in *Bull Durham,* "the guy who has the one-hundred-mile-per-hour fastball but keeps beaning the mascot." You want to give him just enough medicine to establish control, not slow him down to fifty miles per hour.

Even less known is how to treat the mixed states in hypomania, your classic road-rage cases that the *DSM* has overlooked. Think of the pitcher in *Bull Durham* again, this time deliberately beaning the batter. Short of Susan Sarandon rushing out of the stands urging him close his eyes and chant, "Om," psychiatry has no definitive answers.

Long-Term Treatment

The World Federation of Societies of Biological Psychiatry's (WFSBP) *Guidelines for the Biological Treatment of Bipolar Disorders: Maintenance Treatment* (2004) notes: "Although it is of great importance to control these acute manifestations as rapidly and effectively as possible, the real key to treatment of bipolar disorder is successful maintenance treatment." Unfortunately, psychiatry is largely flying in the dark for this phase of treatment. The treatment guidelines are fairly consistent about simplifying the meds regime, generally on the basis that what gets you well does not necessarily keep you well. The APA, for example, takes a dim view of keeping a patient on an atypical antipsychotic, owing to risk of tardive dyskinesia, but does warrant its use to control persistent psychosis or as protection against recurrence.

In what can be regarded as an appalling oversight, these guidelines have nothing to say regarding lowered doses. Virtually all drug studies are based on treating severe mania in the acute phase, which is also the focus of most clinical training. The few maintenance-phase studies have used high doses with alarmingly high dropout rates.

In the old days, psychiatrists had the time to work carefully with hospitalized patients in finding the right dose on one or two meds. These days, clinicians are under pressure to get their patients out the door in a matter of days, if not the next day. Since these are psychiatric emergencies, there is sound rationale for pharmaceutical overkill. But there is a huge difference between medicating a person out of danger and medicating a person into recovery.

Discharged and often disoriented patients then must negotiate their way through the notorious gaps in the health-care system to one of any variety of overworked outpatient providers not equipped to take on the time-consuming challenge of meds changes and dose adjustments. Moreover, many psychiatrists fear landing in professional hot water should their taking a patient off some meds or lowering doses result in another hospitalization.

All too many times, a patient's pleas about feeling like a fat stupid zombie fall on deaf ears. Inevitably, patients quit taking their meds, and then get cruelly blamed for once more landing in the hospital.

You are entitled to challenge your psychiatrist to experiment with low doses, even if they are far lower than what is recommended on the label. In an eye-opening interview, Ross Baldessarini, MD, of Harvard, a pioneer in the treatment of lithium, informed this writer that "Americans tend to be the cowboys of psychopharmacology." Patients, he said, "might feel their wings are being clipped" on too much medication.

"Go lightly on the lithium," he urged. When I put to him the possibility of treating hypomania or the maintenance phase of bipolar disorder with lower than standard doses, he replied: "It is plausible."

Assuming you are acutely attuned to your shifts in moods, it is a fairly simple procedure to bump the dose back up (perhaps temporarily and with your psychiatrist's approval) should you feel yourself cycling into an episode.

Mind you, there are often valid reasons for having as many pills in your medicine cabinet as New England has Red Sox fans. For one, rare is the individual who just has bipolar disorder, and a simplified form of the illness at that. A rapid-cycling bipolar patient, for example, who has breakthrough psychotic episodes, is frequently suicidal, experiences anxiety, has trouble sleeping, needs to lose weight, and has side-effect tremors may need to exchange his medicine cabinet for a walk-in closet.

In the meantime, you need to ask yourself: Do you know why you are taking every medication in your cocktail, what symptom it is treating, in which phase, for how long it is expected to be taken, its benefits versus its risks, and how it complements and interacts with the other drugs? Does your doctor or psychiatrist know?

Treating Rapid-Cycling

Those who rapid-cycle represent a moving target. Seminars on treating rapid-cycling are as plentiful at mental-health conferences as vine-ripened tomatoes in winter. The reason is simple. Psychiatry knows next to nothing.

The treatment guidelines are all uniformly vague on how to treat this aspect of the illness, except for the unequivocal injunction that antidepressants—with their risk of bringing on rapid-cycling—should not be used. This comes as cold comfort to rapid-cyclers, who generally need pharmaceutical support from all points of the compass.

A 1974 study concluded that lithium was a poor agent for treating rapid-cycling, but a 1980 study found that eliminating antidepressants from the mix dramatically enhanced the efficacy of lithium.

Finding the right combination of meds can be a discouraging process, but it is not hopeless. And in getting those meds to work, please don't tempt fate. You are a delicate scale that can easily be tipped in either direction, so ixnay to caffeine and high-sugar foods and bad lifestyle choices.

Bipolar Depression Treatment

We know that Lamictal, Seroquel, and Symbyax (and by implication other atypical antipsychotic-SSRI combos), and to a certain extent lithium, to be reasonably effective for treating bipolar depression, but what about an antidepressant (usually with a mood stabilizer)?

In the December 2003 *Bipolar Disorders*—which was largely devoted to the topic—S. Nassir Ghaemi, MD, of Emory University and others imply that the reward is not worth the risk. Four studies found that the tricyclics did not outperform lithium and another that lithium plus Paxil did no better than lithium alone. Moreover, discontinuing an antidepressant does not appear to pose the same kind of danger as it does for unipolar depression. Finally, Prozac poop-out appears to loom much larger for bipolar patients (a 57.5 percent relapse rate compared to 18.4 percent for unipolar patients, according to another small study).

The picture may change, however, in the case of bipolar II, where mania by definition is not a feature of this shade of the illness, according to an article in the same issue of *Bipolar Disorders* by Jay Amsterdam, MD, and David Brunswick, MD, of the University of Pennsylvania. Moreover, it may be safe to administer an antidepressant to this population without a mood stabilizer, say the authors.

The BAP *Guidelines* recommend an antidepressant plus an antimania agent, while the APA *Practice Guideline* is stricter, recommending an antidepressant (with lithium) as a first option only for severely ill patients. The TIMA *Bipolar Algorithms*, by contrast, advise adding an antidepressant to an antimania agent only after Lamictal, Symbyax, and Seroquel have failed. All three guidelines are vague or tentative in regard to their suggestions for long-term treatment, all three acknowledge the paucity of data to guide them, and none of them distinguish bipolar I from bipolar II.

In a study published in the July 2003 *American Journal of Psychiatry*, Lori Altshuler, MD, and colleagues examined data from the Stanley Foundation Bipolar Network (comprising six treatment locales in the United States and Europe). Less than half of the patients remained on their antidepressants (with mood stabilizers) for two months or more and less than half again responded, which is not exactly a resounding thumbs-up for these meds. But those who did respond were far better off staying on antidepressants, with far fewer relapses into depression.

Basically, according to the study, about 15 percent of bipolar patients may benefit from antidepressants. The problem is we don't know which 15 percent.

Pregnancy and Breast-feeding

At a symposium at the APA's 2003 annual meeting, Zachary Stowe, MD, of Emory University, asked the psychiatrists in the audience how many of them treated women of reproductive age. Just about everyone raised their hands. How many treat these patients with folate? he asked. A minority raised their hands. How many give these patients a pregnancy test? he asked. No one raised their hands.

"You must treat all women patients of reproductive age as if they were pregnant on the first day," Dr. Stowe advised. The rate of birth defects for women on psychiatric meds is 1 in 11, he said, with the danger period in the first trimester, especially for patients on lithium and the antiepileptic mood stabilizers.

In another symposium, Lee Cohen, MD, of Harvard, outlined some of those risks.

For lithium, the risk of fetal heart defects, especially Ebstein's anomaly, is 0.05 percent in the first trimester, ten to twenty times that of the general population. For Depakote, there is a 3 to 8 percent risk of fetal spina bifida in the first trimester, and an unspecified risk of heart defects and behavioral abnormalities. For Tegretol, there is a 0.5 to 1 percent risk of spina bifida in the first trimester and an unspecified risk of craniofacial anomalies and microcephaly. Lamictal is probably the safest of the anticonvulsants, with manufacturer GlaxoSmithKline's registry of 293 pregnancies through September 2002 showing no major birth defects (keeping in mind this symposium was sponsored by GSK).

Dr. Stowe advised that "new and improved" meds means that there is no data. Older-generation antipsychotics, such as Haldol, are considered safe during all phases of pregnancy, while there is little data for the newer atypicals, such as Zyprexa. Factors that need to be considered are obesity and hyperglycemia side effects, which are risk factors for congenital malformations. Risperdal, which can cause hyperprolactinemia (affecting menstrual and sexual function), could be problematic during pregnancy.

No decision is risk free, both speakers observed. Those thinking of going off their meds need to consider that maternal depression can result in higher rates of drug, alcohol, and substance use; poor self-care, nutrition, and sleep; and preterm labor and babies with lower birth weights and developmental deficits.

Planned pregnancy is the safest way to go in terms of fetal risk. For women with bipolar disorder, tapering and discontinuing mood stabilizers is advised prior to conceiving. Stopping mood stabilizers on discovering one is pregnant (say, after five weeks) may be too late, as one is well into the teratogenic (birth defects) phase by this time. For severe bipolar disorder, staying on a mood stabilizer throughout all phases of pregnancy may be considered. Going back on a mood stabilizer is recommended for the second and third trimesters, with this very important proviso: that more than one med increases the chance of birth defects. Dr. Stowe advised that women should not be exposed to a second medication, as there is no data. Monotherapy, he said, at any dose is preferable to two meds, and switching meds at delivery is dumb. One gram of folate is recommended for all women—up to four grams if a woman is on Depakote.

Other options for pregnant women include psychotherapy, ECT, light therapy, calcium channel blockers, and omega-3.

For those wishing to avoid pregnancy, Tegretol, Trileptal, and Topamax accelerate the metabolism of estrogen and progesterone, which can result in birth-control failure.

In its *Practice Guideline,* the APA advises that women who choose to remain on their mood stabilizers should be screened for fetal neural-tube defects before the twentieth week of gestation and go for ultrasound at sixteen to eighteen weeks to detect any cardiac abnormalities in the fetus. Since pregnancy can affect medication levels, periodic monitoring is necessary. At delivery, lithium levels rise dramatically unless care is taken to ensure hydration or lowering the dose or both.

Being stabilized prior to giving birth is critical, as the risk for postpartum relapse for bipolar patients who are ill during pregnancy is nearly 70 percent, according to a 1998 Harvard study, as opposed to 27.8 percent for those who stay well during pregnancy.

Our Right to Remission

The most significant mental-health event of the new millennium thus far may be this sleeper, the inclusion of this sentence in the APA's 2002 *Practice Guideline:* "Treatment is aimed at stabilization of the episode with the goal of achieving remission, defined as a complete return to baseline level of functioning and a virtual lack of symptoms." The *Guideline* goes on to list prevention of future episodes as a goal of long-term treatment.

By contrast, the 1994 APA *Guideline* virtually wrote us off: "The specific goals of treatment are to decrease the frequency, severity, and psychosocial consequences of episodes and to improve psychosocial functioning between episodes. Some patients with severe and chronic impairments will need specific rehabilitative services."

In no uncertain terms, the APA has now put its members on notice that quitting on us is not an option, notwithstanding the severity of our symptoms or past treatment failures. In essence, our right to get well and stay well, with current medications and other treatments, has been codified, and in this era of rising costs and deteriorating services, that's no small feat.

Also implicit in that one sentence in the most recent *Guideline* is the proposition that any trade-off between symptom reduction and medication side effects is unacceptable. Psychiatrists who like to play it safe by oversedating their patients are operating outside the bounds of these new guidelines.

Newer treatments and expanding knowledge will soon render this *Guideline* obsolete. But there is no turning back from its governing principle of "achieving remission . . . return to baseline level of functioning and a virtual lack of symptoms."

This may not be possible in the early and middle going, but in the long term you should not have to settle for anything less.

12

Treating Other Illnesses and Symptoms

Anxiety

Many of the same treatments for depression work well for the different types of anxiety, including cognitive therapy and other talking therapies that focus on coping skills, as well as meds. Right lifestyle choices such as diet, exercise, and sleep are also critical; yoga and meditation are virtually mandatory; and natural treatments such as supplements are also an option.

Principal meds include SSRIs and benzodiazepines (which are potentially habit forming), plus Buspar (buspirone), Neurontin (gabapentin), and Anafranil (clomipramine; for obsessive-compulsive disorder).

Sleep

Benzodiazepines are the most common medication sleep aids, with antianxiety and muscle-relaxant properties. Their major disadvantages include daytime sedation and possible abuse or dependence. The most widely prescribed hypnotic is Halcion (triazolam). Others include Xanax (alprazolam), Valium (diazepam), Ativan (lorazepam), and Klonopin (clonazepam).

Benzodiazepine receptor agonists such as Sonata (zalepon) and Ambien (zolpidem) are said to promote better sleep than the benzodiazepines, but they run a similar risk of dependence, especially after a few weeks on high doses.

Both classes of meds are generally prescribed on a short-term basis, as needed. In 2004, the FDA approved the novel sleep aid Lunesta (eszopiclone) for long-term sleep.

Over-the-counter sleep aids contain antihistamines as their main ingredient, with potentially significant side effects, including sedation, psychomotor impairment, and the blocking of nerve impulses.

Natural sleep agents include melatonin, which is secreted by the pineal gland, and the herb valerian.

One's psychiatric meds may be enrolled in the cause. The following antidepressants have a sedative effect: the tricyclics, plus the novel antidepressants Serzone and Remeron.

Two mood drugs are commonly prescribed in low doses for sleeping. Desyrel (trazodone) is a novel antidepressant very rarely used as such. It is often prescribed as a sleep med, with the advantage that it is nonaddictive and can be taken on as as-needed basis. Low-dose Seroquel, an atypical antipsychotic, also has the advantage of being nonaddictive.

Please ask your physician about the correct time for taking sleep meds. You may be one who is knocked out right away, but in general meds require an hour or more as a head start.

For those having trouble staying awake, there is what some are referring to as the next lifestyle drug, Provigil (modafinil). This drug is being promoted as an agent with a new chemical action that combats fatigue without the jittery highs associated with caffeine and other drugs. Moreover, the manufacturer claims that the drug does not interfere with normal sleep. At present, the drug is only FDA approved for narcolepsy, but it is also being used off-label to treat hypersomnia associated with atypical depression. A 2003 study found Provigil rapidly reduced fatigue and improved wakefulness and concentration in depressed patients, and was well tolerated.

The danger with this drug is that many could abuse it to sustain a dangerous workaholic lifestyle. Please consider it only if you have trouble staying awake during the day.

Then there are the activating antidepressants, which include Wellbutrin, the SSRIs, Effexor, and the MAOIs.

The SSRIs are known to reduce REM sleep (the period of rapid eye movement, when dreaming occurs), but because people who are depressed experience too much REM, this may be a good thing for some individuals.

Pain

Since pain and mood share common neurotransmitters, it is not surprising that antidepressants work reasonably well for pain. One review found that antidepressants worked to a "mild to moderate degree" on headache, migraine, facial pain, nerve pain, rheumatic pain, and probably arthritis and rheumatoid arthritis, though not lower back pain.

Eli Lilly is heavily promoting its new dual-action antidepressant, Cymbalta, as a pain reliever. A 2005 study of depressed patients found the drug lowered overall pain in 25 to 50 percent of the patients, but the effect occurred independently of the resolution of their depression symptoms.

Traditional painkillers from aspirin to Oxycondone (marketed in various strengths as Percocet, Percodan, and OxyContin) are also options. One needs to be mindful that these and other painkillers can be highly addictive and are subject to abuse.

Other options include keeping a pain diary, starting a graduated exercise program, occupational therapy, yoga, stretching, relaxation techniques, acupuncture, chiropractic manipulation, homeopathy, hypnosis, and biofeedback.

Cognitive Dysfunction

A 2003 study of twenty-four patients on low doses of the Alzeimher's drugs Exelon (rivastigmine) and Reminyl (galantamine) found seventeen of them significantly improved their cognitive symptoms after three months.

High doses of vitamins are also an option (more on this shortly). Ginkgo biloba, found to be promising for treating age-related memory problems, may also help.

Apathy

Small studies and clinical experience have found that apathetic patients have responded to meds that activate dopamine and/or enhance what is called cholinergic function (vital to cognition). These include the Parkinson's meds Symmetrel (amantadine) and Parlodel (bromocriptine); the Alzheimer's meds Aricept (donepezil) and Exelon (rivastigmine); amphetamine; Wellbutrin; Ritalin; and selegiline.

Meds Side Effects

Should unwarranted side effects develop, you should alert your psychiatrist and ask for either a new med or to lower the dose or change the scheduling of the dosing. When that doesn't work, the Texas Implementation of Medical Algorithms (TIMA) *Bipolar Algorithms* recommends specific steps for the following side effects.

GI upset. Take medication with food and large amounts of liquid; use histamine blockers such as Tagamet and Zantac.

Mild tremor. Add 20 to 30 mg Inderal (propranolol), a beta-blocker.

Parkinsonian tremor. Divide dosing; add 1 to 2 mg Cogentin (benztropine), or 100 mg Symmetrel (amantadine), both anti-Parkinson's meds, or 25 to 50 mg Benadryl.

Extrapyramidal symptoms (EPS). Add 20 to 30 mg benztropine, amantadine, Benadryl, Catapres (clonidine), an antihypertensive, or Ativan for akathisia; 1 mg benztropine for preventing or managing dystonia, or 1 mg Ativan for managing dystonia.

Tardive dyskinesia. Vitamin E in high doses (1,000 units/day) may help. Note that vitamin E works better with vitamin C. Also, high-dose branched-chain amino acids, vital to muscle tissue maintenance, showed a significant reduction in symptoms in one study.

Sexual Dysfunction

At a symposium at the 2004 APA annual meeting, Anita Clayton, MD, of the University of Virginia, cited these antidotes to sexual dysfunction, all supported by studies: Wellbutrin, Viagra (for men), and Buspar (for women). Other possibilities include hormones (testosterone, estrogen), yohimbine (derived from the bark of an African tree), amantadine, and low-dose psychostimulants.

At another symposium at the same APA meeting, Richard Brown, MD, of Columbia University, noted that although Viagra may improve erection, it doesn't help much with libido and orgasm. The following natural treatments, he said, show promise: rhodiola (an arctic plant that may work on dopamine, which helps libido and boosts energy), which is effective for both men and women; ginkgo biloba (for impotence in men and for the maintenance of an erection); gingseng (which appears to work on dopamine, so woman can benefit, too); maca (a Peruvian root that "can have powerful effects on desire, erections, and orgasms"); horny goat weed (forgive the term; little data is available).

The TIMA *Bipolar Algorithms* also advises adding 4 to 8 mg of the hay-fever drug Periactin (cyproheptadine) shortly before sexual intercourse, or 75 to 300 mg/day of Wellbutrin.

Finally, there is the testosterone patch or gel to replenish depleted testosterone in "grumpy old men."

Overweight

Two drugs are FDA-approved for weight loss. Meridia (sibutramine) was originally developed as an antidepressant that blocks reuptake of serotonin, norepinephrine, and dopamine. The drug results in a loss of 8 percent of body weight over one year. The drug is contraindicated for MAOI antidepressants. The labeling warns that owing to risk of serotonin syndrome, Meridia should not be taken with SSRI antidepressants.

Xenical (orlistat) works in the gut and blocks 30 percent of fat from being absorbed, with improvement in total and LDL cholesterol. The nonabsorbed fat comes out in the stool, with predictable results.

Off-label meds include the diabetic drug Glucophage (metformin), Wellbutrin, Topamax (which may also help reduce binging), and Zonegran.

Drugs in the development pipeline include Axokine, originally developed as an ALS med, and rimonabant, which works as an anti-cannabis to stem the munchies.

Teeth

A recent emergency visit to the dentist served as a forceful personal reminder that our teeth are not to be taken for granted. Many of our meds cause dry mouth, which can lead to tooth decay and gum disease. Drinking lots of water and meticulous dental hygiene are the antidotes.

13

Talking Therapy

Turbocharging Your Antidepressant

A landmark study by Martin Keller, MD, of Brown University, and others in the May 18, 2000, *New England Journal of Medicine* compared the antidepressant Serzone with the talking therapy, cognitive behavioral analysis system of psychotherapy (CBASP). CBASP is largely derivative of other talking therapies such as cognitive, behavioral, and interpersonal therapy. Six hundred eighty-one patients with severe chronic depression were enrolled in the trial, and were assigned to either Serzone, CBASP, or a combination of Serzone and CBASP for twelve weeks. The response rates to either Serzone or CBASP alone were rather underwhelming—55 percent and 52 percent, respectively—for the 76 percent who completed the study, typical of findings for both medications and talking therapy.

The results for the combination drug-therapy group, however, were truly eye-popping, with 85 percent of the completing patients achieving a 50 percent reduction in symptoms or better. Forty-two percent in the combination group achieved remission (a virtual elimination of all depressive symptoms) compared to 22 percent in the Serzone group and 24 percent in the CBASP group.

Clearly, two therapies together represent one of those rare cases of one plus one equals three. In its 2000 *Practice Guideline* for depression, the APA advises that patients with major depression may benefit from combined medication and psychotherapy, while those with minor depression may opt for talking therapy alone. In its 2002 *Practice Guideline* for bipolar disorder, the APA also recommends adding talking therapy to medications therapy for the treatment of bipolar depression.

Manual-Based Therapies

The main talking therapies used for depression are manual based and time limited, generally from ten to twenty sessions, focus on the present, and aim at undoing the type of thoughts, behaviors, and social stressors that conspire against recovery. These therapies include:

- Cognitive therapy, also called cognitive behavioral therapy, which teaches the individual to change his or her distorted negative thoughts into more realistic positive ones, such as turning "It's the end of the world" into "Let's see how we can manage this"
- Behavioral therapy, which can be part of the cognitive behavioral package, focusing on activity scheduling, self-control, and problem solving
- Interpersonal therapy, which assists patients through life's transitions and overcoming deficits in social skills

At the 2002 APA annual meeting, John Markowitz, MD, of Cornell University, one of the coauthors of the Serzone-CBASP study, noted that medications work faster than talking therapy, but talking therapy can remove potential triggers likely to result in relapse. If you are in a terrible marriage, for example, and you take an antidepressant, you may be in a better position to work on that bad marriage. But if you fail to work on that bad marriage, your unresolved situation will catch up to you, he advised.

Another important benefit of talking therapy, said Dr. Markowitz, is that it enhances medications compliance.

At the same symposium, Ellen Frank, PhD, of the University of Pittsburgh, recounted the case of a twenty-eight-year-old graduate student having to deal with the sudden death of her mother, a conflict with her thesis adviser, and a shift in her relationship with her father as a result of her mother's death. Using the skills she learned from interpersonal therapy, the student was able to resolve her dispute with her father, and her depression subsequently remitted.

In 2004, this writer sat down with Dr. Frank, who related the story of her conversation with the then-editor of the *Archives of General Psychiatry,* Daniel Freedman, MD. Dr. Frank had submitted a study demonstrating the efficacy of maintenance talking therapy. "Ellen, why is it you think the treatment works?" asked Dr. Freedman. Dr. Frank had no idea. He said: "I think it's about what it *doesn't* focus on more than what it does focus on."

What he meant, Dr. Frank explained, is that in both cognitive therapy and interpersonal therapy (IPT) there is such an insistent focus on what is going on in the patient's life right now. Ruminating about the past is not part of the program.

When we met, Dr. Frank and her colleagues had just completed a study of women in their childbearing years, when these women may not want to take medication. The average woman in the study had endured four previous experiences of depression and was in her fifth episode. The test subjects received just IPT as their initial therapy, and those who did well continued sessions on either a weekly, bi-weekly, or monthly basis. Dr. Frank and her colleagues found that it made no difference during the maintenance phase whether the women came in weekly, every other week, or monthly.

What they also found was that for those who achieved full remission on IPT, the risk of recurrence when they stayed on maintenance treatment was very low, less than 25 percent over the two years of the study. According to Dr. Frank, "it looks like once again the treatment that gets you well keeps you well."

The caveat here is that not everyone achieves a fully sustained remission on IPT alone (about half of the women in the study), but with meds added to the therapy the rate of remission for those in the study climbed to about 80 percent.

Now it starts getting interesting. "What we're thinking," says Dr. Frank, "is that rather than beginning treatment with the combination, it makes more sense to start the therapy with pharmacotherapy alone or psychotherapy alone and only add the second treatment when the first treatment alone does not bring about remission."

Only about half of individuals need combination treatment, says Dr. Frank. Not achieving remission with either one or the other alone seems to be a good indicator that one needs the combination. The idea is to build on the partial success of the first treatment.

For those wondering how this squares with the Serzone-CBASP study in 2000, Dr. Frank pointed out that Dr. Keller's study involved patients who were chronically depressed, as opposed to patients who suffered from recurrent depression. Recurrent depression is characterized by discrete episodes that come and go, as opposed to an episode that persists over a long time. With chronic depression, the challenge is getting well. With recurrent depression, the challenge is staying well.

In findings released online in December 2003 by the National Academy of Sciences, Keller and others (this time with Charles Nemeroff, MD, PhD, of Emory University, as the lead author) had another look at the Serzone-CBASP study data, and what they discovered was no less startling than their original finding: while there was little difference between antidepressant therapy and talking therapy among the patients with no early childhood trauma, those who had lost their parents at an early age, been physically or sexually abused, and/or been neglected fared significantly better on talking therapy than on an antidepressant, both in terms of response and remission.

Unfortunately, talking therapy has traditionally been the poor relation when it comes to research dollars. That may change, however, as the pharmaceutical industry begins to appreciate how "the competition" can add value to its products. According to Michael Thase, MD, at the 2002 APA meeting, Bristol-Myers Squibb spent $26 million on the Serzone-CBASP study. Hopefully, we will see more studies like this.

Cognitive Therapy

Can you actually *think* your way out of the deep dark pits of despair? Consider this case.

In 1976, David Burns, MD, of the University of Pennsylvania, became a father. The birth was normal, but the boy was blue and gasping for air, and sent into intensive care. Despite the obstetrician's reassurances, Dr. Burns visualized the worst. He imagined a severely brain-damaged son and everything that implied. Feeling his own mental well-being slipping away, Dr. Burns turned to the therapeutic techniques pioneered by his colleague, Aaron Beck, MD.

It didn't take the new father long to identify his negative thoughts and realize that he had jumped to some fairly wild conclusions. Soon his son was breathing just fine, and Dr. Burns was on his way to becoming a leading advocate of Beck's technique, one we know of as cognitive therapy.

Cognitive therapy is fairly new to the mental-health field, but we can actually trace its development back in time twenty-six hundred years to the Buddha and the great emphasis his followers place on watching—and eventually taming—one's thoughts. There, the goal is eventual enlightenment. Here, we are speaking in relatively more modest terms of saving one's own life—of watching how one thinks in certain situations, and making the appropriate adjustments.

Here is how the process works.

Once our brains go down, the mind sends out all kinds of negative thoughts that can keep us trapped in a vicious cycle of depression. Even in more upbeat moods, we all too easily fall into the kind of thinking that can take us on a one-way trip down the elevator shaft, or very close to the edge.

All-or-nothing thinking is one example. Blowing negative events out of proportion is another, and blaming ourselves, no matter what, still another. Typically, we filter out positive feedback and assume the worst based on little or no evidence.

We've all done it. We get stuck in traffic and our day is naturally ruined. We win some praise from the boss, but somehow it doesn't count. It rains on the family picnic and we're the ones who apologize, instead of God.

Sometimes it gets personal. We misplace our keys and assume we're jerks. We forget a person's name and automatically we're stupid.

And sometimes it can get very serious, especially when we don't see life going according to our expectations. In this case, single incidents become part of an unending flow that stands for everything that is wrong with the world or ourselves. Here the mind is working overtime, indiscriminately processing outside information and stamping out negative thoughts on a production-line basis.

To give an extreme, but all too common, example, say you're a mother stuck in traffic. But instead of merely thinking that you are going to be fifteen minutes late, you see this as a situation that never should have happened in the first place had the bright promise of your potential been fulfilled. The world was your oyster, back in your early twenties—degree from a prestigious university, dream job in a Fortune 500 company, the career fast track, chic-and-fabulous size-six dresses. Then what happens? Marriage and kids, no more career fast track, and bulging out of size tens.

And here you are, midway between your dismal cubicle at a thankless job in a company that's going nowhere and the soccer game you're supposed to be picking up your bratty kids from, and your husband doesn't give a shit, and, goddamnit, it just wasn't meant to be this way . . .

Bring on the depression or the screaming raging manic fit.

In cognitive therapy, your therapist is likely to ask you to recall what you were thinking as you plunged into your last depression or flipped into mania—all those stuck-in-traffic thoughts, if you like—and work with you in recognizing them and nipping them in the bud before they can cause future damage.

In essence, you are being asked to become a detached observer of your own nearly automatic worst thoughts. Once you've established breathing room, you can turn these thoughts around and substitute new ones. To stick with the stuck-in-traffic example, the car can become your peaceful inner sanctum rather than your personal torture chamber.

And how does it *feel* being in your inner private sanctum? A hell of a lot better than your personal torture chamber, thank you very much, which is precisely the point of the whole cognitive-therapy exercise.

Establishing a good working relationship with your therapist is vital. When mine greeted me in Hush Puppies, I was ready to do a 180 back out the door. By contrast, a psychiatrist in a leisure suit would be okay with me (go figure). Part of my attitude stemmed from the fact that early in my treatment I just wanted a pill to get me back on my feet, not a know-it-all telling me how to run my life.

But once I realized therapy was about learning valuable coping skills rather than getting inside my head, I became a model (in a manner of speaking) client. But does it work? One of my newsletter readers, FG, reports:

> *If I can be mindful of thoughts, emotions and physical sensations on an ongoing basis then it's an excellent coping mechanism. Negative thoughts, emotions and physical pain become objects of mindfulness instead of drawing me into a downward spiral. In fact, both positive and negative thoughts, emotions and sensations are viewed in the same light of mindfulness and awareness. I find this approach often very liberating.*

According to Monica Basco, PhD, of the University of Texas Southwestern Medical Center and a leading proponent of cognitive behavioral therapy, speaking at the 2000 DBSA annual conference: "I do not believe you should be a passive recipient of care."

And this, perhaps, is cognitive therapy's greatest asset: the simple knowledge that we are not helpless bystanders, that in the unending battle for control of our own brains there is still an "I" that can put up a fight. And where there is "I," there is hope.

Chewing the Fat

Mobster Tony Soprano is grilling meat on the barbecue. Suddenly, as he observes the ducks that frequent his swimming pool head south for the winter, he experiences a panic attack and collapses.

When the doctors can find nothing physically wrong, he goes to psychiatrist Jennifer Melfi and confides that he is feeling depressed. Dr. Melfi assures him: "With today's pharmacology, no one needs to suffer with feelings of exhaustion and depression."

And our overwrought gangster replies: "Here we go. Here comes the Prozac."

But Tony is bleeding on the inside, and the Prozac amounts to nothing more than a Band-Aid. Thus, Tony agrees to open-ended weekly therapy.

The type of therapy is derivative of psychoanalysis. Psychoanalysis is most identified with Freud, who in 1900 began treating a young woman he called Dora. Under psychoanalysis, Dora told Freud of her family's closeness to that of Herr K., how her own father had been having an affair with Frau K. and how Herr K. was turning his attentions on her.

Freud wondered why his patient felt disgust rather than desire, and suddenly one of history's great Archimedes' moments occurred: An "aha!" A "Eureka!" An apple falling from the tree. Freud speculated that Dora *unconsciously* desired Herr K. For good measure, he also claimed that she lusted for Frau K.

A few days later, he confidently wrote to a friend: "The case has smoothly opened to the existing collection of picklocks." Freud was about to make himself famous.

Dora, however, was decidedly less impressed and broke off the treatment. Undoubtedly, a lot of lusting was going on, but it was almost certainly on the part of the doctor fantasizing about his patient.

Nevertheless, in one fell swoop Freud put an end to the notion that we are rational beings governed by rational thinking. At the same time, he also held out hope that the worst inside us could be stripped of its strange dominion simply by bringing it out into the open.

Sexual desire is a strong part of unconscious motivation, but Freud's peculiar take on the topic (think penis envy) would pollute the waters of psychoanalysis for years to come. These days, Freud is as fashionable as polyester, and psychoanalysis occupies a backwater of psychiatry.

Much more practical and accessible than psychoanalysis is psychodynamics, which can be considered a short form of psychoanalysis. Gone is the couch. Sessions are more focused, typically one a week, and may be time limited, tailored to the patient's needs, such as encouraging meds compliance. Various studies, however, indicate that short-term psychodynamics is less effective than cognitive, behavioral, and interpersonal therapy.

As long-term treatment, the APA in its *Practice Guideline* for depression advises that psychodynamics is usually associated with goals beyond that of immediate symptom relief. The therapy is addressed at modifying the underlying psychological conflicts that make patients vulnerable to depression. For bipolar disorder, the APA recommends long-term treatment in the context of illness management.

In *The Sopranos,* Dr. Melfi gamely tries engaging her patient in a therapeutic dialogue: "What's the one thing every woman—your mother, your wife, your daughter—have in common?" she asks.

Tony replies: "They all break my balls."

Eventually, Dr. Melfi notices that meat features in all of Tony's panic attacks, and with her prompting her patient recalls a buried childhood memory of watching his mafioso father chopping off a butcher's pinkie.

"My God!" exclaims Dr. Melfi.

"What," Tony responds, "your dad never cut off anybody's pinkie?"

But an important breakthrough has occurred. By this time, however, Tony is into his third year of therapy. Better late than never.

Finally, after four years, Tony is ready to throw in the towel. "Truth and happiness?" Tony says in reply to Dr. Melfi. "Come on, I'm a fat fucking crook from New Jersey. What truth and happiness?"

But you know Tony will be back. The only thing that is going to stop his therapy from going on forever is a federal indictment.

Tony Soprano is obviously a caricature of a therapist's worst nightmare, but when all is said and done there is little to distinguish a Jersey mob boss struggling with being a good son to a mother who tries to have him whacked from a woman in a bad marriage who is trying to put behind her an abusive relationship with her father.

They have yet to invent a pill that solves these problems, and heaven help us if they ever do. These are the tough issues that our brain keeps under lock and key inside a strongbox inside a safe in a vault under the bottom of the sea. X does not mark the spot. You are in for a long journey.

Many psychiatrists who specialize in medications treatment insist that their patients see a talking therapist on a regular basis. There are no guarantees, but the payoff can be life-changing. The one caveat is that you should not enter any therapy likely to uncover past trauma and abuse until your mood is stabilized, usually with medications or through a less-invasive short-term talking therapy such as cognitive therapy.

Unfortunately, insurance tends to cover only a limited number of sessions, so you may have to hit up your friends at the Bada Bing for a loan.

14

Singing the Brain Electric

Electroconvulsive Therapy

Nothing in the field of mental health is more apt to get a rise out of people than the subject of electroconvulsive therapy (ECT). Movies such as *One Flew Over the Cuckoo's Nest* have portrayed the procedure as nothing less than an instrument of torture, while in *The Bell Jar,* Sylvia Plath wrote that "with each flash a great jolt drubbed me till I thought my bones would break and the sap fly out of me like a split plant."

Yet ECT is fully endorsed by the psychiatric profession, and many patients swear it has saved their lives. Long regarded as a treatment of last resort—after all attempts at medications therapy have failed—more and more ECT is moving up to frontline status. The APA's 2001 task force report, *The Practice of Electroconvulsive Therapy: Recommendations for Treatment, Training, and*

Privileging, maintains that depriving patients from early treatment could "prolong suffering, and may possibly contribute to treatment resistance."

ECT having an 80 percent response rate for acute depression, antidepressants don't come close.

In *Night Falls Fast,* Kay Jamison, PhD, justifies ECT as a first-line treatment for suicidal patients, to stabilize their condition when slow-acting drugs and therapies are not an option.

ECT works on the principle of an electrically induced convulsion, similar to a grand mal epileptic seizure. The concept can be traced back to the Hungarian psychiatrist Ladislaus von Meduna, who, back in the 1930s, ironically had neither depression nor electricity in mind. Dr. Meduna happened to notice that epilepsy and schizophrenia rarely coexist. His bright idea was to use drugs to induce seizures in patients with psychosis.

Shortly after, a pair of Italian psychiatrists, Ugo Cerletti and Lucio Bini, observed that electricity that was used to stun slaughterhouse pigs often resulted in convulsion. Coincidentally, this was around the same time Walter Freeman began performing lobotomies in the United States. The only thing that saved the pioneers of ECT from being held in the same contempt today as Dr. Freeman is that ECT happened to work.

Until very recently, science could offer no credible theory for why an electrical current in the brain could cause a depression to lift. We are still a long way from figuring out the actual chain of events, but PhD Ron Duman's team at Yale has come up with some interesting findings. Dr. Duman, you may recall, is one of the investigators responsible for discovering that antidepressants can result in the regeneration of neurons in rats. He has also discovered similar brain activity as a result of electroshock, leading him to speculate that ECT, as well as antidepressants, may "reverse the atrophy of stress-vulnerable neurons or protect these neurons from further damage."

Back in the bad old days when ECT was overprescribed—often

against a person's will—the patient experienced violent, and sometimes bone-breaking, muscle contractions. Now the patient is given neuromuscular blocking agents, which limit muscular activity to an involuntary twitching in the toe.

Immediately prior to the treatment, the patient is injected with a medication that prevents abnormal heart rhythms, then is given an intravenous barbiturate that acts as the general anesthetic, and then is given the blocking agents. Electrodes are attached to the patient's scalp either on one side of the brain or two. A switch is flipped for a few seconds, the convulsion itself lasts about thirty seconds, and several minutes later the patient wakes up disoriented and groggy, and often with no recollection of the events surrounding the treatment.

The most pronounced side effect is short-term memory loss in about two-thirds of the patients. Some patients can also experience longer-term and permanent memory loss. The psychiatric profession has reacted defensively to the parade of patients who have come forward with their stories, equating their narratives to *Cuckoo's Nest* scare tactics, but the truth is psychiatrists have downplayed this rather disturbing invasion of the brain's hard drive. Part of this can be attributed to the politics of ECT; the opposing camps have waged an absurd campaign of hyperbole and denial for decades.

Only recently has the psychiatric establishment publicly owned up to the possibility of serious memory problems. A 2003 Institute of Psychiatry (London) review of thirty-five studies on ECT published in the *British Medical Journal* found the rate of reported persistent memory loss between 29 and 55 percent, though one reader who responded noted that the findings were based on a lot of old information.

At the 2005 APA annual meeting, Harold Sackeim, PhD, of Columbia University, acknowledged that the cognitive side effects that some patients experience can be persistent and profound. On the other hand, ECT is not the same as it was five years ago. "It is changing as we speak," he assured the gathering. This is largely due to changes in the width of the electrical pulse. Back in the old days of sine-wave stimulation, characterized by a phase duration of 8.3 milliseconds, patients risked a massive reduction in cognitive performance, even at six months. Bilateral administration (with electrodes to both sides of the skull) was especially toxic.

The introduction of brief-pulse stimulation in the 1980s greatly reduced, but hardly eliminated, risk of cognitive impairment and memory loss. The standard pulse width is between 0.5 and 2 milliseconds.

A new generation of machines that produce an ultrabrief pulse (at phase durations that vary from 0.1 to 0.4 milliseconds) promises a kinder and gentler era. A very recent unpublished study found virtually no difference in memory loss between patients on the new machines and the control group. The briefer pulses permit clinicians to calibrate lower seizure thresholds. Right unilateral ultrabrief ECT, said Dr. Sackeim, "appears optimal."

A further refinement in the works is focal electrically applied seizure therapy (FEAST), which concentrates the seizure to the frontal right part of the brain without affecting areas involving memory and related functions.

ECT's effect is generally not long term, so many psychiatrists recommend an occasional "booster charge," every six months or so.

Patients disillusioned by psychiatry's lack of candor in the past are entitled to be skeptical of its claims for an improved ECT. Writes Anita on my Web site:

> *Before the ECT, I was a horticulturalist by trade and a botanist by education. I could give complete names, scientific and common, and all the information about any plant I saw. Now, it is ALL GONE. I have also forgotten huge chunks of my former life. I can't remember things from a week ago.*

Every movie is new to me, because I cannot remember ever seeing it before. Thank god my husband can fill in the missing parts for me, especially about important parts of our children's lives. Please let this stand as a warning.

But Wendy reports: "The ECT was the smartest thing I could have ever done. It got me out of a downward spiraling depressive episode that saved my life."

One psychiatrist told this writer that he has seen such miraculous results with ECT that if he were a patient, he would have instructions tattooed to his forehead to the effect that this treatment should be used should he find himself in a state of crisis. Less dramatic than a tattoo is a legal document called an advance psychiatric directive. This anticipates emergencies when a patient may not be thinking clearly and is being pressured from all sides. Basically, the patient is saying yes or no while he still has his wits about him.

Whether formalizing your wishes in writing or not, this is hardly a decision you want to put off till the last minute. Whichever way you choose to go, turning in your homework early is the best option.

rTMS

A possible alternative to ECT is repetitive transcranial magnetic stimulation (rTMS), described by Mark George, MD, of the University of South Carolina, at the 2005 APA annual meeting as "tickling the cortex," but sending signals into the deeper regions.

A magnetic coil is placed over the patient's scalp (specifically, the left prefrontal cortex). The field passes unimpeded through the skull (unlike ECT) and induces an electrical current in the brain. There have been sixty-two published studies on 1,415 depressed patients showing "a reasonable effect size." Better results corresponded to longer courses, greater pulse intensity, and pulse quantity.

One manufacturer, Neuronetics, is completing a study involving 240 patients. The NIMH is engaging in a four-year trial with the same number of patients. One of the aims of the latter study is to find out where it's best to apply the stimulation. The left prefrontal cortex, Dr. George acknowledged, is "a rule of thumb I literally pulled out of a hat."

The procedure is safe and noninvasive. However, rTMS can cause unintended seizures under the wrong conditions. Accordingly, the International Society for Transcranial Stimulation recommends the procedure be performed in a medical setting with patients continuously monitored. Some patients may experience headaches.

An investigational procedure in the United States, rTMS is not FDA-approved. The treatment is approved in Canada.

MST

An investigational treatment, magnetic seizure therapy (MST), uses rTMS technology to induce seizures. The effect is much like ECT, but because the current passes through the skull unimpeded, Sarah Lisanby, MD, of Columbia University, explained at the 2005 APA meeting, it allows for more precise targeting into the brain. The aim is to induce seizures that do not spread to the motor cortex, thus sparing the memory regions of the brain. A study on primates showed better memory after MST than electroshock. Human subjects reoriented themselves much more quickly after MST than ECT and experienced less retrograde amnesia.

ECT had much better efficacy than MST in treating depression in academic settings, but was about the same in community settings. Dr. Lisanby and her colleagues are currently experimenting with higher doses in primates.

VNS

Vagus nerve stimulation (VNS) has received a lot of attention recently. In July 2005, the treatment was granted an FDA indication for depression in treatment-resistant patients. The treatment is also approved for epilepsy.

A pacemaker-like device is implanted in the chest and sends a current up a wire attached to the vagus nerve at the base of the skull. From there, various pathways into the brain are activated.

The treatment is not without controversy. A major twelve-week double blind study of patients still on their meds carried out by the manufacturer, Cyberonics, proved a disappointing failure. Rather than call it quits, Cyberonics kept the trial going as an open study and used as a comparison group patients receiving treatment as usual. After one year, 30 percent of the VNS patients responded to the treatment (or, to put it another way 70 percent failed to respond).

Cyberonics succeeded in convincing an FDA panel that 30 percent was an excellent result in light of the fact that this was a severely depressed population that had failed on all other treatments. Despite concern about the underwhelming response and the nature of the trial, the panel green-lighted the treatment for approval, with conditions. The FDA, however, rejected the panel's recommendation, then later reversed itself on receiving more data from Cyberonics.

At the 2005 APA meeting, Lauren Marangell, MD, of Baylor University, quoted Dr. George in calling the vagus "the superhighway into the brain." She ruled out that the patients in the study could have improved over time as the result of the natural course of their illness, as those in the treatment-as-usual group had much poorer responses.

The surgery is performed on an outpatient basis. The dose can be adjusted in real time by passing a magnetic wand over the chest. This is performed in the clinician's office. Patients can turn the device on or off at home. There are no major side effects other than hoarseness in some patients and occasional vocal hiccups.

Deep Brain Stimulation

A taste of the future was offered at the 2005 APA meeting by Benjamin Greenberg, MD, PhD, of Brown University. Needlelike leads with four electrodes are inserted into targeted regions of the brain, guided by MRI scans. An extension wire runs from each lead to one or more VNS-like devices implanted in the chest. The treatment is FDA-approved for Parkinson's, and is being investigated for obsessive-compulsive disorder and depression. OCD patients reported changes in mood within two minutes of the device being switched on. A small pilot study on depressed patients had a similar effect. When the device was turned off or the battery failed, the patients got worse.

A 2005 study by Helen Mayberg, MD, of Emory University, identified Brodmann area 25 (not to be confused with Area 52) in the subgenual cingulate region. Four of six treatment-resistant patients remitted when the adjacent white matter was stimulated.

Deep brain stimulation may supplant cingulotomies and capsulotomies, surgeries that have been used for OCD and are being investigated for depression. Guided by brain scans, a "gamma knife" (beams of gamma radiation) cuts lesions in specific areas of the brain. Unlike deep brain stimulation, the surgery is irreversible.

Brain-Scan Therapy

A funny thing happened a few years ago when a technician at McLean Hospital, affiliated with Harvard University, performed routine brain-scans of depressed bipolar patients. The hospital had just installed a new type of MRI machine that creates a specific type of magnetic field. The procedure is called echo-planar magnetic resonance spectroscopic imaging (EP-MRSI).

Researchers typically employ magnetic resonance imagings (MRIs) and other types of imaging to measure volume and activity in discrete areas of the brain in test subjects as they experience a mood episode. Functional MRIs monitor changes in brain activity while subjects are engaged in various cognitive tests.

McLean Hospital had performed more than ten thousand MRIs over the previous ten years, but this time the technician observed something different. One of the first people examined on the new machine, who went in severely depressed, emerged laughing and joking. Similar unexpected results occurred in other subjects.

A follow-up study published in 2004 found that twenty-three of thirty bipolar patients reported significant improvement in their depressions after undergoing EP-MRSI, compared to those receiving sham EP-MRSI. The type of field generated by EP-MRSI is similar to rTMS, but the global reach of the new machine suggests that many more regions of the brain are affected. One of these may be the corpus callosum, a thick cable of nerves deep in the brain that coordinates activity between the two hemispheres.

"In depression, the two halves of the brain may get out of balance, and the electromagnetic pulses may restore the balance," one of the researchers, Bruce Cohen, MD, speculated.

Current machines are far too expensive and cumbersome for widespread use, but tabletop models that could conceivably sit in doctors' offices are in the design stage.

15

Complementary Treatments

Originally, this chapter was paired with the "Lifestyle" chapter. Then I decided that this only served to reinforce the artificial distinction between so-called alternative and mainstream psychiatry. Conceptually, there is little difference between relying on a pharmaceutical product to get you better and one that comes from a health-food store. In the medicine cabinet, they both look the same.

Before we proceed, it pays to keep in mind that *natural* should not be equated with *harmless*. Saint John's wort, for example, has many dangerous interactions with other drugs. Unscrupulous suppliers have been known to mislabel their products or spike them with poisonous substances. According to Todd Cooperman, founder of the independent ConsumerLab.com, which tests nutritional products, in an article in the June 2, 2000, *San Francisco Chronicle*: "On average, we're seeing that one-quarter to one-third of the products do not meet the [claims on the] label, often by a wide margin."

We know that nature's way may be the best way. The catch is we don't know enough about nature itself. Alarming numbers of people are experimenting on themselves with what's out there, often without telling their doctors.

The most "natural" remedy, of course, may be using nothing at all, but many of us need an assist from either nature or pharmaceuticals, or both together. Should you go the natural route, buy only from a reputable supplier and use only under a doctor's guidance.

Nutritional Supplements

Leave your drugs in the chemist's pot if you can heal the patient with food.

—Hippocrates

In a study published in the July 2002 *British Journal of Psychiatry,* 172 young adult prisoners in maximum security were given supplements of vitamins and minerals roughly equating to the U.S. recommended daily allowance (RDA), plus fatty acids. The average time for those staying in the study was 146 days. While there was no change in the placebo group, there was a 35.1 percent drop in antisocial behavior and a 37 percent drop in violent offenses for those taking supplements for at least two weeks.

Speaking at a symposium, "Mineral/Vitamin Modification of Mental Disorders and Brain Function," at the 2003 APA annual meeting, the study's lead author, Bernard Gesch, CQSW, of Oxford, noted that crime has increased severalfold in the last fifty years. Over the same period of time, he reported, the trace-element content in fruits and vegetables appears to have fallen significantly.

The RDA (recommended daily allowance) was never meant to be regarded as optimal, more than one speaker reminded those at the same symposium. Instead, it is the minimum considered to prevent diseases such as scurvy or beriberi. According to a 2002 review article published in *JAMA,* "most people do not consume an optimal amount of all vitamins by diet alone."

At the same session, David Benton, PhD, of the University of

Wales, Swansea, cited his 1995 study in which those who took 50 mg of thiamin (vitamin B1)—nearly fifty times the RDA—reported improved moods and exhibited faster reaction times, with no change in the placebo group. The study population (female undergrads) was well nourished with no mood disorders.

Dr. Benton related that the brain is arguably the most nutritionally sensitive organ in the body, playing a key role in controlling bodily functions. It is the most metabolically active organ, with 2 percent of the body's mass accounting for 20 percent of basal metabolic rate. With millions of chemical processes taking place, he went on to say, if each of these is only a few percent below par, it is easy to imagine some sort of cumulative effect resulting in less-than-optimal functioning.

Added Bonnie Kaplan, PhD, of the University of Calgary: "We know that dietary minerals and vitamins are necessary in virtually every metabolic action that occurs in the mammalian brain."

A 2003 Finnish study of 115 depressed outpatients being treated with antidepressants found that those who responded fully to treatment had higher levels of vitamin B_{12} in their blood at the beginning of treatment and six months later. The comparison was between patients with normal B_{12} levels and higher-than-normal ones, rather than between deficient and normal. The study's authors speculated that one possible explanation could be that B_{12} is needed to manufacture certain neurotransmitters. Another theory is that vitamin B_{12} deficiency leads to the accumulation of the amino acid homocysteine, which has been linked to depression.

Other studies have singled out selenium, chromium picolinate, folate, and other vitamins and minerals.

It isn't just about mood. An article in the March 26, 2004, *Psychology Today* reports that antioxidants scavenge and fight off free radicals, those rogue oxygen molecules that damage cell membranes and DNA. The brain, being the most metabolically active organ in the body, is especially susceptible to free-radical damage. Free-radical damage is implicated in cognitive decline and memory loss, and may be a leading cause of Alzheimer's.

Studies suggest that vitamins C and E may work synergistically to prevent Alzheimer's and to slow memory loss. The RDA for vitamin E is 22 international units (IU) and 75 to 90 mg for vitamin C, but supplements may contain up to 1,000 IU of vitamin E and more than 1,000 mg of vitamin C. In the Alzheimer's study, involving five thousand individuals, the greatest impact occurred among those who took the two vitamins in combination.

In 1969, the Nobel Prize–winning scientist Linus Pauling coined the term *orthomolecular* to describe the use of naturally occurring substances, particularly nutrients, in maintaining health and treating disease. According to Dr. Pauling: "Orthomolecular psychiatry is the achievement and preservation of mental health by varying the concentrations in the human body of substances that are normally present, such as the vitamins."

Orthomolecular medicine was pioneered by Abram Hoffer, MD, PhD, who said in a 1998 interview: "I made a prediction in 1957 that by 1997 our practices would be accepted. I assumed it would take 40 years, since in medicine it typically takes two generations before new ideas are accepted. We're more or less on schedule."

Back near the midpoint in the schedule, a 1973 APA task force report used the word *deplorable* to describe the lack of hard research evidence to back the claims of proponents of high-dose vitamins and orthomolecular treatment. In light of the fact that funding for these kinds of studies is virtually nonexistent, however, the criticism is rather disingenuous. In fact, there is an institutional bias against studying more than one ingredient at a time, which dooms proposals for large-scale randomized control trials for multivitamins and minerals to death by red tape.

To turn the critical spotlight around, the evidence for the three meds combinations most of us find ourselves on is totally lacking, with no studies whatsoever, which would make any polypharmacy claims by the psychiatric profession equally "deplorable" (not that anyone would ever think of using such a term).

Thirty years later, the profession is still a long way from embracing nutritional supplements, but it has probably advanced beyond employing excessive rhetoric to attack its adherents. Having said that, in today's largely unregulated market, quacks with fantastic claims abound, along with suppliers of shoddy goods. Buyer beware is the rule.

Speaking of fantastic claims . . .

In 2000, this writer happened to come across an item in a Canadian newspaper about an Alberta company that was test-marketing a mix of thirty-six supplements based on a formula to calm aggressive hogs. I ran a short item in my newsletter, and next thing, the company was bombarded with inquiries about its product.

Founder Anthony Stephan's story is compelling. After his bipolar wife, Deborah, committed suicide in 1994, he exhausted all medical routes and turned to friend David Hardy for help for two of his bipolar children. David came up with a variation on the formula he used for calming down hogs, and Anthony administered the supplement to his kids, with miraculous results.

Reports Victoria, on my Web site:

I have a friend who I went to school with who is severely bipolar. She was hospitalized for mania about twice a year and could not work for six years since it surfaced. She would fly into rages and destroyed her own car over trivial things. She spent money with wild abandon, had affairs and kept taking off on trips she couldn't afford. Wandered the streets of Toronto psychotic and homicidal. Thanks to the (supplement) she is off disability, working full time teaching, and lost sixty pounds. She is completely medication-free for two years now and is no longer seeing a psychiatrist.

The company has not suffered from lack of controversy, but in December 2001, it received a significant boost to its credibility with a pilot study and accompanying commentary published in the *Journal of Clinical Psychiatry*. In a University of Calgary open trial, fourteen bipolar patients were placed on the supplement, concurrent with their meds. Thirty-three of the thirty-six ingredients in the supplement are vitamins and minerals, most about ten times the RDA. After forty-four weeks, depression scores dropped by 55 percent and mania scores by 66 percent. Most patients were able to lower their meds doses by 50 percent. Two were able to replace their meds with the supplement. Three dropped out after three weeks. The only side effect was nausea, which went away at a lower dose.

In her article, the study's author, Bonnie Kaplan PhD, noted that deficient levels of some nutrients (e.g., B vitamins) are related to brain and behavior disorders as well as poor response to antidepressant medication. Less is known about trace elements, but zinc, magnesium, and copper all appear to play important roles in modulating the brain's NMDA receptor (which is being targeted by at least twenty medications presently in the development pipeline). Bipolar disorder, she speculates, may be an error of metabolism, or those with bipolar may be vulnerable to nutrient deficiencies in the food supply. "There is very good work," she said in an interview, "going back to the 1950s on something called biochemical individuality. For example, your requirements for zinc or B_{12} may be different from another person's. We're not clones. We're really very different biochemically."

In an accompanying commentary to Dr. Kaplan's study, Charles Popper, MD, of Harvard, observed: "In view of the fifty years of experience with lithium, the notion that minerals can treat bipolar disorder is unsurprising. . . . Depending on how this line of research develops, [we] may need to rethink the traditional bias against nutritional supplementation as a potential treatment for major psychiatric disorders." Dr. Popper mentioned using the supplement to treat twenty-two bipolar patients. Of these, nineteen showed a positive response, and eleven remained stable for nine months without drugs.

Some misguided company representatives have advised customers to gradually go off their meds, but just two patients in Dr. Kaplan's study and only half of Dr. Popper's patients achieved this result. You will almost certainly, however, have to reduce your meds, as the supplement has a way of amplifying side effects (and perhaps the meds' efficacy).

If you are considering therapy with vitamins or other nutrients, do so with your psychiatrist in the loop. Since "integrative psychiatrists" are a rarity, it is wise to seek nutritional expertise from another source. It also pays to ensure that your psychiatrist is open-minded about nutritional supplements and would consider adjusting your meds if you responded well to your new regimen. Keep in mind that the final decision regarding lowering meds is one to be made between you and your psychiatrist, not with the person who is advising you on nutrition.

And once more, buyer beware. Nutritional supplements may turn out to be a lifesaver for you, but you may have to negotiate a Wild West marketplace first. If you are highly skeptical of drug-industry claims, maintain that same skepticism for natural products. Live well . . .

Amino Acids

Natural-health advocates are touting amino acids on the basis that certain ones are the building blocks of the neurotransmitters identified with mood. The best supporting evidence we have is that some positive findings from very small studies may contradict some negative ones.

Basically, you are spending your own money to be your own

guinea pig, but the results may justify the investment. The amino acids roll call:

■ Tyrosine, a precursor of both norepinephrine and dopamine, can act as an energizer, and is available over the counter. Phenylalanine, a precursor to tyrosine, is also an option, but is toxic to those with poor phenylalanine metabolism (these individuals are already on notice from phenylketonuria [PKU] tests routinely administered to newborns).

■ Tryptophan, the precursor to serotonin, was removed from the U.S. market in 1989 after a manufacturer produced a highly toxic contaminate. There is still concern that overconsumption may result in eosinophilia-myalgia syndrome. The substance is available by prescription. Less is more, with lower doses (1 to 3 gm) more effective than higher doses. Taking the amino acid with carbohydrates helps in its absorption.

■ The intermediary between tryptophan and serotonin, 5-HTP, is available without prescription.

■ Julia Ross, author of *The Mood Cure,* refers to gamma-aminobutyric acid (GABA) as "our natural valium," and recommends it to her clients for calming down. However, as this neurotransmitter does not easily cross the blood-brain barrier, you may wind up instead with very expensive urine.

■ The November 2003 *Psychology Today* reports that taurine is being investigated for bipolar disorder. Taurine acts as an inhibitory neurotransmitter.

Omega-3

A major epidemiological study published in the July 24, 1996, *JAMA* compared the prevalence of depression across ten nations. The survey yielded eye-opening results in showing how the lifetime and annual rates for depression vary widely from country to country (e.g., 1.5 of every 100 adults in Taiwan experience depression in their lifetimes, while the figure is 19 for every 100 adults in Beirut). A 1999 study by Joseph Hibbeln, MD, of the NIMH, compared this data with fish consumption, finding the higher-consuming populations experienced less depression.

A 2003 study by the same author compared similar cross-national epidemiological data—this time involving bipolar disorder—and seafood consumption, again finding a strong correlation.

The working ingredient of fish oil is omega-3, a polyunsaturated fatty acid that is also found in certain plants such as flaxseeds, pumpkinseeds, and walnuts. According to Dr. Hibbeln, in a September 3, 1998, Reuters article: "In the last century, [Western] diets have radically changed and we eat grossly fewer omega-3 fatty acids now. We also know that rates of depression have radically increased by perhaps a hundred-fold."

In an article in the April 24, 2001, *New York Times,* Dr. Hibbeln noted that omega-3 seems to be critical to the growth and maintenance of brain cells, especially cell membranes. When omega-3 is not available, the body uses omega-6, which produces cell membranes less able to cope with neurotransmitter traffic.

A healthy diet should provide for at least 5 gm daily of essential fatty acids, divided between omega-3 and omega-6. At least two studies show depleted omega-3 levels in the red blood cell membranes in depressed patients.

The 1999 Harvard pilot study that started it all was conducted on thirty patients with bipolar disorder, generally in stable condition but with a history of relapses (all had experienced bipolar episodes over the past year). All but eight of the subjects were on medications, which were left unchanged. Half the subjects were given 9.6 grams of fish oil capsules, the other half received olive oil.

Andrew Stoll, MD, who led the study, admits that the olive oil, which did not have a fishy taste, was not a perfect placebo. In one case, a person's cat actually attacked the fish-oil capsules. But, as he jokingly confessed in a session at the 2000 DBSA annual conference, "you want a flawed study. That way, you get money to do another study."

The trial was supposed to go on for nine months, but was stopped after four due to its outstanding results, with the omega-3 group staying in remission significantly longer than the placebo patients. By two months, half of the placebo group had dropped out, compared to two in the fish-oil group. The omega-3 group actually did less well in lowering their mania scores than those taking placebos, but fared much better in getting their depression down. Some patients experienced nausea, diarrhea, and fishy aftertaste, not surprising considering the extremely high doses.

Currently, Dr. Stoll is conducting a much larger and longer study.

A 2003 Chinese pilot study also found omega-3 worked for unipolar depression.

On my Web site, April reports: "I have been using the omega-3 for about six months after reading a different article on the internet. I have been told by most of my family and friends that my moods are much more stable. This is great. I have been on other medications for nine years and they were not consistent." According to another reader, Cahira: "Not only does it act as a mood stabilizer, it also improves my mental clarity as well."

The two active ingredients of omega-3 fish oil are EPA (eicosapentaenoic acid) and DHA (docosahexaenoic acid). EPA is considered to be the ingredient with the therapeutic effect, so it is important to buy omega-3 that contains more EPA than DHA. How the two chemicals work together has not been determined.

"Less is more" may be the case with EPA. A 2002 study of seventy depressed treatment-resistant patients found those on one gram of EPA fared "dramatically better" than those on 2 and 4 gm. The less-is-more principle is supported in a 2003 Stanley Foundation Bipolar Network study of fifty-nine depressed bipolar patients, which found that those on 6 gm/day of EPA did no better than those taking the placebo over four months.

Less is more may also apply to omega-3. Large doses may result in oxidative stress as the omega-3 is being metabolized. This may explain why some studies using EPA failed at higher doses. Accordingly, Dr. Stoll recommends 1.5 to 3.5 gm a day of omega-3, taken with vitamins C and E.

Any fish you eat, he says, should be ocean fish rather than farm-raised fish. This is because omega-3 travels up the food chain from algae, while farm-raised fished are fed grains, which do not contain omega-3.

There is a possibility of omega-3 causing switches into mania or hypomania, so it is critical to consult your psychiatrist beforehand. Otherwise, the worst side effect appears to be "salmon burps."

Saint John's Wort

The active ingredients in Saint-John's-wort are hypericin, extracted from the flowering tops of the plant, polycyclic phenols, and pseudohypericin. Because it is available in the United States as an over-the-counter herbal remedy rather than as a drug (as in the case in Europe), there is virtually no government oversight. Owing to lack of regulation, consumers cannot be guaranteed evenness in quality or quantity from batch to batch or manufacturer to manufacturer.

Following two NIH-funded studies published in the *Lancet,* the FDA in 2000 issued a public-health advisory warning of the risk of dangerous interactions with Saint John's wort and indinavir, a protease inhibitor used to treat AIDs. The advisory also warns against possible interactions with other protease inhibitors.

In addition, the FDA warned that "St John's wort appears to be an inducer of an important metabolic pathway, cytochrome P450," where as many as 50 percent of prescription drugs are metabolized. Taking the herb while on birth control may result in your naming your unexpected next child Wort.

More than two dozen small trials on mild to moderately depressed populations have turned up positive results. A 2002 study of 375 patients with mild to moderate depression found Saint-John's-wort "produced significantly greater reduction" in depression scores.

But for those whose depression comes supersized, a 2001 study of two hundred adult outpatients with major depression over eight weeks found that Saint John's wort "failed to produce significant differences vs placebo."

Basically, Saint John's wort is to an antidepressant what Tylenol is to OxyContin—that is, reasonably effective as long as you don't ask too much of it. Whether the modest benefit is worth the trouble of potentially dangerous herb-drug interactions is a matter you need to discuss with your psychiatrist.

SAM-e

A 1999 book, *Stop Depression Now,* trumpets on its front cover: "The Breakthrough Supplement That Works As Well As Prescription Drugs, in Half the Time . . . with No Side Effects."

Sound too good to be true? We are told SAM-e has been prescribed in Europe for more than twenty years and that in Italy it outsells Prozac. One of the coauthors of *Stop Depression Now,* Richard Brown, MD, of Columbia University, said at the time of the book's publication that he had used the supplement on his patients with successful results for five years.

SAM-e—short for S-adenosylmethionine—is a molecule found in our bodies and is vital to a process called methylation, in which one molecule passes a methyl group (one carbon and three hydrogen atoms) to another molecule. It is a transaction essential to more than a hundred processes in the body, from the brain to the bones. Levels of SAM-e are notably lower among depressed people of all ages.

In all, there have been some forty studies—virtually all European—involving fourteen hundred depressed patients. They typically show SAM-e working in a matter of days (as opposed to four to six weeks with antidepressants) with virtually no side effects.

One of my readers, Ariadne, reports:

> *Last year, after a couple years of struggling with acute depression, I went off Elavil in anticipation of getting pregnant. I soon fell back into a deep depression despite having weaned very slowly. At my therapist's advice, I began taking SAM-e, 400 milligrams a day, along with a B complex vitamin (SAM-e will rob your body of B's), and got pregnant soon after. With my OB's consent, I continued this dosage throughout my pregnancy. I never had the common mood swings of pregnancy and felt better than I had in years. SAM-e is my miracle "drug"!*

But be advised that Ariadne's miracle drug may do nothing for you. Please buy from a reputable supplier and use only under a doctor's guidance.

Bright-Light Therapy

Bright-light therapy developed out of treating seasonal affective disorder (SAD), and may also serve for other types of depression, especially in situations where meds may not be an option, such as pregnancy. It is the eyes that respond to the light rather than the skin.

A light box is the standard device (in units ranging from 2,500 to

10,000 lux), but light visors are also effective. Patients keep their eyes open and glance toward the light, but avoid staring directly into it. Sessions should start at ten or fifteen minutes a day, and gradually increase to thirty to forty-five minutes a day in the morning or evening. Maximum duration is ninety minutes, though many trials have used durations of two hours or more. The most common side effects are eyestrain and headache. The major disadvantage is the time commitment—that is, unless you can set up your light box at your workstation or while you're eating a meal or reading the paper.

Morning treatment is thought to be more effective than evening treatment, possibly due to coinciding with solar and circadian rhythms. Evening light may keep some people awake at night. People with bipolar disorder respond to light therapy, but need to be mindful of the possibility of the light inducing mania.

Outdoor walks and indoor activities by the window should be considered a form of light therapy. Even an overcast day produces light equivalent to a light box.

A small 1998 study comparing bright-light therapy to Prozac in patients with SAD found similar response rates, but bright light achieves a much quicker result. A 1989 meta-analysis of fourteen studies involving 332 patients with SAD found that low-intensity (2,500 lux) bright-light therapy lasting two hours a day reduced depression scores by 50 percent in the course of a week.

For nonseasonal depression, the results are far more equivocal. A 2004 Finnish review of twenty studies—most of dubious quality—concluded that "bright light therapy offers modest though promising antidepressive efficacy." Hypomania was more evident in the bright-light group compared to the controls.

Light boxes can be purchased for approximately $200 to $250. Some insurance companies may cover the costs.

Whatever you do, don't use a tanning bed as your light source. Let your doctor know what you're doing, and work closely with him or her on your treatment plan.

Acupuncture

Amelia had been taking Zoloft for three years, but was having trouble with its side effects. Serzone didn't help, and Paxil (40 mg) only seemed to get her right back where she started—grateful to feel human again, but not at all happy with her excess sleep, weight gain, and loss of sexuality. Amelia had originally turned to acupuncture for her flu and bronchitis, and found it worked wonders. Now she wondered if acupuncture could help her depression.

In 1998, the NIH's Office of Alternative Medicine funded a pilot study at the University of Arizona. Working with acupuncturist Rosa Schnyer, John Allen, PhD, devised a sixteen-week trial on thirty-eight seriously depressed women. First, the two worked up a standard treatment plan that targeted certain "depression points" on the body. Then they devised a dummy treatment calling for needles in nonspecific places. The acupuncturists administering the treatment had no idea whether they were using the real plan or the dummy plan.

Then the subjects were divided into three groups. The first group received the depression-specific acupuncture, the second group got the dummy treatment, and the third group was put on a wait list before being placed on eight weeks of the real thing.

Following the treatment, the depression-specific groups experienced a 43 percent reduction in their symptoms, compared to a 22 percent reduction for the dummy group. More than half no longer met the criteria for clinical depression. Only five people dropped out of the study—two who moved away, one who became pregnant, and two who didn't like the needles. The dropout rate was much lower than for studies using medications.

As for Amelia, she was able to swap for free sessions by giving piano lessons to the acupuncturist's son. On the advice of her acupuncturist, she did not quit her medication. She began the treatment in May—never going more than once a week—and gradually, she says, she began to recover. "For a few days I felt a little better," she recounts, "then after that I felt bad days. But the better days got better oh so gradually and the bad days less bad."

Amelia would lie on a table as her acupuncturist put some needles into her ear, arm, and leg—always on the right side (except for a few needles in the other leg). One time he put the needles in similar areas on the left side. He would also point a heat lamp at the places in the leg where he left needles. The needles prick, according to Amelia, "just the littlest bit." Then she would remain on the table while her acupuncturist left the room for twenty minutes. Finally, the acupuncturist would take out the needles and rub some areas of Amelia's back and neck.

Amelia thinks the first few visits were critical, but her follow-up visits were important, too. Gradually, she reports, "the better days got better oh so gradually and the bad days less bad."

If you are on medication, don't necessarily expect to flush your pills down the toilet. Amelia slowly weaned off Paxil but switched to Saint John's wort.

Experimental Treatments

There are degrees of experimental. The complementary therapies we have discussed so far can be regarded as experimental but promising. The following should be considered merely experimental.

Negative Ion Therapy

In this context, ions are charged particles of air. Outdoor pollution, hot desert winds, winter, and indoor environments (particularly with the heat and TV going) cause high positive-to-negative ion ratios that may contribute to depression and other bad moods. Negative ions, by contrast, are associated with clean country air and the invigorating mist from nature and fountains.

A small 1995 Columbia University study found that 58 percent of patients with seasonal affective disorder responded to a high-output electronic negative-ion generator. Another Columbia University study is in progress.

Home versions of the generator retail at about $150, but you may want to experiment with taking extra showers or by simply leaving the shower running for five minutes with the bathroom door open.

Air Power

Gunnar Heuser, MD, PhD, of UCLA, has yet to treat patients with depression or bipolar disorder, but his work using a hyperbaric chamber on those exposed to neurotoxins, including several who manifested attention deficit disorder (ADD), may be the beginning of a trend.

The high air pressure inside the chamber forces more oxygen into the body's blood and tissues. Before-and-after SPECT (single photon emission computed tomography) imaging on Dr. Heuser's patients showed marked reduction in blue and violet areas—signifying a return of more normal blood flow—in the brain.

Interactive Metronome Therapy

Chiropractor James Blumenthal, DC, of the Applied Kinesiology Center of Los Angeles, explains that ADHD and other disorders may derive from the brain's failure to adequately process and integrate the functions of both hemispheres. This includes motor as well as cognitive function.

With interactive metronome therapy, kids are hooked up to headphones and a hand or foot trigger and instructed to keep a beat. Immediate feedback cues them when they are slightly off. The theory is that once rhythmic coordination develops in the subject, mental coordination—including academic performance—follows suit.

PART FOUR

SPECIAL POPULATIONS

16

Young and Old

Early Onset Depression

On my Web Site, young Collie writes: "I understand how sometimes the world can seem so terrible, and everything can go wrong, to the point where death is the only way out. I have prayed to God to let me die, because sometimes life seems so hard and complicated that death is the only way to make it better." She goes on to say:

I have so many problems, and everyone knows it. I don't really have any friends to talk about it with because they're part of the reason I have so many problems. They aren't true friends. I mean okay, like I'm in seventh grade and there's the whole popular unpopular stuff I have to deal with, as well as boys, hair, makeup, clothes, and all of the other stupid crap seventh graders have to go through.

Hopelessly behind in her homework, and feeling completely alienated, Collie concludes: "This sucks. Sometimes my problems get so bad I think death is the only way out. I really don't know what to do anymore. It's so hard."

Recalling her adolescence, Sherri writes:

I felt like an "alien" amongst "normal" people during my adolescent years. At age 13, I experienced my first depressive episode and began withdrawing from family and friends. My bedroom became my sanctuary where I lived in a world of my own. I felt truly accepted when praised by teachers and parents. I felt truly superior when I did better than anyone in the class. I felt like pond scum when no one ever asked me out on a date or to the prom. I was truly alone.

Della, a child-abuse survivor, reports: "Depression was my only constant. As a small child, I started to embrace, even welcome it. It was the only thing that was mine, the only thing I could control, or so I thought. I would rhythmically moan and bump my head on the wall at the same time."

One in every 50 Americans under eighteen are seriously depressed, according to estimates, and up to 1 in 12 teens, most who go undiagnosed and untreated.

According to Cynthia Pfeffer, MD, of Columbia University, testifying at a 2004 FDA public hearing into the safety and efficacy of antidepressants in kids: "Since prior to World War II, each successive generation seems to have a higher risk for major depressive disorder."

Dysthymia (chronic minor depression) is often underrecognized, she went on to say. Seventy percent of youth with dysthymia break out into major depression, usually within two to three years of the onset of dysthymia.

Compared to adults, adolescents have more behavioral problems.

Psychotic depression occurs in 30 percent of youngsters with major depression. Co-occurring disorders may be present in up to 90 percent of youth with major depression, including dysthymia, anxiety, disruptive behavior, and substance use.

The personal toll can be enormous: homework not done, lessons not learned, ostracism by peers, alienation from family, run-ins with authority. A typical depressive episode can rage on for nine months or more, the length of a school year, enough time to brand a youth as undesirable and sabotage forever his or her brightest hopes and dreams. Six to 10 percent of kids with major depression have a protracted course, 40 to 60 percent relapse after remission, and 20 to 60 percent have recurring episodes after recovery.

The victim may retreat into his or her inner world or take comfort in alcohol or illegal drugs. Or the opposite may happen in the form of aggressive behavior that has neighbors dialing 911.

If problems are not resolved in youth, they often carry over into adulthood. Writes Dave on my Web site:

I was 5'7", 165 pounds in the third grade and I only got bigger from there. I have always known that I was different from everyone else, and here lately in my life I have become even more so. I feel so alienated from everyone, it's like I'm totally alone. I have been deserted by friends, I am misunderstood by my family, and the weight of trying to relate to me has grown too burdensome for them, so much so that they don't even try to relate to me anymore. I'm just an anomaly that resides in the house and one day I will be gone again.

Ultimately, all too many seek the wrong way out: Dr. Pfeffer cited CDC data from 2001 that found that 19 percent of high-school students had seriously considered attempting suicide, nearly 15 percent had made plans to attempt suicide, and almost 9 percent had made a suicide attempt the preceding year.

A nine-year study released in 1993 found children with major depression had a 74 percent rate of suicidal thinking and a 28 percent rate of suicide attempts. The percentages were about the same for those with dysthymia.

Since the 1950s, youth male suicide rates in the United States increased threefold, making suicide the third-leading cause of death in our youth. Fortunately, there has been a sharp decline in that rate, starting in the United States in 1994 and around the same time in other industrialized nations, possibly related to teens being prescribed SSRIs.

Too often, parents confuse depression with typical child or adolescent behavior. Making matters worse is the fact that kids, ever sensitive to stigma, are not inclined to speak up. According to Harold Koplewicz, MD, of NYU, speaking at a 1999 White House conference on mental illness: "Teenagers are never volunteering to be customers for mental health services."

As to why kids get depressed, all the usual suspects are trotted out: the stresses and strains of modern life, working parents, broken homes. Poor kids are at greater risk due to more environmental stressors, but well-off kids are hardly immune. After a certain age, girls become far more likely victims in much greater numbers, probably due to concerns about their appearance and fitting in.

At a session of the 2002 DBSA annual conference, author Michael Yapko, PhD, referred to an April 22, 2001, *Time* article, "The Quest for a Super Kid," which chronicled childhoods turning into apprentice adulthoods and programs more concerned with building résumés than building character. "I have a niece who is eleven going on fifty-seven," Dr. Yapko revealed. Fully one-quarter of kids in Dr. Yapko's niece's class need chiropractors because of having to drag their book-laden backpacks around.

Antidepressants were designed for adult brains, but in 2003, following two successful trials, the FDA approved Prozac for kids aged seven to seventeen, the first and only antidepressant indicated for such use. Prior to this, the drug had been used off-label for this population. Nevertheless, the FDA was worried about one of the trials, which found that the Prozac kids gained two pounds less and grew half an inch less after nineteen weeks than those on placebos. Eli Lilly has promised to do more studies.

Several of the other antidepressants have failed in clinical trials in children, and have raised concerns over their safety, resulting in two highly publicized FDA public hearings in 2004 and a new black-box warning on the product labeling explicitly linking antidepressant use in kids to the risk of suicidal behavior.

The reported safety data from the FDA and its U.K. counterpart, the Medicines and Healthcare products Regulatory Agency (MHRA), although spotty, revealed that 6.1 percent of the kids in the Prozac trials experienced hyperactivity, 3.1 displayed agitation, and 2.6 had manic or hypomanic reactions (as opposed to hardly any or zero in the placebo groups). Although the FDA did not connect these specific effects to suicidal behavior, in October 2004, it instructed manufacturers to warn on the product labeling that kids on antidepressants need to be carefully monitored, as "there is concern that such symptoms may represent precursors to emerging suicidality."

An FDA analysis of twenty-five pediatric trials involving four thousand patients found: "Out of one hundred patients treated we might expect two to three patients to have some increase in suicidality due to short-term treatment . . . that is beyond the risk that occurs with the disease being treated." But in a study published in the October 2003 *Archives of General Psychiatry,* researchers from Columbia University reviewed 588 case files of kids aged ten to nineteen and found that a 1 percent increase in antidepressant use was associated with a decrease of 0.23 suicides per 100,000 adolescents per year, suggesting that your depressed child is probably a lot safer on antidepressants than off them.

The best way to assess the benefits versus the risks and ensure optimal meds care for your child is to consult a psychiatrist, ideally one with a specialty in pediatric psychiatry. At the FDA hearings, bereaved parents came forward with numerous examples of primary-care physicians who failed to warn them and their children of the potential adverse effects of these drugs and provide proper follow-up care. If a primary-care physician is your only option, make sure he or she has some basic competence in treating kids for depression.

A 1999 University of Michigan study found that only 8 percent of a surveyed group of six hundred family physicians and pediatricians in North Carolina reported having received adequate training in the management of childhood depression. Yet that did not stop 72 percent of the same group from prescribing SSRIs to patients under age eighteen.

An informed parent working closely with a psychiatrist can greatly minimize the risk. Keeping a watchful eye out for strange behavior can be difficult with teens—who are strange by definition—but when in doubt, call your psychiatrist immediately.

A 2004 NIMH study of 439 youths found Prozac helped teens overcome depression far better than talking therapy, and that the greatest success came when the two treatments were combined. After twelve weeks, 43 percent responded to talking therapy, 61 percent to Prozac, and 71 percent to combination of Prozac and talking therapy.

Even though other antidepressants have not been successful in pediatric clinical trials, it may be appropriate to prescribe them off-label to kids in certain situations. The FDA does not forbid the practice, but you are entitled to a clear explanation from your child's psychiatrist.

Early Onset Bipolar Disorder

On my Web site, Geraldine writes:

It is very difficult to be a parent of a child with bipolar. I have a six-year-old son who is diagnosed with ADHD. Doctors will not officially diagnose a child this young with bipolar. With all the articles I have read and the medicine I have recommended to the doctors, I know he is bipolar. He is currently in a class for behavior disorder. I get called at least once or even twice a week to pick him up because he has hit another child or spit on the teacher. I am very close to losing my job and I feel like my world is tumbling down around me.

Demitri Papolos, MD, and Janice Papolos, authors of *The Bipolar Child: The Definitive and Reassuring Guide to Childhood's Most Misunderstood Disorder,* advise that parents with a hyperactive child consider the possibility of bipolar disorder first, rather than ADHD or other disorders. This is especially important in light of the fact that a misdiagnosis with the wrong medications can have a bad impact on a bipolar child. According to Demitri and Janice Papolos, 93 percent of bipolar children meet *DSM-IV* criteria for ADHD.

In 2001, Dr. Papolos, along with parents, researchers, and clinicians, and Janice Papolos, set up the Juvenile Bipolar Research Foundation (www.bpchildresearch.org). The JBRF is aiming to produce an expert consensus on the diagnostic criteria for early onset bipolar. The *DSM-IV*, which is based on our knowledge of the illness in adults, does not explain how the illness manifests in kids, particularly in prepuberty.

Dr. Papolos is developing a "core phenotype" that identifies four mood states—mania/hypomania (including mixed), anger, depression, and anxiety, present most days over twelve months.

The core phenotype also singles out "poor modulation of drives" that result in behaviors that are excessive for age and context, and a number of disturbances that include anger and aggression, extremes in self-esteem, sleeping/waking difficulties, anxiety, easy arousal, and cognitive deficits.

"All of these are basic human behaviors," Dr. Papolos explained to this writer during a phone interview, "but they're writ large." Rages typically go on for hours, leaving families mentally whipped in their wake but unable to let down their guard for fear of yet another Vesuvius erupting without provocation. But outsiders rarely find out because moms and dads—in the words of Papolos's book—"like battered wives present a brighter face to the world and refuse to have themselves picture their child or them that way."

On my Web site, Anonymous writes of her eight-year-old daughter:

I am physically abused by her, biting, pinching, kicking, punching, tearing my clothes, trashing the house and calling the police on me. . . . It has been an emotional and physical journey with searching for the right counselor and doctors because a counselor thought I was abusing her when I would actually be defending myself. The adrenaline of a child in a rage, I feel, is comparable to an adult.

If only mood disorders were just about mood. When I put that observation to Dr. Papolos during our phone interview, I literally felt the receiver resonate in a palpable wave of agreement.

According to Dr. Papolos, bipolar kids generally come alert at about eleven o'clock, and as the day goes on they get more and more energy. This lasts until about four in the afternoon, when, as one parent told Dr. Papolos, "the rocket thrusters go off." Over the course of the evening, the kid is still accelerating, making reentry and bedtime a virtual impossibility.

"Executive functions are probably one of the least studied and most often overlooked contributors to academic and behavioral problems in children," Dr. Papolos told the 2004 JBRF conference. These are the central processes that are most intimately involved in getting organization and order to our action and behavior, he explained.

These kids lack the ability to organize things. Their rooms become landfills, their backpacks black holes. As Janice Papolos put it, parents have to act as their child's frontal lobes.

Many of my Web site readers report a sense of being different as a child. Janet recalls: "I knew that I was different at a very early age. In Catholic school, I questioned religious theories. My questions were met with the 'we have a heretic here' response. Childhood was pretty painful. I was an outsider who was bored constantly. My parents tried to keep me involved in activities, but nothing really kept me interested. My room and books provided my safe haven."

Says Enigma:

My earliest childhood memory is of primary school and the assassination of JFK and wondering why the tears were flowing for someone I had never met. At least then I was "normal" or at least my reactions were. From then on, oh how I wished the aliens would pick me up and place me on the right planet—a place where mood swings are common, ECT and deep sleep were never heard of, medical retirement was not in the dictionary, and "tar and cement" had never been invented.

A 1993 Johns Hopkins study of two generations of bipolar families found that the second generation experienced illness onset 8.9 to 13.5 years earlier and 1.8 to 3.5 times more severe. The authors of the study speculate that this may be attributable to a genetic factor known as anticipation, through which genetic mutations are passed from generation to generation in a form of repeat sequences that are enlarged over the generations.

But the answer could be as simple as what one mother of a nine-year-old bipolar child posted on an Internet message board: "Perhaps we are finally seeing doctors and psychiatrists who are willing to believe it's a real condition, not just a figment of overactive parents' imaginations. Perhaps the professionals are realizing that mothers really DO know their children best."

At the 2001 Fourth International Conference on Bipolar Disorder hosted by the Western Psychiatric Institute in Pittsburgh, Barbara Geller, MD, of Washington University (St. Louis) presented two-year-study findings that showed child-onset mania is not just a milder version of the adult variety. The ongoing study of 268 kids compared 93 who experienced mania to those with ADHD and a population of controls.

Nearly 90 percent of bipolar adolescents have co-occurring ADHD, Dr. Geller said, but bipolar kids can be distinguished by their elation and grandiosity. Children may not have maxed out their credit cards or have had four marriages, she told the conference, but there are strong parallels. A grandiose bipolar disorder adult, for example, called the president to tell him how to run the country, while a manic child repeatedly called school officials to tell them how to run the school.

As well as elation and grandiosity, bipolar kids differ from ADHD kids in flight of ideas. Kids typically say, "I need a stoplight up there," or "My thoughts broke the speed limit."

Most of the kids in the study had mixed mania or psychotic episodes, while 87 percent rapid-cycled, usually continuously, some for three years, with a poor prognosis over eighteen months. The mean age of onset when the study began was seven years, with the kids ill for three years. Surprisingly, less than half had been given an antimania drug. Almost no one had recovered after six months. After eighteen months, half had recovered, and after twenty-four, two-thirds, but half of these relapsed. In families with high maternal warmth, 42 percent of the kids relapsed versus 100 percent in families with low maternal warmth. "A seven-year-old manic child," she concluded, "is sicker than a twenty-year-old manic adult."

Findings published three years later validated her original results.

The clinical view of a raging out-of-control monster in diapers is counterpoised by an admittedly unscientific but forcefully accurate observation of my Web site reader Melody, who deserves the last word for now:

> *There are many extra-sensitive people out there, obviously not enough, and they are the ones that from birth on to school days, teen years and adult life suffer the most in a world that has definitely taken away a lot of their energy instead of giving back what they deserve as spiritual people. I think there are people that are simply born with an extra-sensitive nerve and it is probable that they do have more capacity than normal people to be in contact with the spiritual world. It is just like the artist, the musician and the mathematician.*
>
> *They have certain talents that evolve spirituality through their sensibility. It would be good actually for parents, medics and teachers to become aware of these special children, they are not the same as normal ones and they deserve special attention.*

Treating Early Onset Bipolar Disorder

Meds

Once a correct diagnosis is achieved, medication tends to be a no-brainer, though there will always be people like Zel, who posted: "There is no biological data which supports the hypothesis of biological nature of mood disorders in children. None!" And similarly, from Anonymous: "Stop drugging them and start treating them."

In response, Millie is equally blunt, writing: "If I did not medicate my child he would be dead—his bipolar illness is so severe and so obvious that I challenge anyone who witnesses his symptoms before a hospitalization is required to tell me that bipolar in children does not exist and does not require medication by a psychiatrist."

At the 2004 JBRF conference, Dr. Papolos advised that medications treatment should be based on an informed collaborative partnership between the parent and the psychiatrist. He also thinks that every child should have a neuropsychological assessment by a competent pediatric neuropsychologist.

But treatment can be problematic. At the 2001 Fourth International Conference on Bipolar Disorder, Boris Birmaher, MD, of the University of Pittsburgh, presented an unpublished multicenter study that treated seventy-three bipolar I adolescents and followed them for seventy-six weeks. Despite the fact that 70 to 80 percent of them recovered, approximately 80 percent of each subgroup (mixed, manic, depressed) experienced a recurrence of the illness. Seventy percent of patients required hospitalizations. Forty percent of the time, patients required at least three medications. Furthermore, "most patients continued to have fair to poor social adjustment."

There are only a handful of studies on meds treatment for bipolar kids, all of them small, but generally indicating that mood stabilizers and atypical antipsychotics have some efficacy. But side effects can be a major problem, Melissa DelBello, MD, of the University of Cincinnati, told a symposium at the 2004 APA annual meeting. Lithium and Depakote can result in hair loss, weight gain, and acne—huge issues for kids. Many Depakote users also had polycystic ovary syndrome to contend with. Kids in one Risperdal study gained 4.4 pounds, and in a Zyprexa study they gained 12 pounds in just twenty-eight days. Then there is diabetes and cognitive dulling.

The much-publicized FDA investigation into the risk of suicidality among kids on antidepressants only looked at those with unipolar depression. Moreover, the FDA made no attempt to investigate the hypomanic and similar reactions that are well known to happen in kids and try to link them to potentially harmful behavior. Nevertheless, it did instruct manufacturers to place on their labeling (but not in the black box) a warning that owing to the risk of inducing mania and mixed states in bipolar patients, physicians should "adequately screen" their patients for bipolar disorder before initiating antidepressant treatment.

Unfortunately, "adequately screen" is a far lower standard than "carefully screen."

Our best data is from testimony by the Child and Adolescent Bipolar Foundation (CABF) to the FDA in its February 2004 public hearing. In anticipation of its testimony, the CABF surveyed its members (parents of bipolar kids), and found that 20 percent of the survey responders were convinced that their own children became suicidal due to treatment with an antidepressant. One parent reported her six-year-old son became "hyper" on his first antidepressant, and "very agitated" on the second. Despite this, the doctor increased the dose, sending the boy into a total psychotic state that included hallucinations, severe suicidality, severe paranoia, and homicidality, all new symptoms.

As a general rule, an antidepressant that works unusually fast (such as within a few days) is a universal indicator of trouble ahead.

Because the best that psychiatrists can do for now is cite their own clinical experiences with bipolar medications rather than any convincing studies, parents are entitled to take a skeptical approach and hold the psychiatrist to account for any drug he or she may recommend. This includes asking if the drug has worked well for other kids treated in his or her practice, as well as evidence of any research (such as a pilot study) to show at least some evidence of efficacy and safety.

Parents should also be fully satisfied as to what the drug is being used for—what symptoms or side effects it is supposed to manage, how it works with other drugs in the cocktail, and how long the child is expected to remain on the drug. Since side effects can have a more pronounced effect on kids than adults, parents should not leave the office until the physician has recited the full litany of things that can go wrong and how they apply to their child's individual needs.

Since these side effects may affect your child's development as much as the underlying illness, the parent needs to establish from the beginning that there is no such thing as a fair trade-off between improving mood symptoms and worsening health and deteriorating quality of life.

Talking Therapy

A helpful psychosocial intervention includes family-focused therapy, developed by David Miklowitz, PhD, of the University of Colorado at Boulder. The therapy emphasizes understanding the illness and its triggers and taking preventive action, and creating a stable family environment that promotes recovery and encourages medication adherence.

A 2004 study found that thirty-four bipolar kids (mean age eleven) who participated in twelve sessions of a family-focused therapy and cognitive behavioral therapy combined with their meds significantly reduced their symptoms and improved their functioning, with high levels of treatment adherence.

Parents are encouraged to check out other family therapy programs if family-focused therapy is not available in your area.

Educational Intervention

School performance is an early casualty of childhood bipolar disorder. As if the eruptions of the illness and the meds' side effects aren't bad enough, even in states of wellness, cognition and attention deficits can sabotage learning. Moreover, bipolar kids frequently lack the social skills to get along with others. Accordingly, educational intervention is a necessity.

The second edition of *The Bipolar Child* devotes a full chapter on working with your school system in developing an Individualized Educational Plan or Program (IEP) for your child in a regular school or sending your kid to a special school. At the 2004 JBRF conference, both Janice Papolos and Dr. Papolos stressed the critical need for a comprehensive IEP. For instance, if your child does not perform at his or her best till eleven in the morning, it may be advisable to press for a later start or to see if the school can schedule gym or nonacademic classes before that time.

Janice Papolos observed that she has been very impressed by the dedication of teachers. In a survey for *The Bipolar Child,* parents overwhelmingly reported that the schools did everything to help. The whole school has got to be on board, she stressed. She compared a bipolar kid at school to Kramer, from *Seinfeld,* falling into a room. Only at school, however, teachers and students tend not to be as indulgent as Jerry and Elaine.

Bipolar kids need everything broken down, she went on to say. They generally can't sequence. They need to be taught, for instance, not to barge into a room, to stop and look around first. They need to learn how to cope with their anxiety, which is a huge stressor. Teachers, often in collusion with other teachers, must have on hand a bag of tricks to head off a meltdown.

"It's up to parents and teachers to keep installing the software," she advised, "but eventually it will stick."

Supplements/Diet/Toxins

At the 2003 Non-Pharmaceutical Approaches to Mental Disorders conference staged by Safe Harbor, Cheryl related how her adopted son—we'll call him Andrew—started to unravel at age eight. "It was the scariest thing to happen to a mother," she recalled. Andrew threw things, flew into rages, and jumped out of a van at fifty miles an hour. Andrew was diagnosed with bipolar I and put on meds, but according to his mother he became a vegetable, sleeping all the time, gaining weight, and not engaging in the outdoor activities he once loved. Whereas Andrew had once tested four to six years above grade level, he was now testing two years below. As Cheryl explained: "They felt they had solved my problem. I felt I lost my child."

In desperation, she weaned her child off his meds and started him on a regimen of vitamins and other nutrients. This nearly resulted in Andrew getting kicked out of school, but she stayed the course and was happy to report that her son had just been named the most joyful kid in his class.

As a general rule, supplements and diet should complement rather than replace meds therapy. For supplements or diet, it is advisable to consult a nutritionist and work with an open-minded psychiatrist. Like all aspects of your child's treatment, you will need to become your own expert.

Diet is a matter of common sense. That twenty-ounce Coke your kid may drink at school contains fifteen teaspoons of sugar. And he or she may glug down another fifteen on the way home. Modern diets are turning our kids into obese individuals and future diabetics. No smoking gun has been found making the link to mental health, but researchers are bound to connect the dots sometime soon.

It may also be a good idea to test your child for toxic substances and sensitivities to certain types of food. Dust, mold, various chemicals such as those in fertilizers, and pollens can affect the central nervous system and the brain. Doris Rapp, MD, author of *Our Toxic World: A Wake Up Call,* advises asking: "Was it a pollen season? Had you just moved or started a new job or school? Did you purchase a new mattress, carpet, furnace, furniture? Did you paint or pesticide your home? Did you remodel or repair something in your home? Was there an upset in your health (an infection or operation), life, home, family?"

Conclusion

Finding the right diagnosis for your kid and getting him or her on the right meds with appropriate psychosocial and educational interventions, as well as lifestyle changes, is bound to be a process of heartbreak and frustration. But never abandon the hope that your child can eventually lead an enriching, creative, and productive life. An article in the *South Florida Sun-Sentinel* describes one family's journey through hell, but finally—after finding a psychiatrist who made a correct diagnosis and treated their kid accordingly—the mother, Tina, was able to say of her thirteen-year-old son, Steven: "I don't know this kid. He's a different kid. He's fun. I enjoy being around him. . . . Steven was getting A's where he used to get F's. . . . I never bonded with Steven. Now that he's stable, I'm learning to love him. I'm catching up on nine years."

Kids like Steven have been out of the closet with their diagnosis since day one. Unlike previous generations with the illness, they are growing up refusing to be invisible and demanding to be heard. Please take pride in your kids—they will truly change the world.

Depression in the Elderly

Mildred Reynolds, EdD, MSW, is a longtime educator and advocate. She recently completed her term as vice president of the Depression and Bipolar Support Alliance. In 1960, at the age of thirty, a depression "unbelievably and indescribably painful" struck her. It felt, she wrote, "like a rat was gnawing on my brain." Suicide to her "seemed not like harm to self, but relief for self."

But Dr. Reynolds was living in the dark age of Freud. It wasn't until the late 1970s that her psychiatrist prescribed medications for depression. Several years later, twenty-four years from the time she first sought help, she was finally given a diagnosis, but it took another nine years to find a combination of medications that really worked well.

"Today," Dr. Reynolds writes, "I have fears, but I do not dwell on them. For example, I fear that the medication that 'got me well' will no longer 'keep me well.' If I become depressed in a nursing home, will I be able to get the psychiatric care I need? Throughout the years of living with depression, I have developed many good coping skills. But they will be of no help if I develop dementia—perhaps the greatest fear of all."

Her article appeared as part of a 2002 special issue of *Biological Psychiatry* on late-life mood disorders. For those who qualify for senior-citizen discounts, depression poses its own set of hazards. *Biological Psychiatry* cites a 1994 Indiana University study of 1,711 patients sixty years or older in an academic primary-care practice, which found 292 patients were depressed and 140 remained depressed nine months later. The depressed patients were more likely to rate their health as fair or poor, were more likely to have an emergency-room visit, had more outpatient visits, and had more outpatient charges than nondepressed patients.

Contrary to popular belief, however, depression is not part of the normal aging process. True, older people may seem to have a lot more to be depressed about. Ten to 20 percent of widows and widowers experience depression during the first year of bereavement, but in general the percentage of depressed among the elderly is only marginally higher than in the population as a whole. And with age comes an array of coping skills.

What may be different about some older people with depression is the condition of fine fibers (white matter) that run like wiring beneath the brain cortex. Lesions (hypertensities) in white matter have been identified in age-related illnesses such as dementia, and are a focus of investigation in geriatric depression. A 2003 Duke University study of MRI scans on 133 depressed patients, age sixty and over, on antidepressants found that those who achieved and sustained remission over a two-year period had significantly fewer increases in white-matter hypertensity volume than those who did not achieve or sustain remission.

One cause of these lesions (also found in gray matter) may be vascular disease, hence vascular depression.

Unfortunately, the primary-care physicians who represent the front lines in health care often fail to diagnose depression in their older patients. A 1997 University of Illinois study of 141 family physicians and general internists found that 29 percent reported that "depressed elderly patients frustrated them," and 24 percent were too pressured to routinely investigate depression.

Ironically, *Biological Psychiatry* noted, it is easier for most physicians to order expensive and often unnecessary tests for a patient with a vague physical complaint than to spend the extra time necessary to make a more accurate diagnosis or provide education and counseling.

Symptoms of late-onset depression—which may include agitation, anxiety, and irritability—often differ from the rest of the population. They are often ignored or confused with Parkinson's or Alzheimer's or dementia—not to mention thyroid disorders or strokes or heart disease—or taken as side effects of medication, which they sometimes are. Depression frequently co-occurs with these and other disorders, blending into the landscape of the victim's usual aches and pains, and tending to become difficult to spot.

The problem is compounded by the unwitting patient, conditioned to the stigmas of an earlier era. The very same person who would not hesitate to reveal to his doctor his darkest personal secrets—his incapacitating injuries, his difficulty breathing, those embarrassing memory lapses and humiliating no-shows in the bedroom—would seemingly rather be struck down by lightning or make a speech in public while naked than admit in confidence to the simple fact of feeling down in mood.

If only doctors would talk to their patients. In Chapter 5, we discussed a 2000 study that found depressed elderly patients had a 26 percent higher mortality rate compared to those who did not have depression in their age group. (Here, once again, I should remind you that this is not the same as saying your depressed mother or grandmother has a fatal illness.)

We can only guess at how many extra beds in the hospital—not to mention days inside—are the result of hidden depression. How many heart and other operations and their complications, how many prescriptions written, how many hours spent in the care of a health professional, are an unnecessary drain on our health-care system? All those Medicare and Medicaid dollars, all those HMO premiums, all that money that ultimately comes out of our own pockets—how many billions or tens or hundreds of billions of that is wasted due to unseen depression?

All because we are too stingy to invest a dime up front on depression.

Deteriorating health, a sense of isolation and hopelessness, and difficulty adjusting to new life circumstances often combine to create a hell on top of a hell that demands ultimate release. It's one of those bitter facts of death that tend to get swept under the carpet—suicide in the elderly far exceeds the population as a whole. Among elderly white males, the suicide rate is six times the national average. Amazingly, 75 percent of these had seen a doctor within the last month. And as the baby-boomer generation starts trading in their Walkmans for walkers, the overall statistics will go through the roof, initiating a public-health problem of major proportions.

The sad part is much of this can be avoided, for elderly people have the same response to antidepressants and other therapies as the rest of the population. Accordingly, if you are an older person, or are caring for one, it pays to be mindful of the following points:

▋ Depression is not a natural condition of old age and should not be tolerated as part of the process of aging. Older people are as responsive to treatment as the young.

▋ Have your doctor administer a routine depression screening test.

▋ Take any talk or idea of suicide very seriously. Elderly people are far more likely than the rest of the population to follow through.

▋ Support matters. Depression is twice as rampant in nursing homes as elsewhere.

▋ There may be physical or other causes of actual depressive symptoms, including low blood pressure, hypothyroidism, Parkinson's disease or the side effects from its medications, as well as grieving the loss of loved ones.

The Sexes and Relationships

Depression in Women

In an article on my Web site, Barbara Sebranek compares her depression to the lyrics in an REM song, "The Great Beyond": "I'm pushing an elephant up the stairs."

When she was a kid, she and her younger sister were sent to a foster home and forced to do backbreaking labor. As she describes it:

I remember vividly how comforting the idea of dying was: I could go to sleep one night and just never wake up. I was not a particularly precocious child and for that reason I had no way of knowing that in order to escape by death, it would likely be necessary for me to have an active hand in my demise. I wanted to die, yet I had no real concept of suicide. All

*I knew was that I was hurting, big time, and that I would
continue in agony until death intervened.*

Barbara attributes her adult depression to the horrors of her
childhood "state-sanctioned hell." At age twenty-eight, she got
treated for depression, but:

*While the meds lessened the frequency and severity of depres-
sive episodes and thus relieved much of my pain, they did little to diminish guilt. But I had no idea that my guilt feelings
were related to my depression. To me, it was a separate issue.
After all, I had always been and continued to be a poor excuse for a human being, so I had plenty to feel guilty about!*

Part of her guilt was that she "would never be Mother-of-the-
Year material." As she describes her daughter's upbringing: "With
one parent absent physically and the other parent absent mentally,
she had been left to fend for herself emotionally during her forma-
tive years. Add to that a genetic predisposition for depressive disorders, and you have the ingredients for some very serious latent
mental health issues."

At the time she submitted her story to my Web site, Barbara was
not yet ready to relate what had happened to her daughter, now
grown. Shortly after her article was published, however, it all
poured out of her, leading to the awful moment of truth: " 'I regret
having to tell you this,' came the voice over the line. 'Your daughter
attempted to take her life with a handgun.' "

The bullet had rendered her face an unrecognizable pulp. Emergency surgeries followed. She was expected to die, but languished in
the hospital for two years, unable to speak as doctors kept delaying
reconstructive surgery.

As Barbara concluded in her first article: "While my guilt hovers like a mammoth beast near the first riser, my daughter is faced with the monumental task of hoisting an entire herd of elephants."

Depression affects 1 in 5 women over the course of a lifetime, double the number in males. In addition to classical depression, women are also subject to specific types related to their ability to bear children, such as postpartum depression and depression brought on by PMS.

With the onset of puberty, women begin suffering far more than boys, which carries over into adulthood and peaks at peri-menopause, the transition into menopause. Thereafter, the numbers gradually recede back to the levels of men.

In October 2000, the American Psychological Association (the other APA) convened a summit of more than thirty-five experts on women and depression, chaired by Carolyn Mazure, PhD, of Yale University. In April 2002, the APA released a fifty-nine-page report based on that summit, *Summit on Women and Depression*, which provides a useful indication of what we know and what we don't know.

As many as 75 percent of women experience some premenstrual emotional and behavioral problems, the report notes. Meanwhile, pregnancy and delivery produce dramatic changes in estrogen and progesterone levels, as well as major changes in the HPA axis, while perimenopause results in critical fluctuations in estrogen and other hormones.

Summit on Women and Depression is quick to point out that these changes have not yet been definitively linked to mood disorders, though the onset of puberty, when girls start experiencing depression in greater numbers than boys, may be the nearest thing to a smoking gun. "Biology clearly affects the risk of depression and biology is changed by depression," this part of the report concludes.

Concerning life stress and trauma, the report is decidedly less ambiguous: "Serious adverse life events are clearly implicated in the onset of depression," the report says. Eighty percent of depression cases are preceded by a serious life event, with women three times more likely than men to experience depression in response to stressful events. Childhood sexual abuse, adult sexual assault, and male-partner violence have been "consistently linked" to higher rates of depression in women.

Other stressors include poverty, inequality, and discrimination.

Making matters worse is the fact that women engage in "ruminative thinking," that is, "a mental focus on symptoms of distress and their possible causes and consequences, repetitively and passively." Ruminative behavior, explains the report, is associated with longer and more severe episodes of depression. "Unmitigated communication," a tendency in women to base their self-worth on relationships and their external environment and take on other people's problems as their own, is also linked to depression.

To add insult to injury, depressed women appear to nongenetically transmit their depression to their offspring. Women with histories of depression, the report notes, tend to be more critical toward their adolescent children. Depressed women also experience more marital discord and divorce. Even women in remission are vulnerable. Thus, depressed mothers raised in dysfunctional families risk raising future mothers of dysfunctional families.

None of these factors operates in isolation. Instead, biology, psychology, and social factors work together in "complex and reciprocal interactions."

Postpartum Depression

The "baby blues" affect some 50 to 70 percent of new moms, with onset occurring within three days to a month after delivery and a duration of less than ten days.

At the other extreme is postpartum psychosis, affecting 1 in 500 births, accompanied by hallucinations, delusional thoughts, and agitated behavior. The mother cannot care for her baby, and there is serious risk of both suicide and infanticide. Women with bipolar disorder are at particular risk (with odds of 1 in 5).

Postpartum depression occupies the middle ground, affecting some 10 to 15 percent of deliveries. The term *postpartum* merely refers to the triggering event. This is major depression, pure and simple. The *DSM-IV* specifies that the depression must occur within four months of the child's birth to be truly postpartum, but many experts feel that life is more complicated than that.

On my Web site, Anne, whose one-and-a-half-pound daughter Melissa was born after twenty-six weeks of gestation, reports: "I dared not break down. I was all this child had and I knew that if I succumbed once, it would be all over." For months, she did not shed a tear. "It was like well, I'll schedule the breakdown for later, I don't have time now."

Several months after taking Melissa home, Anne's grandmother died, "and suddenly I literally collapsed in a heap. I was a blubbering, jabbering wreck, a total emotional mess." Her niece came over and took Melissa for the night. "I cried for hours and hours until I eventually fell asleep. That was the start of many nights like this."

Her life essentially felt over, and she began to convince herself that her kids would be better off without her. This went on until Melissa was almost eighteen months old.

Postpartum depression can ambush hopeful new mothers at the time when they least expect it and turn their dreams of parenthood into the worst of nightmares. Reports Pamela Gerhardt in the *Washington Post*: "Bookstores file postpartum depression under psychology. And how many women, giddy with the thought of becoming a mother, are perusing the mental illness section of Barnes and Noble?" One guidebook cited in her article offered this advice: "Treat yourself to a dinner out . . . put on makeup." Another recommended a little mascara.

Ms. Gerhardt confessed to putting her weeks-old son in his crib, then throwing her vacuum cleaner up a tree and onto the front lawn, where it remained in pieces for weeks. Clearly, putting on mascara was out of the question.

If you are a mom-to-be or a new mom (or her significant other):

- Treat postpartum depression as a potential part of the birthing and parenting process, and learn as much as you can.
- Have your doctor screen you for depression, whether you feel you need it or not.
- Don't overburden yourself. You don't have to keep up appearances.
- Get help from friends and family. Make friends with other parents.
- If you suffer from bipolar disorder, prepare yourself for the possibility of postpartum psychosis, and have your support systems well in place.
- Postpartum depression responds to antidepressants, talking therapy, and group support. Do not be afraid to get help.
- If you are breast-feeding, you should remember that small amounts of SSRI antidepressants find their way into baby's milk, but not enough to be considered unsafe.

Male Depression

Ray Bradbury's 1953 short story "The Playground" says it all. A father drops off his boy at nursery school for the first time and observes the following with increasing trepidation: "The rushing children were hell cut loose in a vast pinball table colliding and banging and totaling of hits and misses, thrust and plunging to a grand and yet unforeseen total of brutalities." The father's sister assures him everything will be fine: "He's got to take a little beating and beat others up; boys are like that."

This being science fantasy, the father makes the ultimate sacrifice and switches places with his son, finding himself in the body of a boy at the top of a slide: "He shrieked, he covered his face, he felt himself pushed, bleeding, to the rim of nothingness. Headfirst, he careened down the slide, screeching, with 10,000 monsters behind. One thought jumped through his mind a moment before he hit bottom in a nauseous mound of claws. 'This is hell,' he thought, 'this is hell.' "

Terrence Real, author of *I Don't Want to Talk About It: Overcoming the Secret Legacy of Male Depression*, offers some important insights into how fragile we actually are.

The author was physically and emotionally abused by his father. He was a D student, a drug addict, and a petty criminal before eventually finding his calling as a family therapist in the Boston area, with clients typically sharing similar patterns of abuse and dysfunction.

It's a jungle out there, make no mistake about it, even for men with idyllic childhoods, with rites of passage as brutal as those found in any rain forest. There is nothing new about this, of course, but the depression aspect adds a novel spin.

Boys and men internalize their hurt into what Terrence Real calls "covert depression," a psychic band around the heart sufferers respond to by engaging in destructive addictive behaviors—from classic alcohol and drug use to affairs outside the marriage to workaholism to neglecting or abusing their own children. Typically, they are incapable of making the emotional investment necessary to sustain a lasting loving relationship, either with their wife or kids.

Overt depression erupts when a man's addictive behaviors no longer assuage the hurt. Sometimes it occurs in the middle of therapy, after the client's defenses have been unmasked. Often medication is part of the treatment, but in Terrence Real's view it represents at best a partial response, as "an unhappy, immature, relationally unskilled man on medication becomes, at best, a happier immature, relationally unskilled man."

Terrence describes depression as an "auto-aggressive disease," one in which the self attacks the self. Recovery is about connecting with the hurt and trauma that lies beneath. Boys feel as much as girls, but this is hardly the message we send them. Ultimately, in Terrence's words, "boys become men by lopping off, or having lopped off, the most sensitive parts of their psychic and, in some cases, physical selves."

Terrence's own healing came at age thirty-seven, when his father finally opened up to the horrors of his own poverty-stricken childhood. "Don't let the way I talk fool you," the author's father confides, as he admits, probably for the first time, how precious his son is to him.

"Healing," Terrence Real concludes, "interrupts the legacy of depression's transmission from parent to child. . . . Depressed men, by healing themselves, bring peace to their ancestors and protection to their offspring."

Why Psychiatry Fails Men

Jed Diamond, a therapist and author of *Male Menopause* and *The Irritable Male Syndrome,* and his wife, Carlin, both took depression tests as part of a drug-treatment program involving their son. Jed's wife scored high on the test, while he scored low. As a result, Carlin sought and received help for her depression, while Jed lived in a hellish fool's paradise of believing there was nothing wrong with him.

Years later, in response to Carlin's persistent suggestions that he, too, may be suffering from depression, Jed kept insisting, "I'm not depressed, damn it, leave me alone," clinging to his score from that depression test as "proof" that he was okay.

But all was not well. As Jed told this writer: "I was irritable and angry all the time. But there were reasons for that. I had a lot of stresses on my job, raising kids was not easy, and my wife was going through menopause and having her own problems. 'Who wouldn't be angry,' I would bellow to anyone who would listen." Carlin received the brunt of his anger, which she fought to deflect. But what did she expect? Jed thought. She kept doing all these things that irritated him.

"I was worried most of the time," Jed reported. "But wasn't that normal?" Money problems, family worries, aging parents, getting old, the state of the world. It never stopped.

It failed to dawn on Jed that his worry was a symptom of an inner problem, not a response to problems that someone else was causing in his life. It never occurred to him that his irritability, anger, and blaming were symptoms of a type of depression psychiatry is only beginning to wake up to. "My insistence that I wasn't depressed," he finally acknowledged, "nearly ended my marriage and came close to ending my life."

Do men actually manifest depression differently than women? Consider Neal Conan's intro to NPR's *Talk of the Nation,* which in late October 2002 aired a show on male depression: "There are many theories about men and depression. Some researchers argue that men experience depression differently than women. Men are more likely to describe depression as feeling burnt out, for example, rather than excessive sadness. And men are more likely to deny or forget feelings of depression . . ."

According to Neal Conan's main guest, William Pollack, PhD, a psychologist at Harvard Medical School and the director of the Center for Men and Young Men at McLean Hospital, and the author of *Real Boys: Rescuing Our Sons from the Myths of Boyhood*: "A lot of men get angry, irritable, mean, impulsive, and we say they're . . . SOBs and they're a pain, and let's get rid of them, let's fire them, let's divorce them, when, in fact, behind that mask of masculinity is actually the same sadness, hurt and pain expressed in a male-based fashion."

Says Jed: "We are missing millions of men who suffer from depression because we are not asking the right questions."

The *DSM-IV*'s first and perhaps most important symptom for major depression is "depressed mood most of the day," and its only example is the unfortunate one of "appears tearful."

Skipping down to symptom three, we find: "Significant weight loss when not dieting or weight gain." Think of who runs to the fridge for Ben & Jerry's when feeling low, and now reflect on what men go to the fridge for.

Then we come to symptom seven, "feelings of worthlessness or inappropriate guilt." You may recall that when we discussed depression in women, Barbara had these thoughts in abundant supply. The male equivalent is probably closer to Dr. Pollack's irritable and angry SOBs.

The ninth and final symptom concerns suicidality. More men commit suicide, and they may or may not think about suicide as often as women. But because women make far more attempts, they are much more likely to come to the attention of the psychiatric profession.

Lest we get tempted to split depression into Hamlet and Ophelia subtypes, we need to be reminded that many men suffer from "female" symptoms and vice versa. It is far more useful, instead, to think of depression as a beast of many faces, ranging from feeling sad to being anxious to expressing anger to exhibiting out-of-character aggression. It is an illness that engages all processes of the mind and body, from not being able to think straight to throwing our eating and sleeping out of whack to setting us up for cardiac failure. It is more an illness of not being our usual self than simply being depressed, and hopefully one day the name will reflect that fact.

Unfortunately, psychiatry ghettoizes men, all too often tagging the ones who seek help as antisocial or substance users, and shunting them off to treatment that may not be appropriate or is, at best, only a partial answer. Fortunately, thanks to an emerging awareness among therapists and psychiatrists, it appears likely that male depression will get at least a partial airing in preparation for the next *DSM*.

As for Jed: "Fortunately, I listened to my wife's entreaties that I get help. Too many men die, never realizing they are depressed, never recognizing they have a treatable illness. If you're one of those men, don't wait as long as I did. Your decision may be a matter of life and death."

Midlife Crisis

Men who reach fifty are often at the peak of their careers and are generally in excellent health, but they are also entering a period of life-threatening and quality-of-life illnesses including cardio- and cerebrovascular illnesses, sexual dysfunction, hypogonadism, and suicide. According to Stephen Roose, MD, of Columbia University, writing on Medscape: "It is striking that vascular disease, erectile dysfunction, decreased testosterone, and suicide are all strongly associated with depression."

Starting at age thirty, testosterone levels decline 1 percent a year. By age sixty, 25 percent of men are clinically "hypogonadal." Symptoms include decreased libido, erectile dysfunction, fatigue, irritability, dysphoria, and confusion. Testosterone replacement (such as a transdermal patch) can reverse most of these symptoms. Unfortunately, too many men over sixty take what they think is the only way out. According to Dr. Roose: "In the United States the suicide cohort is overwhelmingly white, male, and older than the age of 60. Strikingly, the relationship between age, gender and suicide is consistent throughout the world and across cultures."

Innocent Bystanders

On my Website, Viola writes:

> *My husband is bipolar. I've watched him stare down kitchen knives tying to decide what to do with them, watched him smash chairs, punch cabinets, be so depressed he couldn't get out of bed, and treat me with such contempt I was convinced I was a horrible wife. I've also seen him playing with our kids with great joy and laughter, work through his anger problems until he rarely raises his voice, treat me with such love and giving I wonder if I had imagined it was as bad as it was.*
>
> *I feel so guilty. He was born this way, he never asked for this. When he tells me he loves me, I know he means it. And when he tells me again how I'm the biggest mistake of his life, he's going to mean that, too. I care deeply and I don't want to add to his pain, but I don't know how other wives stay sane and feel good about themselves and stay on the roller coaster.*
>
> *Now I'm faced with the decision to stay or go. Is it kinder to put my three- and one-year-old through a divorce or stay together and have them grow up thinking love is this weird mix of affection, abuse, and codependence? Would he be better off away from all the parts of my personality that trigger his anger and irritation? Would I be happier alone or just standing tough where I am?*
>
> *I honestly don't know what to do and every choice hurts someone.*

A parent doesn't have the luxury of considering leaving a child. A 2001 Child and Adolescent Bipolar Foundation poll of 723 of CABF's members (parents of bipolar children) found that the levels of stress were "off the charts."

Then there are the innocent kids. Anonymous writes: "I was raised by a bipolar mother who was very abusive, mentally and physically. She never sought help for her problems while I was young, not until I was an adult and moved out of the house. I have never forgiven her for this."

The Burden of Sympathy: How Families Cope With Mental Illness, by David Karp, PhD, tells of mental illness from the point of view of the families. Listen to this candid admission from one distraught mom: "Sometimes I think it would be easier if he had cancer. His disease is so dreadful."

And from a wife: "There are times when I feel like, God, maybe my life would be better off if I wasn't with him."

Heroic measures are possible in the early going, Dr. Karp tells us, because "sympathy margins remain wide and caregivers often believe that once an emotionally ill person realizes how much he or she is cared about, they will get better."

And a few pills, they assume, will fix everything.

Some families turn out to have this kind of good fortune—or at least achieve a result everyone can live with—but these weren't the people Dr. Karp talked to. "The realization that a family member's mental illness may never go away is a crucial identity turning point in the caregiver's career," he writes, "because it forces to the surface of consciousness an array of emotions that previously may have been dimly felt."

As time drags on, Dr. Karp tells us, "caregivers nearly always come to feel greatly frustrated by the persistent, ongoing trauma of mental illness. They find it harder to muster the compassion felt during the early stages of the illness. It is also harder for them to avoid feelings of anger and resentment."

Ultimately, though, comes acceptance, for when all is said and done—for kids, anyway—there is no other choice.

Saving the Relationship

On my Web site, Beatrice writes:

> *I have never experienced the depth of pain in watching some-*
> *one I love suffer so. The only thing that I can compare it to*
> *was watching my beloved father die of pancreatic cancer and*
> *witness him lash out at those of us around him who loved him*
> *as he experienced his pain and frustration.*
>
> *To love someone fills us so completely, but to watch the*
> *one you love suffer a disease such as bipolar illness . . . it just*
> *defies any kind of logic. My mind is clear and very rational as*
> *I hear the words of anger, rage, hate—all leveled at me. I love*
> *this man—I hate the disease.*

Ben reports:

> *My wife, after two and three-quarters years of marriage, five*
> *years together, and a new baby, left, and stated that it wasn't*
> *the "real her" that I married. She got an apartment in a neigh-*
> *boring state, and made plans to go to art college, while setting*
> *up a new life. When she left, I had to take care of all of the re-*
> *sponsibilities, and the bills, and most importantly, my daugh-*
> *ter. She has set up visitation, but states that she no longer*
> *wants to be married, and that she hasn't felt anything for a*
> *long time. But, it's like she pulled a 180 degree turn. I don't*
> *know what to do next.*

Anne Sheffield, author of *Depression Fallout: The Impact of De-*
pression on Couples and What You Can Do to Preserve the Bond
(which is also applicable to bipolar disorder), is a veteran of both
her own and her mother's depression. "There is no way properly to
describe the anguish a depressive can put his family through," says

depression survivor Mike Wallace, of *60 Minutes,* in the book. "Gloom, doom, no love, no real communication, short temper, and leave me alone, fault finding."

Telling Mr. or Ms. Hyde that something is wrong, however, can be as delicate a procedure as diffusing a bomb. Avoid the straight-out "You many be clinically depressed," Ms. Sheffield advises, and try something along the lines of "I've been noticing lately that you're not sleeping well at night. Are they working you too hard at the office?" From there, one looks to gradually break down the elaborate defenses and nudge Cleopatra, Queen of Denial, into an open discussion. Personal presentation helps, Ms. Sheffield adds— for example, hair in place, good shoes. "Selling" depression to an unwilling partner, after all, is pure marketing.

Fine, you've got your partner to talk. Now what? Ms. Sheffield suggests starting with a list of four specific items, such as "No arguing or angry displays in front of the children." Nonspecific instructions to lighten up or think positive, she warns, "might as well be issued in Chinese." When being verbally abused, it is better to leave the room, she advises, than joining battle, which is self-defeating.

Once your partner has bought into his or her diagnosis, there are many ways of assisting with his or her recovery. But depression can be contagious, a result of the loss of self-esteem and stress that comes from living with Miss or Mr. Congeniality. For both your own good and your partner's, then, Ms. Sheffield advises, it is crucial to put yourself first. "To whatever extent possible," she urges, "put some psychological and physical distance between you and your sad mate."

That psychological and physical distance may ultimately involve sleeping in a single bed in another state, but there is life after depression fallout, Ms. Sheffield concludes. Bailing out on Hamlet doesn't mean ending up like Ophelia.

Julie Fast and John Preston, PsyD, authors of *Loving Someone with Bipolar Disorder: Understanding and Helping Your Partner,* encourage partners to collaborate on putting together their own lists of behavioral symptoms, such as anger or excessive spending. Once the two of you know what you're up against, they advise, it may be possible to respond to the first signs of unusual behavior before they spin out of control.

Then the significant other needs to learn to respond rather than react, such as saying "I can see that you're angry. How can I help you?" instead of "What's your problem?" This can become a bit problematic when your partner has just blown $5,000 on a stupid chair and you're the one seething with anger, but these situations—and other bipolar catastrophes—can often be avoided by strict daily adherence to ironclad check-in procedures.

The authors devote a whole chapter to mood triggers, and place strong emphasis on partners working together to reduce the stress in the living environment, from keeping work and social obligations under control to more discriminate TV viewing to proper diet, sleep, and exercise. "Root trigger" is a term they have come up with to define a trigger that may set off other triggers, such as—bad news from work followed by a poor night's sleep resulting in a miserable day at work building into anger that leads to a serious domestic quarrel and triggers thoughts of life not worth living.

Recognizing the root trigger as it occurs and mobilizing quickly can spare both partners a lot of grief.

Ultimately, the authors acknowledge, you may have to make some very tough decisions. "Maybe you have lived in crisis for so long," they write, "you haven't had the chance to examine what your future will look like realistically, if you stay with your partner. What do you need to do to create the life you want?"

That's a question only you can answer.

Getting Along with Our Families

In an article on my Web site, Flora writes: "Sometimes I am amazed that the worst stigma I can face comes from my own extended family." Soon after her diagnosis, she was invited to a family get-together. As she describes it: "There is nothing worse than going to a family function where mothers with small children hang back. They offer the baby to everyone old enough but me. They don't ask me about my plans, my aspirations. I get pity looks and although they want all the details of my illness, they won't ask me directly."

All too often, our illness reduces us to outcasts among our own kin, the living skeleton in the family closet, cast as the classic nutty aunt or crazy uncle. With loving relationships, it can be worse. Where once we were someone's soul mate, now we find ourselves strangers in our own homes, exiled to our domestic gulags, prisoners of ignorance and stigma.

Ironically, our loved ones and family members may be the real nut cases, in denial about their own illness, refusing to talk about it, to even think about it. Chances are you aren't the only one splashing around in your end of the family gene pool. At least we had the courage to acknowledge something was wrong and get treatment. For this, we face ridicule and contempt.

How many of us can relate to Isabelle? "My husband still does not understand the way depression affects the person that is suffering. He thinks I can snap out of it or get over it."

Just snap out of it. If only we broke out in spots when an episode struck, or our skin turned green. Then our families could at least see that the illness was real. Spots they could relate to. And green—it would be like a papal bull absolving us of all guilt. Green would definitely command respect—sympathy, even.

It isn't easy being green—they learned that much from Kermit.

But try being invisible. Says William: "Even my own blood family doesn't understand what I have! They never will and they never could anyway."

You may as well be telling them that Jupiter's Great Red Spot is making you hypersensitive to gravity. Realistically, your family can never understand. It's like asking someone who has never had a headache to imagine having a headache.

My grown daughter, who is my pride and joy, knows all about my illness and tries hard to understand me. Her questions are intelligent and penetrating, and I am good at explaining. But then she makes a comment that makes me realize that she is an outsider looking in. I am saddened, of course, but the realist in me says the only way you can understand this illness is to have it.

One night, I found myself praying to God that my daughter, and any children she may have, never understand me.

But your family can be there for you, and William recognizes this: "My second wife has learned how to recognize what particular mood I'm in as well as which one I'm headed for next. I thank God for her—at least she understands me!"

Probably not exactly understands, but we get the point. No doubt William's wife does more for his wellness than any med in his meds cocktail. A supportive family can have that effect. Here's a few simple guidelines.

■ Keep your expectations realistic. The one difference between your loved ones comprehending your illness and them performing Rachmaninoff's Third Piano Concerto from memory is that performing the Rachmaninoff is a lot easier.

■ Establish a dialogue. Take responsibility for being the initiator.

■ Educate your family. Hand out books and brochures. Print articles from Web sites. Encourage them to get involved with the National Alliance for the Mentally Ill (NAMI);

(www.nami.org), which is very supportive of families. Develop your own thirty-second standard presentation. Although it is not entirely accurate, you can explain you have a chemical imbalance of the brain. If you're doing well, it will be easy for them to accept this explanation. If you're struggling, you will need to explain why Rome wasn't built in a day and thank them for their understanding.

■ Acknowledge the suffering you may have caused others. You may not know it, but your illness-related behavior has probably generated a lot of bad will in the family. A heartfelt act of contrition (even if your illness was the cause rather than you) can help win back the people you may have alienated.

■ Form partnerships. If you are married or living in a loving relationship, your partner needs to be a player in managing your illness. He or she needs to know your triggers and how to help you avoid them, needs to be involved in any contingency planning, and needs to keep reminding you to remain compliant with your treatments and lifestyle regimens. If you're headed into a crisis, this is the person who is likely to be making the executive decisions, from taking away your credit cards and hiding the kitchen knives to calling a doctor.

■ Communicate. Our bad-hair days can equate with Medusa's. Even if you're just feeling a bit grumpy, let your loved one know. This can help you avoid unnecessary confrontations.

Hopefully, your family or loving relationship will turn into your greatest asset. But don't be afraid to selectively disengage. Giving Thanksgiving a miss may be a good idea (but do not interpret this as an excuse to isolate yourself). If you're used to being put up at the house of a family member during the holidays, you might find $80 or $90 a night at a hotel is a good investment in your sanity. And always acknowledge that both you and your loved one need plenty of space apart, sometimes in separate time zones.

Your illness can often bring you closer to your family and your loved one, with your shared hardships forging a stronger bond. But it can also drive you apart, leaving you feeling unloved and unwanted and embittered. Ultimately, your final option may be breaking off all ties with your family or loved one.

Such events are never pleasant. You are in for an extended spell of loneliness, and the aftereffects will remain with you for years—just ask anyone who has experienced a bust-up. But you are also embarking on the first stage of a healing journey. Just make sure you get plenty of support along the way.

Protecting the Kids

On my Web site, Terry writes:

The earliest memory I have is my dad trying to take care of my older sister, younger brother, and I. I think I was only four years old because my sister was in primary school and I was in kindergarten. I knew it wasn't easy for him while my mum was off at a mental hospital a hour away, and I knew it was never easy for him to take her there either.

She started to show she was getting ill by yelling at neighbors she never would have arguments with, and asking us kids to do stupid things. Then was always a call to my aunty and uncle to look after us while my dad grabbed a travel bag and put clothes in it for Mum to wear at the hospital while my brother, sister and I huddled under the covers of beds and cried at the known fact that Mum wasn't coming back for a couple of months.

When she died I was crushed like the rest of my family. I think people who have never had someone in their family with bipolar will never know the pain that these people go through,

*and the family go through while they see their loved ones suf-
fering. My mum said we were never to talk about her illness
to others, ever. I'm sorry, Mum, but now that you are gone I
don't want your suffering to be unnoticed.*

William Beardslee, MD, of Harvard University and Children's
Hospital, Boston, has worked with families for more than twenty
years, and has authored one landmark study on the effect of
parental mood disorders on children, plus numerous other studies.
He also lived through the trauma of his sister's severe depression
and suicide. In his 2002 book, *Out of the Darkened Room: When a
Parent Is Depressed: Protecting the Children and Strengthening the
Family* (which also applies to bipolar disorder), he writes: "When
parents become depressed, they bear a double burden. Even as they
wrestle with the darkness that clouds their lives, they must struggle
to maintain their roles as guardians of their children's future. Making matters worse, depression is often mystifying both to the suf-
ferer and those around them."

Depression, says Dr. Beardslee, is a family illness that psychiatry
still treats as an individual illness. The children who are kept in the
dark must cope with the disruptions their parents undergo, themselves becoming an at-risk population. What is at stake starts with a
consideration of three factors: (1) depression in one or both parents;
(2) other problems parents face, such as alcoholism or anxiety; and
(3) difficulties earlier in the child's life, such as problems with learning to read.

With none of these factors present, says Dr. Beardslee, 6 percent
of children get depressed. The number doubles to 12 percent with
one factor present, but with all of them in play an alarming one half
of all children become depressed. In Dr. Beardslee's words: "The
message is: Get help for yourself before depression can lead to the
'negative chain' of other events that, together, can harm your child.
Build your child's protective resources and do not let your depres-

sion cascade into the multiple risk factors that can undermine your child's health."

"Breaking the silence" is Dr. Beardslee's term for getting a parent's depression out into the open, where the illness is freely discussed among all the family members. Given that one aspect of depression is to make one uncommunicative, this is often easier said than done. Together with your partner, Dr. Beardslee advises, decide what should be discussed and not discussed. Try to show your children that the two of you are united in caring for them. Keep in mind that kids at different ages will deal with the matter very differently. One six-year-old, for instance, was afraid she might catch her father's depression by using his toothbrush.

Reassure your kids, Dr. Beardslee goes on to say, that you will be okay and the illness will not overwhelm your family. Emphasize that no one is guilty or to blame. Speak to the positives, and talk about the illness and its treatment. Tell your children what actions you're taking (such as getting treatment), discuss events your children have witnessed, talk about things that are unusual or upsetting, and help your children feel comfortable enough to talk about things that frighten them.

"Open, ongoing communication," Dr. Beardslee concludes, "is the foundation of the resilience we want in our kids." This is not always easy because kids tend to be kids, but that's the point—family adversity may result in our children growing up fast, but it shouldn't rob them of their innocence and childhoods.

Should We Have Kids?

What if I had known I had bipolar disorder back in 1977, when I was twenty-seven? My first wife and I had assumed we would start having kids sometime after we completed law school and established ourselves in our careers, but then I thought, why wait? Yes, agreed my wife, once we had very carefully weighed all the pros and cons, why wait? A few months later, we found out that we both passed our first-year final exams with flying colors, but we had much better news to report to our families.

But what if I knew then what I know now—that I was a walking train wreck waiting to happen, stoked by runaway mutant genes from both sides of the family? Would I have been so confident in raising the topic of having a kid with my wife? Would I even have a wife?

Had I known that I was male heir to the family gene pool from hell, I would have been decidedly less sanguine about my future, make no mistake about it. The prospect of getting my degree would have been pie in the sky, and how long could my illness have held up to the pressures of a career in law, anyway? So much for being a good provider. As for being a good father, let alone a good husband, what would crazy do to that? And God help me, what if I should pass down what I had to any child of mine?

Heaven forbid, but had I known then what I know now, this branch of the McManamy family tree would have unequivocally stopped with me.

But I was living in a fool's paradise, and every day I thank God for the choice I made. But every day I also live with the guilt and heartbreak over the fact that I failed to turn out to be the father I had expected to be. My daughter has every reason in the world to disown me. Thankfully, owing to her courage and compassion and her seemingly limitless power to forgive, we enjoy an excellent relationship. But no one should have had to go through what she went through. She deserved a much better father. She deserved a real father.

I would be the very last person to discourage anyone with a mood disorder from having a child, but my own experience indictates the folly in not first seriously reflecting on all the things that can possibly go wrong. At the same time, I know many excellent mothers and fathers. They have all been very open in acknowledging that their illness poses special challenges to domestic life, but the one thing they all seem to have in common is a strong partner or the right partner. Raising children is a team effort, and nowhere is this truer than in the case of a parent who has a chronic illness.

If one parent has bipolar disorder, the probability of passing on the illness to your child is 1 in 5. The child of a bipolar parent also has a 1 in 5 chance of having unipolar depression. If these seem like high odds, one needs to be reminded that the deck is stacked in favor of your child turning out mentally sound.

Be fruitful and multiply, but think first.

Postscript: Healing

Perhaps the worst thing about having a mood disorder is the uneasy feeling of no escape. Having fallen victim once, twice, several times, you almost know there will be a reoccurrence. You may be short on specifics, but you are quite certain it will sneak up on you as you're sleeping, in a manner not far removed from this:

While you are under the covers, a crew of 112 roustabouts with their heavy machinery will quietly tiptoe into your room, dismantle a few walls, and lay down five miles of high-speed electrogravitational rail track that runs right under your bed. This is sort of Publishers Clearing House sweepstakes in reverse. God has singled out you and you alone for the visitation that is about to eventuate.

The next day you unwittingly arise, only to find your brain rendered into sushi by the Tokyo Express hurtling out of your closet and through the back of your skull and out over the horizon, your sanity receding in the Doppler blare of the engineer's horn, the clanging crossing bells mocking your weakness and stupidity.

You eventually find a new head to pop onto your shoulders, and pick yourself up, only to be mowed down by the Hoboken Local, then the Chattanooga Choo-Choo, a tram, a trolley, and finally little Puffer Bellies all lined up in a row.

It's hopeless now. The kid down the street and his Cocoa Puffs train can crush what's left of your brain simply by looking in your direction. And this is perhaps the cruelest part of depression or mania—there is no train to finish the job. The final deed is up to you, and you alone.

I had survived my worst round of depressions yet, and was still in a state of shell shock from the experience. One of the first things I did when I crawled out from under the covers was get to the computer. I was new to the Internet, and I was new to finally acknowledging depression, and I was also coming to grips with my diagnosis as a manic-depressive, something I had somehow known all my life but up till now had steadfastly refused to accept.

I bounced from Web site to Web site, reading about what devastating illnesses both depression and bipolar disorder were, but I also found that I didn't have to be a helpless bystander. Then I discovered various mental-health bulletin boards, and even started replying to messages, once I worked up the courage. Over the next few weeks, I found myself gravitating to one particular board that was frequented by bipolars. This was at Bipolar World (www.bipolarworld.net) hosted by Colleen Sullivan.

Someone there had posted ten reasons that you know you're bipolar. Reason number ten, as I recall, was that you know you're bipolar if you think Robin Williams should stop being so laid-back.

Somehow I knew I had found a home of sorts. A few weeks later came a cryptic posting calling for writers. I was a writer. I replied. It turned out thats Colleen Sullivan, also happened to be the mental-health managing editor at Suite101.com, as well as the bipolar editor. She was looking for someone to write on depression for Suite 101. I told her I was good for maybe four articles.

Unbelievably, she did not break off the correspondence.

So I sat down at the keyboard and typed: "Depression isn't the word for it. We're talking about a condition that can take over your mind, rob you of your dignity, deprive you of all the joyful offerings of life, and leave you nose down in two inches of water, feeling totally abandoned by man and God."

Next thing I know, I was the Suite's depression editor. I would write as I learned, I decided, one article at a time. It would all be tied into my recovery. In the space of one week, I banged out three articles, then another three in another week, all backed up and waiting to go. There was no question in my mind now—I would have plenty to write about. It wasn't long after that that I had my first newsletter out. My first e-mailing went out to all of about ten people. I was in the publishing business. Then came my Web site. Through my Web site, I would meet my second wife.

Writing is what helped bring me back from the dead. For me, it is a healing activity. If I were a basketball player, I'd be shooting hoops; if I were a gardener, I would be out with the petunias. Healing is about finding something that makes you feel alive and doing it. When I'm in full flight there is no time and space. The sun takes its leave, booming music falls mute, and the steaming hot cup of tea by my side is stone cold when I pick it up a minute later.

After six months in the land of the living dead, and a good two or three years before that in the land of the quasi-living dead, I was writing again, and really writing. I was still writing in the shadow of depression and manic depression, but I was writing. I was reclaiming my life, one page at a time.

RESOURCES

Patients' and Families' Organizations

Anxiety Disorders Association of America
8730 Georgia Avenue, Suite 600
Silver Spring, MD 20910
(240) 485-1001
www.adaa.org

Child and Adolescent Bipolar Foundation (CABF)
1000 Skokie Boulevard, Suite 425
Wilmette, IL 60091
(847) 256-8525
www.bpkids.org

Depression and Bipolar Support Alliance (DBSA)
730 N. Franklin Street, Suite 501
Chicago, IL 60610-7224
(800) 826-3632
www.dbsalliance.org

*Depression and Related Affective Disorders Association
(DRADA)*
8201 Greensboro Road, Suite 300
McLean, VA 22102
(410) 583-2919 or (888) 288-1104
www.drada.org

Dual Recovery Anonymous (DRA)
PO Box 8107
Prairie Village, KS 66208
(877) 883-2332
www.draonline.org

Families for Depression Awareness
300 Fifth Avenue
Waltham, MA 02451
(781) 890-0220
info@familyaware.org
www.familyaware.org

Juvenile Bipolar Research Foundation (JBRF)
550 Ridgewood Road
Maplewood, NJ 07040
(866)333-JBRF
info@jbrf.org
www.bpchildresearch.org

National Alliance for the Mentally Ill (NAMI)
Colonial Place Three
2107 Wilson Boulevard, Suite 300
Arlington, VA 22201-3042
(800) 950-NAMI
www.nami.org

National Mental Health Association
2001 N. Beauregard Street, 12th Floor
Alexandria, VA 22311
(800) 969-NMHA (6642)
www.nmha.org

National Mental Health Consumers'
Self-Help Clearinghouse
1211 Chestnut Street, Suite 1207
Philadelphia, PA 19107
(800) 553-4539
info@mhselfhelp.org
www.mhselfhelp.org

Professional Organizations

American Academy of Child and Adolescent Psychiatry
3615 Wisconsin Ave NW
Washington, DC 20016-3007
(202)966-7300
www.aacap.org

American Psychiatric Association
1000 Wilson Boulevard, Suite 1825
Arlington, VA 22209-3901
(703) 907-7300
www.psych.org

American Psychological Association
750 First Street, NE
Washington, DC 20002-4242
(800) 374-2721
www.apa.org

International Society for Bipolar Disorders
PO Box 7168
Pittsburgh PA 15213-0168
(412) 605-1412
www.isbd.org

Government Organizations

Center for Mental Health Services
U.S. Department of Health and Human Services
200 Independence Avenue, SW
Washington, DC 20201
www.mentalhealth.samhsa.gov/cmhs

Centers for Disease Control
1600 Clifton Road, NE
Atlanta, GA 30333
(800) 311-3435
www.cdc.gov

Food and Drug Administration (FDA)
5600 Fishers Lane
Rockville, MD 20857-0001
(888)INFO-FDA (463-6332)
www.fda.gov

National Institute of Mental Health (NIMH)
6001 Executive Boulevard
Bethesda, MD 20892-9663
www.nimh.nih.gov

Substance Abuse and Mental Health Services Administration
U.S. Department of Health and Human Services
200 Independence Avenue, SW
Washington, DC 20201
www.samhsa.gov/index.aspx

U.S. Surgeon General
U.S. Department of Health and Human Services
200 Independence Avenue, SW
Washington, DC 20201
www.surgeongeneral.gov

Disabilities

National Disability Rights Network
900 Second Street, NE, Suite 211
Washington, DC 20002
(202) 408-9514
www.napas.org/aboutus/default.htm

Social Security Administration
Office of Public Inquiries
Windsor Park Building
6401 Security Boulevard
Baltimore, MD 21235
(800) 772-1213
www.ssa.gov/disability

U.S. Department of Justice
Civil Rights Division
Disability Rights Section
950 Pennsylvania Avenue, NW
Washington, DC 20530
(800) 514-0301
Online USDJ Technical Assistance for Americans with Disabilities
Act (ADA) www.usdoj.gov/crt/ada/adahom1.htm

Free Meds

*Pharmaceutical Research and Manufacturers of America
(PhRMA)*
1100 Fifteenth Street, NW
Washington, DC 20005
(202) 835-3400
www.phrma.org

Suicide/Crisis

American Association of Suicidology
5221 Wisconsin Avenue, NW
Washington, DC 20015
(202) 237-2280
www.suicidology.org

National Suicide Hotlines
(800) SUICIDE
(800) 273-TALK

Suicide Awareness Voices of Education (SAVE)
9001 E Bloomington Fwy, Suite #150
Bloomington, MN 55420
(952) 946-7998
www.save.org/prevention/friends_depression.html

Suicide Prevention Action Network USA (SPAN USA)
1025 Vermont Avenue, NW, Suite 1066
Washington, DC 20005
(202) 449-3600
info@spanusa.org
www.spanusa.org/C_contact.html

Finding a Professional

Psychiatrist

*American Psychiatric Association District Branch/State
Association Directory*
www.psych.org/dbs_state_soc/db_list/db_info_dyn.cfm

Psychiatrist or Therapist

Psychology Today—The Therapy Directory
http://therapists.psychologytoday.com/verizon

Mental Health Providers Recommended by Patients
Depression and Bipolar Support Alliance—Search
www.dbsalliance.org/referral/search.asp

Psychologist

American Psychological Association State and Provincial
Associations
www.psych.org/dbs_state_soc/db_list/db_info_dyn.cfm

Nutritionist

FindaNutritionist.com
www.findanutritionist.com

Alternative/Integrative Practitioner

Safe Harbor
www.alternativementalhealth.com/directory/search.asp

Acupuncturist

Acufinder.com
www.acufinder.com

Informational Web Sites Specializing in Mood

McMan's Depression and Bipolar Web
www.mcmanweb.com

About.com—Bipolar
bipolar.about.com

About.com—Depression
depression.about.com

Bipolar World
www.bipolarworld.net

Depression Central
www.psycom.net/depression.central.html

DepressioNet
www.depressionet.com.au

Mental Health Infosource
www.mhsource.com

Mental Health Sanctuary
www.mhsanctuary.com

MH Today
www.mental-health-today.com

Psych Central
http://psychcentral.com

PsychEducation.org
www.psycheducation.org/index.html

Wing of Madness
www.wingofmadness.com

E-mail Newsletter

McMan's Depression and Bipolar Weekly
www.mcmanweb.com

Online Support

Mood Garden
www.moodgarden.org

Walkers in Darkness
www.walkers.org

Bipolar Significant Others
www.bpso.org

Medical Web Sites

Doctor's Guide
www.docguide.com

Mayo Clinic
www.mayoclinic.com

Medscape
www.medscape.com

REFERENCES

Chapter 1

Cassano GB et al. "The mood spectrum in unipolar and bipolar disorder: arguments for a unitary approach." *Am J Psychiatry*. 2004 Jul;161(7):1264–9.

DePaulo R. "*Genetic Evidence for a Bipolar Spectrum*," 2004 APA annual meeting. May 4, 2004. New York.

Judd LL, and HS Akiskal. "The prevalence and disability of bipolar spectrum disorders in the U.S. population: reanalysis of the ECA database taking into account subthreshold cases." *J Affect Disord*. 2003 Jan;73(1–2):123–31.

McManamy J. "A Companion Called Fred: My Story of Struggle, Acceptance, and Healing," closing address to the 2002 DBSA annual conference. August 11, 2002. Orlando.

Shaw J, Baker M. "Expert patient—dream or nightmare?" *BMJ*. 2004 Mar 27;328(7442):723–4.

Solomon A. *The Noonday Demon: An Atlas of Depression*. Scribner, 2001.

Chapter 2

Akiskal H (2000) "Beyond the Conventional Subtypes of Bipolar Disorder." Medscape. www.medscape.com/viewarticle/420293?src=search.

American Psychiatric Association. *Diagnostic and Statistical Manual of Mental Disorders,* 4th ed., text rev. *(DSM-IV-TR).* American Psychiatric Association 2000.

Billingsley J. "Bradshaw and Williams go public with depression, anxiety stories. Football stars talk about downs off the gridiron." *HealthDayNews,* May 2, 2003.

Chopin F. *Chopin's Letters.* Dove Publications, 1988.

Dally P. *The Marriage of Heaven and Hell: Manic Depression and the Life of Virginia Woolf.* St. Martin's Press, 1999.

Depression and Bipolar Support Alliance. "Beyond Diagnosis: Depression and Treatment: A Call to Action to the Primary Care Community and People with Depression." 2000.

Frederick Chopin Society in Warsaw. www.chopin.pl/spis_tresci/index _en.html.

Fountoulakis KN et al. "Thyroid function in clinical subtypes of major depression: an exploratory study." *BMC Psychiatry.* 2004 Mar 15; 4(1):6.

Kessler RC et al. "National Comorbidity Survey Replication." *JAMA.* 2005 Jun 18;289(23):3095–105.

Klerman GL, and MM Weissman. "Increasing rates of depression." *JAMA.* 1989 April 21; 261(15):2229–35.

Koukopoulos A. "Treating the Complex Patient," interactive session, Fourth International Conference on Bipolar Disorder, June 16, 2001. Pittsburgh.

Goodwin D. "The man in our memory." *New York Times,* February 17, 2003.

Matza J et al. "Depression with atypical features in the National Comorbidity Survey classification, description, and consequences." *Arch Gen Psychiatry.* 2003;60:817–826.

Murray CJL, and AD Lopez, eds. *The Global Burden of Disease and Injury Series, vol. 1: A Comprehensive Assessment of Mortality and Disability from Diseases, Injuries, and Risk Factors in 1990 and Projected to 2020.* Harvard School of Public Health on behalf of the World Health Organization and the World Bank. Harvard University Press, 1996.

Nierenberg AA et al. "Course and treatment of atypical depression." *J Clin Psychiatry.* 1998;59 Suppl 18:5–9.

Oquendo MA et al. "Instability of symptoms in recurrent major depression: a prospective study." *Am J Psychiatry.* 2004 Feb;161(2):255–61

Roper-Starch Worldwide. "America's Mental Health Survey." National Mental Health Association, 2001. www.nmha.org/pdfdocs/mental-healthreport2001.pdf.

Rosenthal N. "Diagnosis and treatment of seasonal affective disorder." *JAMA.* 1993 Dec 8;270(22):2717–20.

Satcher D. *Mental Health: A Report of the Surgeon General.* Office of the Surgeon General, 1999. www.surgeongeneral.gov/library/mental health/home.html.

Van Gogh V. "Complete Letters of Vincent van Gogh." Vincent van Gogh Gallery. www.vangoghgallery.com/letters/main.htm.

van Praag HM. "Anxiety/aggression-driven depression: a paradigm of functionalization and verticalization of psychiatric diagnosis." *Prog Neuropsychopharmacol Biol Psychiatry.* 2001 May;25(4):893–924.

Chapter 3

Bearden CE et al. "The neuropsychology and neuroanatomy of bipolar affective disorder: a critical review." *Bipolar Disord.* 2001 Jun;3(3):106–50.

Begley CE et al. "The lifetime cost of bipolar disorder in the US: an estimate for new cases in 1998." *Pharmacoeconomics.* 2001;19(5 Pt 1):483–95.

Carey B. "Hypomania's up side distinct but linked to bipolar disorder." NY Times News Service, April 5, 2005.

Cassidy F et al. "Subtypes of mania determined by grade of membership analysis." *Neuropsychopharmacology.* 2001 Sep;25(3):373–83.

Dickerson FB. "Association between cognitive functioning and employment status of persons with bipolar disorder." *Psychiatr Serv.* 2004 Jan;55(1):54–8.

Dunner DL. "Rapid-cycling bipolar disorder." *Bipolar Disorders: Clinical Course and Outcome,* 199–217. American Psychiatric Press, 1999.

Gartner J. *The Hypomanic Edge: The Link Between (a Little) Craziness and (a Lot) of Success in America.* Simon & Schuster, 2005.

Goodwin F, Jamison K. *Manic-Depressive Illness.* Oxford University Press, 1990.

Goodwin G. *Evidence-Based Guidelines for Treating Bipolar Disorder: Recommendations from the British Association for Psychopharmacology.* British Association for Psychopharmacology, 2003.

Heckers S. "Neuroimaging Findings in Bipolar Disorder," symposium, 2004 APA annual meeting. May 4, 2004. New York.

Hershman J, and J Lieb. *Manic Depression and Creativity.* Prometheus Books, 1998.

Hirschfeld RM. "Impact of bipolar depression compared to unipolar depression and healthy controls." Poster presented at 2003 APA annual meeting.

———. "Perceptions and impact of bipolar disorder: how far have we really come? Results of the national depressive and manic-depressive association 2000 survey of individuals with bipolar disorder." *J Clin Psychiatry.* 2003 Feb;64(2):161–74.

Hirschfeld RM et al. "Screening for bipolar disorder in the community." *J Clin Psychiatry.* 2003 Jan;64(1):53–9.

Jamison K. *Touched with Fire: Manic Depressive Illness and the Artistic Temperament.* Free Press, 1996.

Judd LL. "The comparative clinical phenotype and long term longitudinal episode course of bipolar I and II: a clinical spectrum or distinct disorders?" *J Affect Disord.* 2003 Jan;73(1–2):19–32.

Lagace D et al. "Mathematics deficits in adolescents with bipolar I disorder." *Am J Psychiatry.* 2003 Jan;160(1):100–4.

Lish JD et al. "The National Depressive and Manic-Depressive Association (DMDA) survey of bipolar members." *J Affect Disord.* 1994 Aug;31(4):281–94.

Mayo Clinic. "Keeping health in mind: ten steps to keep your memory sharp." MayoClinic.com, April 30, 2003. www.mayoclinic.com/invoke.cfm?objectid=8D8E1F5F-9013-47CF-A5F09A59F23CC286.

McElroy S. "New Treatments in Mania," grand rounds lecture UCLA. Neuropsychiatric Institute, Webcast, March 11, 2003. Los Angeles.

Mondimore F. "Bipolar Depression," presentation, 2002 DRADA annual conference, April 27, 2002. Baltimore.

Narrow WE. "One-year prevalence of depressive disorders among adults 18 and over in the US: NIMH ECA prospective data. Population estimates based on U.S. Census estimated residential population age 18 and over on July 1, 1998." Unpublished table cited by the NIMH. www.nimh.nih.gov/publicat/numbers.cfm.

National Institute of Mental Health. Schizophrenia Web page. www.nimh.nih.gov/publicat/schizoph.cfm#schiz1.

Post RM et al. "Morbidity in 258 bipolar outpatients followed for 1 year with daily prospective ratings on the NIMH life chart method." *J Clin Psychiatry.* 2003 Jun;64(6):680–90.

Schneck CD et al. "Phenomenology of rapid-cycling bipolar disorder: data from the first 500 participants in the Systematic Treatment Enhancement Program." *Am J Psychiatry.* 2004 Oct;161(10):1902–8.

Suppes T. "The Stanley Foundation Bipolar Treatment Outcome Network. II. Demographics and illness characteristics of the first 261 patients." *J Affect Disord.* 2001 Dec;67(1–3):45–59.

————. "Bipolar II Disorder: The Concept of Dysphoric Hypomania," UCLA Neuropsychiatric Insitute Webcast, grand rounds, April 15, 2003, Los Angeles.

Swann A. "Biological Specificity of Bipolar Depression," symposium, 2000 APA annual meeting. May 20, 2000. Chicago.

Tillman R, and B Geller. "Definitions of rapid, ultrarapid, and ultradian cycling and of episode duration in pediatric and adult bipolar disorders: a proposal to distinguish episodes from cycles." *J Child Adolesc Psychopharmacol.* 2003 Fall;13(3):267–71.

Tohen M et al. "The McLean-Harvard first-episode mania study: prediction of recovery and first recurrence." *Am J Psychiatry.* 2003 Dec;160(12):2099–107.

Chapter 4

American Psychological Association. "Controlling anger before it controls you." www.apa.org/pubinfo/anger.html.

Anonymous. "Nigeria tops happiness survey." *BBC News,* October 2, 2003.

Benazzi F. "Major depressive disorder with anger: a bipolar spectrum disorder?" *Psychother Psychosom.* 2003 Nov–Dec;72(6):300–6.

Fisher HE. "The Brain in Love," lecture, APA, May 5, 2004. New York.

Fisher HE et al. "Defining the brain systems of lust, romantic attraction, and attachment." *Arch Sex Behav.* 2002 Oct;31(5):413–9.

Fisher HE, and PR Muskin. "Sex, Sexuality, and Serotonin," symposium, APA, May 1, 2004. New York.

Jamison K. "Exuberance," lecture, 2002 DRADA annual conference. April 27, 2002, Baltimore.

———. *Exuberance: The Passion for Life.* Knopf, 2004.

Janowsky DS. "Introversion and extroversion: implications for depression and suicidality." *Curr Psychiatry Rep.* 2001 Dec;3(6):444–50.

Janowsky DS et al. "Relationship of Myers-Briggs Type Indicator personality characteristics to suicidality in affective disorder patients." *J Psychiatr Res.* 2002 Jan–Feb;36(1):33–9.

———. "Myers-Briggs Type Indicator personality profiles in unipolar depressed patients." *World J Biol Psychiatry.* 2002 Oct;3(4): 207–15.

Kessler RC et al. "Prevalence, severity, and unmet need for treatment of mental disorders in the World Health Organization World Mental Health Surveys." *JAMA.* 2004 Jun 2;291(21):2581–90.

Mammen OK et al. "Anger attacks in bipolar depression: predictors and response to citalopram added to mood stabilizers." *J Clin Psychiatry.* 2004 May;65(5):627–33.

Mao WC et al. "Coping strategies, hostility, and depressive symptoms: a path model." *Int J Behav Med.* 2003;10(4):331–42.

McElroy SL. "Recognition and treatment of DSM-IV intermittent explosive disorder." *J Clin Psychiatry.* 1999;60 Suppl 15:12–6.

McManamy J. "Taking It Personally—Depression, Bipolar, Myers-Briggs." *McMan's Depression and Bipolar Weekly* (Web site), www.mcmanweb.com/article235.htm. June 27, 2003.

Picardi AJ. "Higher levels of anger and aggressiveness in major depressive disorder than in anxiety and somatoform disorders." *Clin Psychiatry.* 2004 Mar;65(3):442–3.

Putnam RD. *Bowling Alone: The Collapse and Revival of American Community.* Simon & Schuster, 2000.

Tucker-Ladd C. "Anger and Aggression," *Psychological Self-Help*, Mental Help Net (www.mentalhelp.net/psyhelp).

Chapter 5

Arias E, et al. *National Vital Statistics Reports Deaths: Final Data for 2001.* CDC, 2003. September 18;52(3).

Billingsley J. *Depression's Symptoms Often Physical, Aches and Pains Can Signal Emotional Upset.* HealthScoutNews, March 15, 2002.

Bridges KW, and DP Goldberg. "Somatic presentation of DSM III psychiatric disorders in primary care." *J Psychosom Res.* 1985;29(6):563–9.

Caspi A. "Influence of life stress on depression: moderation by a polymorphism in the 5-HTT gene." *Science.* 2003 Jul 18;301(5631): 386–9.

DiMatteo R. "Depression is a risk factor for noncompliance with medical treatment, meta-analysis of the effects of anxiety and depression on patient adherence." *Arch Intern Med.* 2000 July 24;160: 2101–2107.

Epstein J et al. *Serious Mental Illness and Its Co-Occurrence with Substance Use Disorders.* Substance Abuse and Mental Health Services Administration, 2002.

Fels A. "Cases: mending hearts and minds," *New York Times,* May 21, 2002.

Frank E. "Treatment Resistance in Mood and Anxiety Disorders: Evidence from Clinical Trials," Symposium, APA. May 1, 2004. New York.

Frasure-Smith N et al. "Depression following myocardial infarction: impact on 6-month survival." *JAMA.* 1993 Oct 20;270(15): 1819–25.

Frasure-Smith N et al. "Depression and 18-month prognosis after myocardial infarction." *Circulation.* 1995 Feb 15;91(4):999–1005.

Fletcher A. *Sober for Good: New Solutions for Drinking Problems—Advice from Those Who Have Succeeded.* Houghton Mifflin, 2002.

Freeman MP et al. "The comorbidity of bipolar and anxiety disorders: prevalence, psychobiology, and treatment issues." *J Affect Disord.* 2002 Feb;68(1):1–23.

Golden S. "Depressive symptoms and the risk of type 2 diabetes: the Atherosclerosis Risk in Communities study." *Diabetes Care.* 2004 Feb;27(2):429–35.

Hariri AR et al. "Serotonin transporter genetic variation and the response of the human amygdala." *Science.* 2002 Jul 19;297(5580): 400–3.

Heim C et al. "Pituitary-adrenal and autonomic responses to stress in women after sexual and physical abuse in childhood." *JAMA.* 2000 Aug 2;284(5):592–7.

Heim C, "Overview of the Relationship Between Stress, Depression, and Anxiety." symposium, 2003 APA annual meeting. May 26, 2003. San Francisco.

Katon W et al. "Medical symptoms without identified pathology: relationship to psychiatric disorders, childhood and adult trauma, and personality traits." *Ann Intern Med.* 2001 May 1;134(9 Pt 2): 917–25.

Kessler RC et al. "Lifetime and 12-month prevalence of DSM-III-R psychiatric disorders in the United States: results from the National Comorbidity Survey." *Arch Gen Psychiatry.* 1994 Jan;51:8–19.

———. "The epidemiology of co-occurring addictive and mental disorders: implications for prevention and service utilization." *Am J Orthopsychiatry.* 1996 Jan;66(1):17–31.

———. "Comorbidity of DSM-III-R major depressive disorder in the general population: results from the US National Comorbidity Survey." *Br J Psychiatry.* 1996;168 June Suppl 30:17–30.

Kroenke K, and RK Price. "Symptoms in the community: prevalence, classification, and psychiatric comorbidity." *Arch Intern Med.* 1993 Nov 8; 153(21):2474–80.

Lopes Cardozo B et al. "Mental health, social functioning, and attitudes of Kosovar Albanians following the war in Kosovo." *JAMA.* 2000 Aug 2;284(5):569–77.

McCauley J. "Clinical characteristics of women with a history of childhood abuse: unhealed wounds." *JAMA.* 1997 May 7;277(17): 1362–8.

Murray C. *Global Health Statistics: A Compendium of Incidence, Prevalence and Mortality Estimates for over 200 Conditions* (Global Burden of Disease and Injury, No 2). World Health Organization, World Bank, and Harvard School of Public Health, December 1, 1996.

Nemeroff CB. "Childhood Trauma and the Neurobiology of Mood Disorders." Symposium, 2003, APA annual meeting. May 20, 2003. Philadelphia.

Nemeroff CB et al. "Differential responses to psychotherapy versus pharmacotherapy in patients with chronic forms of major depression and childhood trauma." *Proc Natl Acad Sci USA.* 2003 Nov 25; 100(24):14293–6.

Penninx BW et al. "Chronically depressed mood and cancer risk in older persons." *J Natl Cancer Inst.* 1998 Dec 16;90(24):1888–93.

Ramrakha S. "Psychiatric disorders and risky sexual behaviour in young adulthood: cross-sectional study in birth cohort." *BMJ.* 2000 29 July;321:263–266.

Regier DA et al. "Comorbidity of mental disorders with alcohol and other drug abuse: results from the Epidemiologic Catchment Area (ECA) Study." *JAMA.* 1990 Nov 21;264(19):2511–8.

Sachs G. "STEP-BD Update." Session, Fifth International Conference on Bipolar Disorder. June 12, 2003. Pittsburgh.

Salama P et al. "Mental health and nutritional status among the adult Serbian minority in Kosovo." *JAMA.* 2000 Aug 2;284(5):578–84.

Sapolsky R. "Taming stress." *Scientific American.* Sept 2003.

Schulz et al. "Association between depression and mortality in older adults: the Cardiovascular Health Study." *Arch Intern Med.* 2000; 160(12):1761–1768.

Simon N et al. "Pharmacotherapy for bipolar disorder and comorbid conditions: STEP-BD data." Poster presented at 2004 APA annual meeting.

Substance Abuse and Mental Health Services Administration. *Report to Congress on the Prevention and Treatment of Co-occurring Substance Abuse Disorders and Mental Disorders.* U.S. Department of Health and Human Services, 2002.

Tennant C, and L McLean. "Mood disturbances and coronary heart disease: progress in the past decade. Psychological factors are increasingly being identified as important contributors to the onset and course of coronary heart disease." *MJA.* 2000;172:151–2.

Wulsin L. "Does depression kill?" *Arch Intern Med.* 2000;160: 1731–2.

Chapter 6

Barchas J. "Adventures in Psychiatric Research: Neurobiology to Public Policy," lecture, APA annual meeting. May 4, 2004. New York.

Cotter D et al. "Reduced glial cell density and neuronal size in the anterior cingulate cortex in major depressive disorder." *Arch Gen Psychiatry.* 2001 Jun;58(6):545–53.

Diamond MC et al. "Increases in cortical depth and glia numbers in rats subjected to enriched environment." *Comp Neurol.* 1966 Sep; 128(1):117–26.

———. "On the brain of a scientist: Albert Einstein." *Exp Neurol.* 1985 Apr;88(1):198–204.

Dreshfield-Ahmad LJ et al. "Enhancement in extracellular serotonin levels by 5-hydroxytryptophan loading after administration of WAY 100635 and fluoxetine." *Life Sci.* 2000 Apr 14;66(21):2035–41.

Drevets WC. "Subgenual prefrontal cortex abnormalities in mood disorders." *Nature.* 1997 Apr 24;386(6627):824–7.

Duman RS et al. "Chronic antidepressant treatment increases neurogenesis in adult rat hippocampus." *J Neurosci.* 2000 Dec 15;20(24): 9104–10.

———. "Regulation of adult neurogenesis by antidepressant treatment." *Neuropsychopharmacology.* 2001 Dec;25(6):836–44.

Eriksson PS et al. "Neurogenesis in the adult human hippocampus." *Nat Med.* 1998 Nov;4(11):1313–7.

Manji HK. "Research Update." Session 2002 NAMI annual convention, June 29, 2002. Cincinnati.

———. "Neurobiology of Bipolar Disorder: Neuroplasticity and Cellular Resistance," grand rounds lecture UCLA Neuropsychiatric Institute, Webcast, 2003.

———. "Enhancing neuronal plasticity and cellular resilience to develop novel, improved therapeutics for difficult-to-treat depression." *Biol Psychiatry.* 2003 Apr 15;53(8):707–42.

Manji HK et al. "Lithium-induced increase in human brain grey matter." *Lancet.* 2000 Oct 7;356(9237):1241–2.

———. "Regulation of cellular plasticity cascades in the pathophysiology and treatment of mood disorders: role of the glutamatergic system." *Glutamate and Disorders of Cognition and Motivation.* Ann NY Acad Sci. 2003;1003:273–91.

Mitterauer B. "Imbalance of glial-neuronal interaction in synapses: a possible mechanism of the pathophysiology of bipolar disorder." *Neuroscientist.* 2004 Jun;10(3):199–206.

Rajkowska G et al. "Reductions in neuronal and glial density characterize the dorsolateral prefrontal cortex in bipolar disorder." *Biol Psychiatry.* 2001 May 1;49(9):741–52.

Sanacora G. "Increased occipital cortex GABA concentrations in depressed patients after therapy with selective serotonin reuptake inhibitors." *Am J Psychiatry.* 2002 Apr;159(4):663–5.

————. "Increased cortical GABA concentrations in depressed patients receiving ECT." *Am J Psychiatry.* 2003 Mar;160(3):577–9.

Sanacora G et al. "Subtype-specific alterations of gamma-aminobutyric acid and glutamate in patients with major depression." *Arch Gen Psychiatry.* 2004 Jul;61(7):705–13.

Sapolsky R et al. "Glucocorticoids exacerbate insult-induced declines in metabolism in selectively vulnerable hippocampal cell fields." *Brain Res.* 2000 Jul 7;870(1–2):109–17.

Schoepp D, and H Manji. "Glutamate: An Exciting Neurotransmitter," symposium, 2003 APA annual meeting. May 20, 2003. San Francisco.

Chapter 7

Ananthaswamy A. "Undercover genes slip into the brain." *New Scientist.* March 20, 2003. www.newscientist.com/news/news.jsp?id=ns 99993520.

Cosmides L, and J Tooby. "Evolutionary psychology: a primer." Web paper, 1997. www.psych.ucsb.edu/research/cep/primer.html.

Dobzhansky T. "Nothing in biology makes sense except in the light of evolution." *American Biology Teacher.* 1972;35:125–129.

Freedman R et al. "Alpha-7 nicotinic receptor agonists: potential new candidates for the treatment of schizophrenia." *Psychopharmacology (Berl).* 2004 June;174(1) 54–64.

Gibbs W. "The unseen genome: gems among the junk." *Scientific American,* November 2003.

———. "The unseen genome: beyond dna." *Scientific American*, December 2003.

Hagen E. "The functions of postpartum depression." Web paper, 1999 www.anth.ucsb.edu/faculty/hagen/working.html.

Horrobin D. *The Madness of Adam and Eve: How Schizophrenia Shaped Humanity*. Bantam Books, 2002.

Hudson JI et al. "Family study of affective spectrum disorder." *Arch Gen Psychiatry*. 2003 Feb;60(2):170–7.

Insel T. "Mental Health: The Best of Times and the Worst of Times," research plenary, 2003 NAMI annual convention. July 1, 2003. Minneapolis.

———. "NIMH Update" Fifth International Conference on Bipolar Disorder, lecture. June 12, 2003. Pittsburgh.

Insel T, and F Collins. "Psychiatry in the genomics era," *Am J Psychiatry*. 2003 Apr;160(4):616–20.

Kelsoe JR, TB Barrett et al. "Evidence that a single nucleotide polymorphism in the promoter of the G protein receptor kinase 3 gene is associated with bipolar disorder." *Mol Psychiatry*. 2003 May;8(5):546–57.

McKie R. "Schizophrenia 'helped the ascent of man.' Scientist says gene mutation is key to genius and despair." *Sunday Observer*. March 18, 2001.

MacKinnon DF et al. "Comorbid bipolar disorder and panic disorder in families with a high prevalence of bipolar disorder." *Am J Psychiatry*. 2002 Jan;159(1):30–5.

McLean Hospital. "Common gene could link multiple psychiatric, medical disorders." Press release, February 10, 2003. www.hms.harvard.edu/news/pressreleases/mcl/0203commongene.html.

McMahon FJ et al (2001). "Linkage of bipolar disorder to chromosome 18q and the validity of bipolar II disorder." *Arch Gen Psychiatry*. 2001 Nov;58(11):1025–31.

Nemeroff C, and R Lenox. 2000 DBSA annual conference remarks, reported in "Nonsense, Sense, and Antisense," *McMan's Depression and Bipolar Weekly* 2000 Aug 21; 2(30).

Nesse RM. "Is depression an adaptation?" *Arch Gen Psychiatry.* 2000 Jan;57(1):14–20.

Nesse RM. "What is Darwinian medicine?" Web paper. 1997 www.chester.ac.uk/~sjlewis/DM/TEXTS/TEXT1.HTM.

Niculescu AB et al. "Identifying a series of candidate genes for mania and psychosis: a convergent functional genomics approach." *Physiol Genomics.* 2000 Nov 9;4(1):83–91.

Pardridge WM. "Targeting neurotherapeutic agents through the blood-brain barrier." *Arch Neurol.* 2002 Jan;59(1):35–40.

Petronis A. "Epigenetics and bipolar disorder: new opportunities and challenges." *Am J Med Genet.* 2003 Nov 15;123C(1):65–75.

Phelps D. "Bipolar genetics." Web paper, 1997. www.psycheducation.org/depression/fitness.htm.

Potash JB et al. "Suggestive linkage to chromosomal regions 13q31 and 22q12 in families with psychotic bipolar disorder." *Am J Psychiatry.* 2003 Apr;160(4):680–6.

Sapolsky RM. "Gene therapy for psychiatric disorders." *Am J Psychiatry.* 2003 Feb;160(2):208–20.

Scolnick E. "Mental Health Research," research plenary, 2003 NAMI annual convention. July 1, 2003. Minneapolis.

Torrey EF. "A federal failure in psychiatric research: continuing NIMH negligence in funding sufficient research on serious mental illnesses." Treatment Advocacy Center, Public Citizen, Nov. 19, 2003, www.citizen.org/documents/AFC636D.pdf.

Freedman R. "Rethinking the Concept of Phenotype in Psychiatry" symposium, 2003 APA annual meeting. May 19, 2003. San Francisco.

Williams GC, and RM Nesse. "The dawn of Darwinian medicine." *Q Rev Biol.* 1991 Mar;66(1):1–22.

Chapter 8

American Heart Association, "Nutrition Facts." www.american-heart.org/presenter.jhtml?identifier=855.

Marlin Company/Gallup. "Attitudes in the American Warplace VI," 2000.

Anonymous. "Depression sufferers fear stigma at work." New York Times News Service, March 29, 2004.

Benson H, and M Stark. *Timeless Healing.* Repr. Scribner, 1997.

Blumenthal JA et al. "Effects of exercise training on older patients with major depression." *Arch Intern Med.* 1999 Oct 25;159(19):2349–56.

Conti D. "Depression in the Workplace," seminar, 2002 DBSA annual conference. August 10, 2002, Orlando.

Crowley K. "Procovery Primer," *The Power of Procovery: Just Start Anywhere.* www.procovery.com. 2000. procoveryprimer.htm

Davidson RJ et al. "Alterations in brain and immune function produced by mindfulness meditation." *Psychosom Med.* 2003 Jul–Aug; 65(4):564–70.

Depression and Bipolar Support Alliance. *Support Groups: An Important Step on the Road to Wellness.* Brochure.

Depression and Bipolar Support Alliance. "Sleepless in America campaign." Media release, June 14 2004. www.dbsalliance.org/Media/NewsReleases/Sleep.html.

Duke University. "Duke study: exercise may be just as effective as medication for treating major depression." Press release, October 23, 1999, www.sciencedaily.com/releases/1999/10/99102707/1931.htm.

Elkins R. *Solving the Depression Puzzle: The Ultimate Investigative Guide to Uncovering the Complex Causes of Depression and How to Overcome It.* Woodland Publishing, 2001.

Ellison M, and Z Russinova. "A national survey of professionals and managers with psychiatric conditions: a portrait of achievements and challenges." Boston University Center for Psychiatric Rehabilitation, 1999. www.bu.edu/cpr/research/recent/rtc1999/si_3.html.

Fava M et al. "Fluoxetine versus sertraline and paroxetine in major depressive disorder: changes in weight with long-term treatment." *J Clin Psychiatry*. 2000 Nov;61(11):863–7.

Fernstrom JD et al. "Effects of aspartame ingestion on the carbohydrate-induced rise in tryptophan hydroxylation rate in rat brain." *Am J Clin Nutr*. 1986 Aug;44(2):195–205.

Frank E. "Interpersonal and Social Rhythm Therapy." workshop, Fourth International Conference on Bipolar Disorder, June 16, 2001. Pittsburgh.

Gartner J et al. "Spirituality: perspectives in theory and research." *Jnal Psychol and Theol.*" 1991 Spring;19(1).

Hedaya R. *The Antidepressant Survival Guide: The Clinically Proven Program to Enhance the Benefits and Beat the Side Effects of Your Medication.* Three Rivers Press, 2001.

Hedley AA. "Prevalence of overweight and obesity among U.S. children, adolescents, and adults, 1999–2002." *JAMA*. 2004 Jun 16; 291(23):2847–50.

Houston T et al. "Internet support groups for depression: a 1-year prospective cohort study." *Am J Psychiatry*. 2002 Dec; 159:2062–8.

International Center for the Integration of Health and Spirituality. www.nihr.org/programs/researchreports/spiritualitybuffersstress.cfm.

International Center for the Integration of Health and Spirituality. Gallup and USA Today Polls.

Kempermann G et al. "Activity-dependent regulation of neuronal plasticity and self repair." *Prog Brain Res*. 2000;127:35–48

Koenig HG. "Spirituality as a Relevant Clinical Factor," workshop 2002 APA annual meeting. May 20, 2002, Philadelphia.

Koenig HG et al. "Religious attitudes and practices of hospitalized medically ill older adults." *Int J Geriatr Psychiatry*. 1998 Apr;13(4):213–24.

———. "Depressive symptoms and nine-year survival of 1,001 male veterans hospitalized with medical illness." *Am J Geriatr Psychiatry*. 1999 Spring;7(2):124–31.

Koenig HG, ME McCullough, and DB Larson. *Handbook of Religion and Health*. Oxford University Press, 2000.

Korner J. "How to Shrink Obesity," symposium, 2004 APA annual meeting. May 6, 2004. New York.

Kwang-Soo et al. "The impact of religious practice and coping on geriatric depression recovery." Poster presented at the 2002 APA annual meeting.

Larson D et al. "Physicians and patient spirituality: professional boundaries, competency, and ethics." *Ann Intern Med*. 2000 Apr 4; 132(7):578–83.

Lawlor D, and S Hopker. "The effectiveness of exercise as an intervention in the management of depression: systematic review and meta-regression analysis of randomised controlled trials." *BMJ*. 2001 Mar 31;322(7289):763–7.

McGrath-Hanna NK et al. "Diet and mental health in the Arctic: is diet an important risk factor for mental health in circumpolar peoples? A review." *Int J Circumpolar Health*. 2003 Sep;62(3):228–41.

Morselli PL, and R Elgie. "GAMIAN-Europe/BEAM survey I—global analysis of a patient questionnaire circulated to 3450 members of 12 European advocacy groups operating in the field of mood disorders." *Bipolar Disord*. 2003 Aug;5(4):265–78.

Mulready P. "Healing," presentation, Advocacy Unlimited conference. Sept 22, 2001. Hartford, CT.

Noble K. "You really are what you eat." *Time International*, Feb 17, 2003.

Oman D. "Religious attendance and cause of death over 31 years." *Int J Psychiatry Med.* 2002;32(1):69–89.

Pizza Hut. "Pizza hut nutrition calculator." www.yum.com/nutrition/menu.asp?brandID_Abbr=1_PH. 2003.

Pizzaware.com. "Pizza industry facts." http://pizzaware.com/facts.htm.

Roth T. "Sleep and Psychiatric Illness," symposium, 2002 APA annual meeting. May 17, 2002. Philadelphia.

Satcher D. *The Surgeon General's Call to Action to Prevent and Decrease Overweight and Obesity.* Office of the Surgeon General, 2001. www.surgeongeneral.gov/topics/obesity.

Seiden RH. "Where are they now? A follow-up study of suicide attempters from the Golden Gate Bridge." *Suicide Life Threat Behav.* 1978 Winter;8(4):203–16.

Sonawalla SB. "Elevated cholesterol levels associated with nonresponse to fluoxetine treatment in major depressive disorder." *Psychosomatics.* 2002 Jul–Aug;43(4):310–6.

Szabo A et al. "Phenylethylamine, a possible link to the antidepressant effects of exercise?" *Br J Sports Med.* 2001 Oct;35(5):342–3.

van Praag H et al. "Running increases cell proliferation and neurogenesis in the adult mouse dentate gyrus." *Nat Neurosci.* 1999 Mar;2(3):266–70.

Wallis C. "Faith and healing: can prayer, faith and spirituality really improve your physical health? A growing and surprising body of scientific evidence says they can." *Time,* June 24, 1996.

Walsh J et al. "Modafinal Treatment of Chronic Shift Work Sleep Disorder," report session, APA, May 6, 2004. New York.

Walton RG et al. "Adverse reactions to aspartame: double-blind challenge in patients from a vulnerable population." *Biol Psychiatry.* 1993 Jul 1–15;34(1–2):13–7.

Watson R. "The new patient power." *Newsweek,* 2001 June 25; 137 (26) 54–8.

Weintraub A. *Yoga for Depression: A Compassionate Guide to Relieve Suffering Through Yoga.* Broadway, 2003.

Westover AN, and LB Marangell. "A cross-national relationship between sugar consumption and major depression?" *Depress Anxiety.* 2002;16(3):118–20

Woolery A et al. "A yoga intervention for young adults with elevated symptoms of depression." *Altern Ther Health Med.* 2004 Mar–Apr;10(2):60–3.

World Health Organization. "Obesity and Overweight." Global Strategy on Diet, Physical Activity, and Health. Diet and physical activity: a public health priority. 2004. http://www.who.int/dietphysical activity/publications/facts/obesity/en/index.html.

Wurtman JJ. "Depression and weight gain: the serotonin connection." *J Affect Disord.* 1993 Oct–Nov;29(2–3):183–92.

Wurtman JJ, and S Suffes. *Serotonin Solution.* Ballantine, 1996.

Wurtman RJ, and JJ Wurtman. "Brain serotonin, carbohydrate-craving, obesity and depression." *Obes Res.* 1995 Nov;3 Suppl 4:477S–80S.

Chapter 9

Young AS et al. "The quality of care for depressive and anxiety disorders in the United States." *Arch Gen Psychiatry.* 2001 Jan;58(1): 55–61.

Chapter 10

Anderson IM et al. "Evidence-based guidelines for treating depressive disorders with antidepressants: a revision of the 1993 British Association for Psychopharmacology guidelines." *J Psychopharmacol.* 2000 Mar;14(1):3–20.

Anonymous. "The trick to putting Paxil behind: proceed slowly, under a doctor's care." *Washington Post,* August 27, 2002.

Boseley S. "Murder, suicide: a bitter aftertaste for the 'wonder' depression drug antidepressant Seroxat under scrutiny as firm pays out $6.4m." *Guardian,* June 11, 2001.

Brown WA, and W Harrison. "Are patients who are intolerant to one serotonin selective reuptake inhibitor intolerant to another?" *J Clin Psychiatry.* 1995 Jan;56(1):30–4.

Cohen J. *Over Dose: The Case Against the Drug Companies: Prescription Drugs, Side Effects, and Your Health.* Penguin Putnam, 2001.

Davis J. "Drug vs. Talk Therapy for Depression." WebMD, September 7, 2004 http://www.webmd.com/content/article/93/102491.htm.

DeBattista C et al. "Adjunct modafinil for the short-term treatment of fatigue and sleepiness in patients with major depressive disorder: a preliminary double-blind, placebo-controlled study." *J Clin Psychiatry.* 2003 Sep;64(9):1057–64.

Depression and Bipolar Support Alliance. "Most patients report troublesome side effects, modest improvement using current antidepression treatments." Press release, 1999.

Geddes JR et al. "Relapse prevention with antidepressant drug treatment in depressive disorders: a systematic review." *Lancet.* 2003 Feb 22; 361(9358):653–61.

Harvey H. " 'Prozac robber' sent to maximum security psychiatric hospital." *New Haven Register,* June 20, 2000.

Healy D, and C Whitaker. "Antidepressants and suicide: risk-benefit conundrums." *J Psychiatry Neurosci.* 2003 Sep;28(5):331–7.

Hedaya R. "A psychiatrist argues for treating the side effects of today's antidepressant medications." *Washington Post,* February 29, 2000.

Hirschfeld R, chair. *Practice Guideline for the Treatment of Patients with Bipolar Disorder.* 2nd ed. American Psychiatric Association, 2002.

Jahn H et al. "Metyrapone as additive treatment in major depression: a double-blind and placebo-controlled trial." *Arch Gen Psychiatry.* 2004 Dec;61(12):1235–44.

Keller MB et al. "A comparison of nefazodone, the cognitive behavioral-analysis system of psychotherapy, and their combination for the treatment of chronic depression." *N Engl J Med.* 2000 May 18;342(20):1462–70.

Kirsch I, and G Sapirstein. "Listening to Prozac but hearing placebo: a meta-analysis of antidepressant medication." *Prevention and Treatment.* 1998 June 26;1. http://journals.apa.org/prevention/volume1/pre0010002a.html.

Kirsch I et al. "The emperor's new drugs: an analysis of antidepressant medication data submitted to the U.S. Food and Drug Administration." *Prevention and Treatment.* 2002 July 15;5. http://journals.apa.org/prevention/volume5/pre0050022i.html.

Karasu T, chair. *Practice Guideline for the Treatment of Patients with Major Depressive Disorder. 2nd ed.* American Psychiatric Association, 2000.

Mann J. Testimony to an FDA panel in 2004.

McManamy J. "Second time lucky." *McMan's Depression and Bipolar Weekly.* 2003 Feb 19;5(4). www.mcmanweb.com.

"Prozac Mania—The Dark Side of Antidepressants." *McMan's Depression and Bipolar Weekly.* Forsyth Prozac and Schell Paxil cases reported. www.mcmanweb.com/article-19.htm.

Parker G. "Evaluating treatments for the mood disorders: time for the evidence to get real." *Aust NZ J Psychiatry.* 2004 Jun;38(6): 408–14.

Paykel ES. "Remission and residual symptomatology in major depression." *Psychopathology.* 1998;31(1):5–14.

————. "Achieving gains beyond response." *Acta Psychiatr Scand.* Suppl 2002;(415):12–7.

Quitkin FM et al. "When should a trial of fluoxetine for major depression be declared failed?" *Am J Psychiatry.* 2003 Apr;160(4): 734–40.

Stahl S, and N Muntner. *Essential Psychopharmacology of Depression and Bipolar Disorder.* Cambridge University Press, 2000.

Thase ME et al. "Fluoxetine treatment of patients with major depressive disorder who failed initial treatment with sertraline." *J Clin Psychiatry.* 1997 Jan;58(1):16–21.

————. "Citalopram treatment of fluoxetine nonresponders." *J Clin Psychiatry.* 2001;62:683–7.

————. "Double-blind switch study of imipramine or sertraline treatment of antidepressant-resistant chronic depression." *Arch Gen Psychiatry.* 2002 Mar;59(3):233–9.

Markowicz J, A Nierenberg, and ME Thase. "Recovery from Depression: New Perspectives to Improve Outcomes." 2002 APA conference. May 20, 2002. Philadelphia.

Wolf CR et al. "Pharmacogenetics." *BMJ.* 2000;320:987–90.

Chapter 11

Allison DB, and JL Mentore. "Antipsychotic-induced weight gain: a comprehensive research synthesis." *Am J Psychiatry.* 1999 Nov;156 (11):1686–96.

Altshuler L et al. "Impact of antidepressant discontinuation after acute bipolar depression remission on rates of depressive relapse at 1-year follow-up." *Am J Psychiatry*. 2003 Jul;160(7):1252–62.

American Diabetes Association, American Psychiatric Association, American Association of Clinical Endocrinologists, North American Association for the Study of Obesity. "Consensus Development Conference on Antipsychotic Drugs and Obesity and Diabetes Diabetes Care." *Diabetes Care*. 2004 Feb;27(2):596–601.

Amsterdam JD, and DJ Brunswick. "Antidepressant monotherapy for bipolar type II major depression." *Bipolar Disord*. 2003 Dec;5(6): 388–95.

Angst J et al. "Mortality of patients with mood disorders: follow-up over 34–38 years." *J Affect Disord*. 2002 Apr;68(2–3):167–81.

Bauer MS, and L Mitchner. "What is a 'mood stabilizer'? An evidence-based response." *Am J Psychiatry*. 2004 Jan;161(1):3–18.

Beasley CM et al. "Olanzapine versus haloperidol: acute phase results of the international double-blind olanzapine trial." *Eur Neuropsychopharmacol*. 1997 May;7(2):125–37.

Bowden CL et al. "Efficacy of divalproex vs lithium and placebo in the treatment of mania: the Depakote Mania Study Group." *JAMA*. 1994 Mar 23–30;271(12):918–24.

———. "A randomized, placebo-controlled twelve-month trial of divalproex and lithium in treatment of outpatients with bipolar I disorder: Divalproex Maintenance Study Group." *Arch Gen Psychiatry*. 2000 May;57(5):481–9.

Calabrese JR. "Research and Treatment Update on Bipolar Disorder," update, 2001 DBSA annual conference. August 11, 2001. Cleveland.

———. "A placebo-controlled eighteen-month trial of lamotrigine and lithium maintenance treatment in recently depressed patients with bipolar I disorder." *J Clin Psychiatry*. 2003 Sep;64(9):1013–24.

———. "A randomized, double-blind, placebo-controlled trial of queti-apine in the treatment of bipolar I or II depression." *Am J Psychiatry*. 2005 Jul;162(7):1351–60.

Chengappa KN et al. "Changes in body weight and body mass index among psychiatric patients receiving lithium, valproate, or topiramate: an open-label, nonrandomized chart review." *Clin Ther*. 2002 Oct;24(10):1576–84.

Cohen L. "Treatment of Bipolar Illness During Pregnancy, Postpartum, and Lactation," symposium, APA annual meeting. May 16, 2003. San Francisco.

Deutschman D et al. "Levetiracetam: efficacy, tolerability, and safety in bipolar disorder in 200 patients." Poster presented at 2004 APA Meeting.

Dunner DL, and RR Fieve. "Clinical factors in lithium carbonate prophylaxis failure." *Arch Gen Psychiatry*. 1974 Feb;30(2):229–33.

Frye MA. "The increasing use of polypharmacotherapy for refractory mood disorders: 22 years of study." *J Clin Psychiatry*. 2000 Jan;61 (1):9–15.

Galvin PM et al. "Clinical and economic impact of newer versus older antipsychotic medications in a community mental health center." *Clin Ther*. 1999 Jun;21(6):1105–16.

Geddes J et al. "Atypical antipsychotics in the treatment of schizophrenia: systematic overview and meta-regression analysis." *BMJ*. 2000 Dec 2;321(7273):1371–6.

Ghaemi SN et al. "Antidepressants in bipolar disorder: the case for caution." *Bipolar Disord*. 2003 Dec;5(6):421–33.

Goldberg JF, and CJ Truman. "Antidepressant-induced mania: an overview of current controversies." *Bipolar Disord*. 2003 Dec;5(6):407–20.

Goodwin FK et al. "Suicide risk in bipolar disorder during treatment with lithium and divalproex." *JAMA*. 2003 Sep 17;290(11):1467–73.

Goodwin FK. "The Rationale for Combined Psychotherapy," symposium, 2003 APA annual meeting. May 19, 2003. San Francisco.

Grunze H et al. *Guidelines for the Biological Treatment of Bipolar Disorders*. Pt. 1–3. World Federation of Societies of Biological Psychiatry, 2002–2004.

Hirschfeld RM et al. "The safety and early efficacy of oral-loaded divalproex versus standard-titration divalproex, lithium, olanzapine, and placebo in the treatment of acute mania associated with bipolar disorder." *J Clin Psychiatry*. 2003 Jul;64(7):841–6.

Jamison K. *An Unquiet Mind: A Memoir of Moods and Madness*. Vintage, 1997.

Kukopulos A et al. "Course of the manic-depressive cycle and changes caused by treatment." *Pharmakopsychiatr Neuropsychopharmakol*. 1980 Jul;13(4):156–67

Lehman A, chair. *Practice Guideline for the Treatment of Patients with Schizophrenia*. American Psychiatric Association, 2004.

Lepkifker E et al. "Renal insufficiency in long-term lithium treatment." *J Clin Psychiatry*. 2004 Jun;65(6):850–6.

Lykouras L, and J Hatzimanolis. "Adjunctive topiramate in the maintenance treatment of bipolar disorders: an open-label study." *Curr Med Res Opin*. 2004 Jun;20(6):843–7.

Mech A. "Use of zonisamide in depressed and bipolar adults: a chart review study." Poster presented at the 2004 APA annual meeting.

Mullen J, and D Sweitzer. "Mania remission rates and euthymia with quetiapine combination therapy." Poster presented the 2004 at APA annual meeting.

National Institute of Mental Health. "Child and adolescent bipolar disorder: an update." 2000. www.nimh.nih.gov/publicat/bipolarupdate .cfm.

Perkins D. Citation of 2000 FDA briefing document at the 2004 APA annual meeting.

Perugi G et al. "Adjunctive dopamine agonists in treatment-resistant bipolar II depression: an open case series." *Pharmacopsychiatry.* 2001 Jul;34(4):137–41

Post R. Fourth International Conference on Bipolar Disorder, 2001.

Potkin SG et al. "Predicting suicidal risk in schizophrenic and schizoaffective patients in a prospective two-year trial." *Biol Psychiatry.* 2003 Aug 15;54(4):444–52.

Rosenheck R et al. "Effectiveness and cost of olanzapine and haloperidol in the treatment of schizophrenia: a randomized controlled trial." *JAMA.* 2003 Nov 26;290(20):2693–702.

Retail Price of Zyprexa and other psychiatric meds listed on RxUSA, Web site listing retail price of Zyprexa and other psychiatric meds, www.rxusa.com.

Sachs GS et al. "Combination of a mood stabilizer with risperidone or haloperidol for treatment of acute mania: a double-blind, placebo-controlled comparison of efficacy and safety." *Am J Psychiatry.* 2002 Jul;159(7):1146–54.

Stahl S, and N Muntner. *Essential Psychopharmacology of Antipsychotics and Mood Stabilizers.* Cambridge University Press, 2002.

Stowe Z. "Depression in Pregnancy and Lactation: Making Informed Decisions to Protect the Mother and Infant," APA 2003 annual meeting. May 17, San Francisco. 2003.

Swann AC et al. "Depression during mania: treatment response to lithium or divalproex." *Arch Gen Psychiatry.* 1997 Jan;54(1):37–42.

Tohen M et al. "Efficacy of olanzapine in combination with valproate or lithium in the treatment of mania in patients partially nonresponsive to valproate or lithium monotherapy." *Arch Gen Psychiatry.* 2002 Jan;59(1):62–9.

————. "Efficacy of olanzapine and olanzapine-fluoxetine combination in the treatment of bipolar I depression." *Arch Gen Psychiatry.* 2003 Nov;60(11):1079–88.

Tondo L, and RJ Baldessarini. "Reduced suicide risk during lithium maintenance treatment." *J Clin Psychiatry.* 2000; 61 Suppl 9:97–104.

Tondo L, RJ Baldessarini, and G Floris. "Long-term clinical effectiveness of lithium maintenance treatment in types I and II bipolar disorders." *Br J Psychiatry.* 2001 Jun;178(Suppl 41):S184–90.

Weisler et al. "Carbamazepine extended release treatment of manic and mixed symptoms." Poster presented at the 2004 APA annual meeting.

Chapter 12

Benca R. "Current Therapeutic Approaches to Sleep," symposium, 2002 APA annual meeting. May 18, 2002. Philadelphia.

Brannan SK et al. "Duloxetine 60 mg once-daily in the treatment of painful physical symptoms in patients with major depressive disorder." *J Psychiatr Res.* 2005 Jan–Feb;39(1):43–53.

Brown R. "Better Sex: Naturally," medical update, 2004 APA annual meeting. May 5, 2004. New York.

Clayton A. "Effects of Psychiatric Illness and Medication on Sexual Function," symposium, 2004 APA annual meeting. May 1, 2006. New York.

Hussain M. "Rivastigmine and galantamine in neurocognitive deficits in bipolar mood disorder." Poster presented at the 2003 APA annual meeting.

Lynch M. "Antidepressants as analgesics: a review of randomized controlled trials." *J Psychiatry Neurosci.* 2001 Jan;26(1):30–6.

Ninan PT et al. "Adjunctive modafinil at initiation of treatment with a selective serotonin reuptake inhibitor enhances the degree and onset of therapeutic effects in patients with major depressive disorder and fatigue." *J Clin Psychiatry.* 2004 Mar;65(3):414–20.

O'Malley PG et al. "Antidepressant therapy for unexplained symptoms and symptom syndromes." *J Fam Pract*. 1999 Dec;48(12):980–90.

Chapter 13

Beck A et al. *Cognitive Therapy of Depression*. Guilford Press, 1987.

Billig M. "Freud and Dora: repressing an oppressed identity." Massey University Web page. www.massey.ac.nz/~alock/virtual/dora4.htm.

Burns D. *Feeling Good: The New Mood Therapy*. Rev. ed. Avon, 1999.

Gloaguen V et al. "A meta-analysis of the effects of cognitive therapy in depressed patients." *J Affect Disord*. 1998 Apr;49(1):59–72.

Jarrett RB, and AJ Rush. "Short-term psychotherapy of depressive disorders: current status and future directions." *Psychiatry*. 1994 May;57(2):115–32.

Miklowitz DJ. "Family Intervention and Pharmacotherapy in the Post-Episode Phase of Bipolar," 2003 APA annual meeting. May 17, 2003. San Francisco.

Miklowitz DJ et al. "Integrated family and individual therapy for bipolar disorder: results of a treatment development study." *J Clin Psychiatry*. 2003 Feb;64(2):182–91.

———. "A randomized study of family-focused psychoeducation and pharmacotherapy in the outpatient management of bipolar disorder." *Arch Gen Psychiatry*. 2003 Sep;60(9):904–12.

Chapter 14

Duman RS, and VA Vaidya. "Molecular and cellular actions of chronic electroconvulsive seizures." *J ECT*. 1998 Sep;14(3):181–93.

George M, et al. "Brain Stimulation: New Treatments for Mood Disorders." symposium, 2005 APA meeting. May 22, 2005. Atlanta.

Jamison, K. *Night Falls Fast: Understanding Suicide.* Vintage, 2000.

Mayberg H et al. "Deep brain stimulation for treatment-resistant depression." *Neuron.* 2005 Mar 3;45(5):651–60.

Plath S. *The Bell Jar.* Perennial, 2000.

Rohan M et al. "Low-field magnetic stimulation in bipolar depression using an MRI-based stimulator." *Am J Psychiatry.* 2004 Jan;161(1): 93–8.

Rose D et al. "Patients' perspectives on electroconvulsive therapy: systematic review." *BMJ.* 2003 Jun 21;326(7403):1363.

Weiner RD. *Practice of Electroconvulsive Therapy: Recommendations for Treatment, Training, and Privileging.* A Task Force Report of the American Psychiatric Association. American Psychiatric Association, 2001.

Chapter 15

Allen J. "Depression and acupuncture: a controlled clinical trial." *Psychiatric Times,* March 2000.

Alpert JE, and M Fava. "Nutrition and depression: the role of folate." *Nutr Rev.* 1997 May;55(5):145–9.

Benton D, and R Cook. "The impact of selenium supplementation on mood." *Biol Psychiatry.* 1991 Jun 1;29(11):1092–8.

Benton D et al. "The impact of long-term vitamin supplementation on cognitive functioning." *Psychopharmacology (Berlin).* 1995 Feb;117(3):298–305.

———. "Vitamin supplementation for 1 year improves mood." *Neuropsychobiology.* 1995;32(2):98–105.

Benton D et al. "Mineral/Vitamin Modification of Mental Disorders and Brain Function," symposium, 2003 APA annual meeting. May 20, 2003. San Francisco.

Brown R, T Bottiglieri, and C Coleman. *Stop Depression Now: Sam-E, the Breakthrough Supplement That Works As Well As Prescription Drugs, in Half the Time . . . with No Side Effects.* Berkeley, 2000.

ConsumerLab.com. "St John's Wort—Beware of Contamination, Insufficient Ingredient, and Drug Interaction." ConsumerLab.com. www.consumerlab.com.

Davidson JR et al. "Effectiveness of chromium in atypical depression: a placebo-controlled trial." *Biol Psychiatry.* 2003 Feb 1;53(3):261–4.

Fletcher RH, and KM Fairfield. "Vitamins for chronic disease prevention in adults: clinical applications." *JAMA.* 2002 Jun 19; 287(23):3127–9.

Food and Drug Administration. "Risk of drug interactions with St. John's wort and indinavir and other drugs." Public health advisory. February 10, 2000.

Gesch B, and A Eves. "Food provision and the nutritional implications of food choices made by young adult males, in a young offenders' institution." *Br J Psychiatry.* 2002 July;181: 22–28.

Hakkarainen et al. "Is low dietary intake of omega-3 fatty acids associated with depression?" *Am J Psychiatry.* 2004 Mar;161(3):567–9.

Hibbeln JR. "Fish consumption and major depression." *Lancet.* 1998 Apr 18;351(9110):1213.

Hintikka J et al. "High vitamin B_{12} level and good treatment outcome may be associated in major depressive disorder." *BMC Psychiatry.* 2003 Dec 02;3(1):17.

Hoffer A. Interviewed by P.B. Chowka in "On orthomolecular medicine, 1997. http://members.aol.com/pbchowka/hoffer.html.

Horrobin D et al. "Depletion of omega-3 fatty acid levels in red blood cell membranes of depressive patients." *Biol Psychiatry.* 1998 Mar 1; 43(5):315–9.

Howe K. "Herb remedies: panacea or problem? Health officials look to improve safety, labeling in $14 billion industry." *San Francisco Chronicle,* June 2, 2000.

Kaplan BJ et al. "Effective mood stabilization with a chelated mineral supplement: an open-label trial in bipolar disorder." *J Clin Psychiatry.* 2001 Dec;62(12):936–44.

Lecrubier Y et al. "Efficacy of St. John's wort extract WS 5570 in major depression: a double-blind, placebo-controlled trial." *Am J Psychiatry.* 2002 Aug;159(8):1361–6.

Lewy AJ et al. "Morning vs. evening light treatment of patients with winter depression." *Arch Gen Psychiatry.* 1998 Oct;55(10):890–6.

Lipton M et al. *Task Force Report on Megavitamin and Orthomolecular Therapy in Psychiatry.* American Psychiatric Association, 1973.

Marangell LB et al. "A double-blind, placebo-controlled study of the omega-3 fatty acid docosahexaenoic acid in the treatment of major depression." *Am J Psychiatry.* 2003 May;160(5):996–8.

Marano H. "Managing bipolar disorder," *Psychology Today,* November 2003.

———. "Vitamins: boost for the brain," *Psychology Today,* March 26, 2004.

Markowitz JS et al. "Effect of St John's wort on drug metabolism by induction of cytochrome P450 3A4 enzyme." *JAMA.* 2003 Sep 17; 290(11):1500–4.

Morris MS et al. "Depression and folate status in the U.S. population." *Psychother Psychosom.* 2003 Mar-Apr;72(2):80–7.

Noaghiul S, and JR Hibbeln. "Cross-national comparisons of seafood consumption and rates of bipolar disorders." *Am J Psychiatry.* 2003 Dec;160(12):2222–7.

Pauling L et al. "On the orthomolecular environment of the mind: ortho-molecular theory." *Am J Psychiatry*. 1974 Nov;131(11):1251–67.

Peet M, and DF Horrobin. "A dose-ranging study of the effects of ethyl-eicosapentaenoate in patients with ongoing depression despite apparently adequate treatment with standard drugs." *Arch Gen Psychiatry*. 2002 Oct;59(10):913–9.

Piscitelli SC. "Indinavir concentrations and St John's wort." *Lancet*. 2000 Feb 12;355(9203):547–8.

Popper CW. "Do vitamins or minerals (apart from lithium) have mood-stabilizing effects?" *J Clin Psychiatry*. 2001 Dec;62(12):933–5.

Post RM. "An overview of recent findings of the Stanley Foundation Bipolar Network." Part 1. *Bipolar Disord*. 2003 Oct;5(5):310–9.

Robbins J. "Research suggests positive effects from living off the fat of the sea." *New York Times*, April 24, 2001.

Ross J. *The Mood Cure: The 4-Step Program to Rebalance Your Emotional Chemistry and Rediscover Your Natural Sense of Well-Being*. Viking, 2002.

Ruhrmann S et al. "Effects of fluoxetine versus bright light in the treatment of seasonal affective disorder." *Psychol Med*. 1998 Jul;28(4):923–33.

Shelton RC et al. "Effectiveness of St John's wort in major depression: a randomized controlled trial." *JAMA*. 2001 Apr 18;285(15):1978–86.

Stoll AL. 2000 DBSA annual conference.

Stoll AL et al. "Omega-3 fatty acids in bipolar disorder: a preliminary double-blind, placebo-controlled trial." *Arch Gen Psychiatry*. 1999 May;56(5):407–12.

Su KP et al. "Omega-3 fatty acids in major depressive disorder: a preliminary double-blind, placebo-controlled trial." *Eur Neuropsychopharmacol*. 2003 Aug;13(4):267–71.

Terman M et al. "Light therapy for seasonal affective disorder: a review of efficacy." *Neuropsychopharmacology.* 1989 Mar;2(1):1–22.

Terman M, and JS Terman. "Treatment of seasonal affective disorder with a high-output negative ionizer." *J Altern Complement Med.* 1995 Jan;1(1):87–92

Truehope. "About Truehope." www.truehope.com/_about/aboutus.asp.

Tuunainen A et al. "Light therapy for non-seasonal depression." *Cochrane Database Syst Rev.* 2004;(2):CD004050.

Weissman MM et al. "Cross-national epidemiology of major depression and bipolar disorder." *JAMA.* 1996 Jul 24–31;276(4):293–9

Chapter 16

Birmaher B, Geller B. Fourth International Conference on Bipolar Disorder, 2001.

Callahan CM et al. "Longitudinal study of depression and health services use among elderly primary care patients." *J Am Geriatr Soc.* 1994 Aug;42(8):833–8.

Conan N. "Analysis: Male depression." *Talk of the Nation,* NPR, October 10, 2002.

DelBello M. "Balancing the Efficacy and Tolerability for Pediatric Bipolar Disorder," symposium, 2004 APA annual meeting. May 5, 2004. New York.

Food and Drug Administration Center for Drug Evaluation and Research. Summary Minutes of the CDER Psychopharmacologic Drugs Advisory Committee and the FDA Pediatric Advisory Committee. Public hearing, September 13–14, 2004. www.fda.gov/ohrms/dockets/ac/04/transcripts/4006T1.htm.

Food and Drug Administration Center for Drug Evaluation and Research Psychopharmacologic Drugs Advisory Committee with the Pediatric Subcommittee of the Anti-Infective Drugs Advisory Committee. Public Hearing, February 2, 2004. www.fda.gov/ohrms/dockets/ac/04/transcripts/4006T1.htm.

Food and Drug Administration Psychopharmacologic Drugs Advisory Committee and the Anti-Infective Drugs Advisory Committee. Briefing Information, February 2, 2004. www.fda.gov/ohrms/dockets/ac/04/briefing/4006b1.htm.

Geller B et al. "Two-year prospective follow-up of children with a prepubertal and early adolescent bipolar disorder phenotype." *Am J Psychiatry.* 2002 Jun;159(6):927–33.

————. "Relationship of parent and child informants to prevalence of mania symptoms in children with a prepubertal and early adolescent bipolar disorder phenotype." *Am J Psychiatry.* 2004 Jul;161(7): 1278–84.

Glasser M, and JA Gravdal. "Assessment and treatment of geriatric depression in primary care settings." *Arch Fam Med.* 1997 Sep–Oct; 6(5):433–8.

Harakas M. "Tempered hope for years, bipolar disorder put Steven Feldman and his parents in a world of hurt: only now are they rebuilding their lives and looking forward to the future." *South Florida Sun-Sentinel,* October 22, 2000.

Kluger J, Park A. "The quest for a superkid: geniuses are made, not born—or so parents are told. But can we really train baby brains, and should we try?" *Time,* April 22, 2001.

Koplewicz H. White House Conference on Mental Illness, 1999.

Kowatch RA, et al. "Combination pharmacotherapy in children and adolescents with bipolar disorder." *Biol Psychiatry.* 2003 Jun 1;53 (11):978–84.

March J. Kids' antidepressant-talking therapy study revealed in testimony to the Food and Drug Administration, September 2004, www.fda.gov/ohrms/dockets/ac/04/transcripts/4006T1.htm

McInnis MG et al. "Anticipation in bipolar affective disorder." *Am J Hum Genet*. 1993 Aug;53(2):385–90.

Mendlewicz J, and JD Rainer. "Morbidity risk and genetic transmission in manic-depressive illness." *Am J Hum Genet*. 1974 Nov;26(6): 692–701.

Miklowitz D et al. "Family-focused treatment for adolescents with bipolar disorder." *J Affect Disord*. 2004 Oct;82 Suppl 1:S113–28.

Miller M and et al. Testimony to FDA. February 2, 2004 and September 13–19, 2004 www.fda.gov/ohrms/dockets/ac/04/transcripts/4006T1.htm.

Olfson M et al. "Relationship between antidepressant medication treatment and suicide in adolescents." *Arch Gen Psychiatry*. 2003 Oct;60(10):978–82.

Papolos D, and J Papolos. *The Bipolar Child: The Definitive and Reassuring Guide to Childhood's Most Misunderstood Disorder*. Rev. and exp. ed. Broadway, 2002.

———. "Juvenile Bipolar Disorder," 2004 JBRF conference. September 8, 2004. Maplewood, NJ.

Rapp D. "Symptoms and Causes; Understanding Environmental Sensitivity." www.drrapp.com/toxicplaces.html.

Reynolds MM. "Mood disorders in late life: a patient's perspective." *Biol Psychiatry*. 2002 Aug 1;52(3):148–53.

Rushton JL et al. "Pediatrician and family physician prescription of selective serotonin reuptake inhibitors." *Pediatrics*. 2000 Jun;105 (6):E82

Schulz R. "Association between depression and mortality in older adults: the Cardiovascular Health Study." *Arch Intern Med*. 2000; 160(12):1761–68.

Schwenk T. "Diagnosis of late life depression: the view from primary care." *Biol Psychiatry.* 2002 Aug 1;52(3):157–63.

Taylor W. "White matter hyperintensity progression and late-life depression outcomes." *Arch Gen Psychiatry.* 2003 Nov;60(11): 1090–6.

Chapter 17

Beardslee W. *Out of the Darkened Room: When a Parent Is Depressed: Protecting the Children and Strengthening the Family.* Little, Brown, 2002.

Bradbury R. "The Playground." In *The Stories of Ray Bradbury.* Knopf, 1990.

Diamond J. E-mail correspondence with the author, 2002.

Fast J, and J Preston. *Loving Someone with Bipolar Disorder: Understanding and Helping Your Partner.* New Harbinger Publications, 2004.

Gerhardt P. "Momma, this isn't just 'the baby blues'; why I threw our vacuum up the tree, and other insights about postpartum depression." *Washington Post,* March 14, 2000.

Karp D. *The Burden of Sympathy: How Families Cope with Mental Illness.* Oxford University Press, 2001.

Real T. *I Don't Want to Talk about It: Overcoming the Secret Legacy of Male Depression.* Scribner, 1998.

Roose S. "Men over 50: an endangered species." Medscape, October 3, 2001. www.medscape.com/viewprogram/597.

Sheffield A. *Depression Fallout: The Impact of Depression on Couples and What You Can Do to Preserve the Bond.* Perennial Currents, 2003.

INDEX